Memorial Days

A History of Community Partnerships 1897-2007

Cullom Davis
and
Kathryn Wrigley

Memorial Health System
Springfield, Illinois
2007

Table of Contents

Table of Vignettes

Foreword

When new leaders assume responsibility for an organization, their emphasis is upon developing a sense of direction. The focus is on the future, not the past. People and practices that historically made valuable contributions can be overlooked; not intentionally, but for lack of information and awareness.

When I joined Memorial in 1983, veteran board members like Norman P. Jones, Robert C. Lanphier III, Walter R. Lohman, Robert B. Oxtoby, William R. Schnirring and A. D. Van Meter helped me develop an appreciation for the institution's prior achievements and leaders. I am grateful to them and to others for opening me to Memorial's history, even as we charted its future.

In 1985, the president and CEO of Decatur Memorial Hospital, Tony Perry, gave us a copy of that organization's history, *The Vigil Never Ceases Two Miles North: An Update History*. With Memorial's centennial only 12 years away, I realized that this milestone would afford an ideal opportunity to enable future generations to discover our interesting past.

The Decatur president recommended that we appoint an "impeccable committee" of knowledgeable and respected people who could "weather any criticism which might result from the publication of the book." This seemed like very sound advice and led to the appointment of a blue ribbon group: Bob Oxtoby (chairman), John Denby, M.D., Richard Herndon, M.D., Howard Humphrey, Grant Johnson, M.D., Bud Lohman, Ann Pearson, M.D., Don Ross, M.D., D. W. Sherrick, M.D., Ed Curtis and Mitch Johnson. For six years, they faithfully monitored the drafting of the first edition.

Cullom Davis is a well-known historian and author not only in central Illinois, but far beyond. By consensus, the board agreed to invite him to write Memorial's centennial history and now to update it. We could not have been more pleased when he and (in the instance of the first edition of *Memorial Days*) Kathryn Wrigley accepted the assignments. This second edition provides insight into an additional decade of progress from 1997-2007.

Memorial is more than a hospital or health system. It is not only a response to disease and pestilence, but a reflection of community pride. It has evolved from the hospital vision of our founder, Martin Luecke, to an expansive, regional, community-owned health system affiliated with the Southern Illinois University School of Medicine.

As I prepare to end a twenty-four-year career as Memorial's President and Chief Executive Officer in December, 2007, I look back with pride at all that we have accomplished together. Memorial is recognized as a national leader in "maintaining, restoring and improving the health of the people and communities we serve."

I would like to express my personal appreciation to the Boards of Directors, the medical staffs, the employees, volunteers, Friends of Memorial, donors, management, other organizations and—most importantly—our community. You gave me a great career opportunity and assisted me in ensuring Memorial's success. I wish you all the best of success as you lead Memorial into the future.

This book is about you. You are Memorial.

Robert T. Clarke
President and Chief
   Executive Officer
Memorial Health System
August, 2007

Preface

It is singularly appropriate for an institution with the word "memorial" as its distinguishing name to honor its past by publishing a centennial history (1997) and now a second edition (2008). Just as it was renamed Memorial Hospital in 1943 to acknowledge its debt to civic supporters, now it celebrates an important milestone by recounting its evolution from a struggling Lutheran infirmary to a sprawling health system. The story is one of remarkable growth and success, but the path it followed was uneven and often tortuous. Greatness came to Memorial Health System neither easily nor swiftly, but it eventually came, and a candid account of that progress should be instructive for citizens of the region it serves and students of modern American medical care.

The authors of this study spent more than five years locating, supplementing, sifting and analyzing a substantial volume of hospital records and other sources, in order to write a history that is comprehensive, critical and contextual. This account tells the story in some detail, but it also attempts to identify certain broad traits and impulses that have permeated Memorial's history. Some of these themes are characteristic of community hospitals generally, while others reflect the unique circumstances and personalities that converged to shape Memorial. Vital to appreciating the institution's character, they bear previewing here.

Like many of its peers throughout the country, Springfield (later Memorial) Hospital experienced dramatic growth through the 20th century, transforming from a cottage industry to a conglomerate. Through most of these years the emphasis was upon physical and horizontal expansion: the addition of buildings, beds and market share. In recent years Memorial has concentrated on vertical and ancillary growth: the development of outpatient health care services and an ever widening regional market. Administratively it mushroomed from a "peculiar bureaucracy" consisting simply of a matron, receptionist and clerk to a corporate hierarchy of president, vice presidents, management specialists and staff. The organizational payroll grew from less than a dozen to more than 5,400. In this sense Memorial Medical Center has mimicked the dynamic expansion of the entire health care industry, and indeed most private and public institutions in the United States.

Similarly, the hospital's changing fortunes and character over the years have mirrored national trends. Its near-bankruptcy and recovery in the

1930s paralleled the country's experience during the Great Depression. Like many of the nation's hospitals and charitable institutions, it began life as a sectarian facility but later became secular. The role of women at Memorial is a story in itself. Through most of its early years they predominated, not only as nurses but also as superintendents. Notable among the civic leaders who rescued the institution in the 1930s and spearheaded its rebuilding were women like Mildred Bunn. During the postwar years when society redefined women as homemakers, leadership at the hospital likewise fell exclusively to men. Later, as the feminist movement broke down other barriers, women regained some administrative and governance positions at Memorial.

Perhaps less common have been certain other conspicuous qualities. One has been a steadfast commitment to education, though the focus has changed over the years. At the outset and for many years, the words "Training School" were part of Springfield Hospital's name and integral to its mission. Nursing education continued for more than 75 years. By the time Memorial Hospital stopped training nurses, it already was deeply involved in educating physicians, through its close association with SIU School of Medicine. As the hospital transformed into a "medical center" and later Memorial Health System, it broadened its educational focus to include patients and the general public. Moreover, inservice training programs have added employees to the institution's educational clientele. No longer limited to producing registered nurses, education at Memorial today is comprehensive in scope and (together with patient care and research) a primary institutional mission.

Another distinguishing tradition has been Memorial's charitable impulse. Its founders contributed long hours, considerable effort and scarce funds to create a second general purpose hospital for area citizens. Their dedication, supplemented by nearby and distant Lutheran parishes, kept the institution going for more than 30 years. Their successors were civic leaders and lay volunteers who governed wisely, repeatedly raised funds for additional construction, and provided collateral goods and services. The advent and growth of private insurance and federal aid programs significantly altered but did not erase Memorial's charitable heritage. In modern times the Friends organization and the Foundation have greatly broadened the variety and scope of free services to patients and the general public. No longer a charitable institution in the traditional and narrow sense, Memorial Medical Center today serves an entire region's health needs in countless and important ways. Its lay directors, like their Lutheran fore-bears, volunteer their time and talent as a public service.

One key to the institution's growth and success has been its ability to forge community ties and partnerships. In the early years these included Trinity Lutheran Church, Concordia Seminary, a regional Lutheran hospital association, and many neighboring Lutheran churches.

Later the connections broadened to include the Masons, Jewish temples and organizations, and numerous Protestant churches. Today Memorial Health System is a complex collection of subsidiaries, affiliates, community alliances and cooperative agreements. In Springfield and more than a dozen central Illinois communities it maintains working partnerships with local health care organizations and groups. Its relationship with SIU School of Medicine is so integral that visitors to Memorial's campus scarcely can distinguish where one's property and activity end and the other's begin. St. John's Hospital, once its arch-rival, is now a partner on various initiatives and programs.

Through much of its first century, Memorial Medical Center was engaged in a determined and at times desperate quest for success and stature. Founded on narrow and insecure footings, Springfield Hospital spent decades seeking institutional stability, financial solvency and community credibility. Following its reorganization and rebuilding, the aspiration shifted higher, to parity with its senior and larger rival, St. John's Hospital. This dream animated Memorial directors and staff for another 40 years. By the 1980s, with parity achieved, new goals arose to challenge hospital leaders. Creating medical "centers of excellence," adding premier ancillary services, widening the system's regional market, and adapting proactively to a rapidly changing health care environment now taxed Memorial's energy and resources. Today the quest, put simply, is to reinforce Memorial Health System's stature as "the health care system of choice for central and southern Illinois." Amidst all of the tangible evidence of success, system officials are as determined as their predecessors to overcome all obstacles and reach new heights.

A key to the foregoing drive has been Memorial's final trait, a sturdy resilience in the face of adversity. Repeatedly, almost chronically in its early years, the struggling hospital seemed on the brink of closure or sale, only to survive for the next challenge. Directors and staff met incessant crises much like episodes of the then-popular "Perils of Pauline" serial. Meeting monthly and sometimes weekly, board members confronted cash shortfalls, equipment failures, physician ultimatums, staff resignations, and accreditation warnings. Their successors faced different but no less daunting challenges, including space crises, a nurses' revolt, executive turnover, and an abortive early experiment with prepaid health care. What saved and ultimately strengthened the institution was an abiding tenacity on the part of hospital officials, employees, volunteers and physicians. Among Memorial's various early legacies, both good and bad, this habit of fortitude and resilience has been an extraordinary asset.

It was characteristic of President Robert T. Clarke's executive style that planning for Memorial Health System's centennial began six years in advance. He approached this opportunity with the same foresight and mental focus that he and his associates marshaled for a new hospital building or health care venture. Never before had he or the institution he has headed for 14 years conducted an anniversary, so he solicited advice and model ideas from industry peers.

Clear from the outset was Clarke's determination to make the centennial a milestone of high quality, professional effort and enduring value. He persuaded board members to name a representative panel of directors, physicians and administrators to oversee the planning. Uppermost in his mind was the preparation of a carefully researched, interpretive history. Accordingly, he engaged two professional historians to survey the scattered records, produce oral histories with key figures from all areas of hospital activity, and conduct the necessary research. The product of this effort would be a book that recounted Memorial's history with candor and within the larger context of parallel events and trends in the nation's and the community's histories. Complementing this long term endeavor would be a week-long series of ceremonies and celebrations, each one designed expressly for a segment of the system's broad constituency: employees, retirees, volunteers, physicians, the general public and civic leaders. The combination of festive events and an interpretive history would produce a birthday party of enduring value.

In the course of their work the authors had the benefit of much assistance and cooperation. Memorial executives, especially Robert Clarke and Mitchell Johnson, generously accommodated all requests and consistently affirmed their commitment to an objective, critical history that would recount the institution's setbacks and embarrassments as fully as its achievements. Members of the special centennial task force that met periodically and provided valuable advice included chairman Robert Oxtoby,

Robert Clarke, Edgar Curtis, Dr. John Denby, Dr. Richard Herndon, Howard Humphrey, Dr. Grant Johnson, Mitchell Johnson, Walter Lohman, Dr. Ann Pearson, Dr. Donald Ross and Dr. William Sherrick.

Previous historical studies supplied a useful foundation for the work. Dr. Floyd S. Barringer, who practiced neurosurgery at Memorial for 35 years, also exercised his lifelong hobby in history to gather evidence and compile a brief chronicle of the hospital. Stuart Fliege, who has written extensively on the history of Trinity Lutheran Church, generously shared his findings and sources on the early years. He also recruited church volunteers to assist with an English transcription of the Lutheran board's minutes. Gerlinde Coates and Christine Purtell faithfully translated from German the voluminous board proceedings that spanned the hospital's first quarter century.

Other individuals provided access to important records. At Memorial Medical Center, Andrea Ferrero-Violet, Kathy Bird, Luisa Van Roekel, Cindy Appenzeller and Becky Garretson helped ensure that all hospital records were available for examination. The appointment in 1996 of archivist James Ladd consolidated the files in one location. At Springfield's Lincoln (public) Library, Edward Russo and his colleagues in the Sangamon Valley Collection responded to numerous requests, as did personnel in the reference and periodicals departments. Sandy Vance, librarian at the **State Journal-Register,** helped locate old newspaper files on microfilm. Librarians at the SIU School of Medicine also cooperated generously.

Crucial to the authors' approach were the reminiscences of more than 30 current and former Memorial physicians, nurses, administrators, other employees and directors. Their oral histories, comprising several thousand transcript pages, offered invaluable assessments and anecdotes, particularly for the postwar period. There is a complete list of these individuals in the book's essay on sources. Martha Benner accurately transcribed the tapes.

The latter stages of work also drew valuable assistance. Members of the editorial panel which patiently reviewed successive drafts of the text were Robert Clarke, Edgar Curtis, Becky Garretson, Mitchell Johnson, Scott Kiriakos, Robert Oxtoby, and Dr. Ann Pearson. Other volunteers who corrected mistakes and made suggestions were William Boyd, Wilma Fricke, Dr. William Sherrick and Dr. James Singleton. Andrea Ferrero-Violet coordinated this effort, and Carmen Morgan typed the numerous chapter drafts. Becky Garretson took special pains to locate illustrations, while Gary Carter and Memorial's photography staff expertly copied them. Mary Hempstead compiled the index.

The authors have worked hard to be both accurate in their description and reasonable in their assessment of Memorial's first century of service. While this book leaned heavily on the help of individuals identified above, we and not they are responsible for any mistakes of fact and judgment. Our fondest hope is to have produced a narrative that honestly portrays and fairly interprets a proud institution's legacy for the 21st century.

Springfield, Illinois

February, 1997

Cullom Davis is Professor of History Emeritus at the University of Illinois in Springfield, and former director of the Lincoln Legal Papers. He is author or editor of five books and numerous articles.

*Kathryn Wrigley is a medical librarian and historian. A former editor of the **Papers of Abraham Lincoln**, she also published a history of the Sangamon County Historical Society.*

This updated edition carries Memorial's history through 2007, the conclusion of Robert Clarke's extraordinary 24-year service as president and CEO. Both his retirement and the appointment of his highly regarded successor, Ed Curtis, mark a pivotal transition for Memorial Health System.

Cullom Davis was the sole author of revisions and new text for this edition. Helping with access to system minutes, reports, press files, and archival records were Kathy Bird, Andrea Ferrero-Violet, Susan Friedman, Pam Hinckley, Mitch Johnson, and Jim Ladd. Oral history interviews with thirteen people (cited by name in the essay on sources) added valuable information and perspectives.

December, 2007

Memorial Milestones

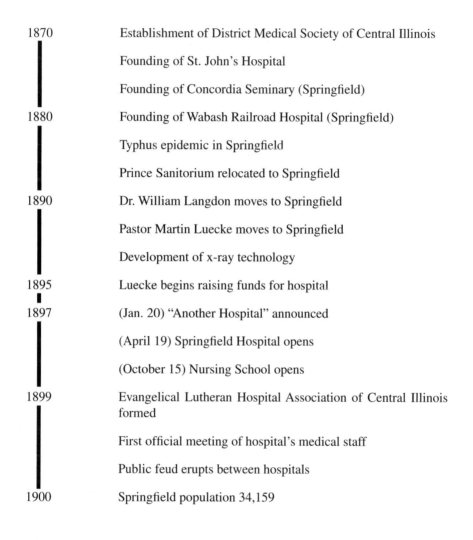

1870	Establishment of District Medical Society of Central Illinois
	Founding of St. John's Hospital
	Founding of Concordia Seminary (Springfield)
1880	Founding of Wabash Railroad Hospital (Springfield)
	Typhus epidemic in Springfield
	Prince Sanitorium relocated to Springfield
1890	Dr. William Langdon moves to Springfield
	Pastor Martin Luecke moves to Springfield
	Development of x-ray technology
1895	Luecke begins raising funds for hospital
1897	(Jan. 20) "Another Hospital" announced
	(April 19) Springfield Hospital opens
	(October 15) Nursing School opens
1899	Evangelical Lutheran Hospital Association of Central Illinois formed
	First official meeting of hospital's medical staff
	Public feud erupts between hospitals
1900	Springfield population 34,159

Chapter One

An Act of Faith and Courage

The day after Easter Sunday, 1897, brought residents of Springfield, Illinois both a new mayor and a new hospital. The latter event, after several months of anticipation and delays, seemed almost anticlimactic, drawing only two paragraphs of press attention. The **Illinois State Journal,** one of two local dailies, reported that on Monday, April 19, 1897, the Springfield Hospital and Training School "has been thrown open." The account was not of ribbon cuttings or any civic fanfare, but simply of the successful use of x-ray equipment to locate bullet fragments in a shooting victim.

From such "a humble beginning" was launched an institution that a century later would be unrecognizable to its original sponsors. They were a small band of devout German Lutherans and dedicated physicians who yearned to bring a second charitable private hospital to their burgeoning central Illinois city. With scant capital, expert advice, or planning, they were animated more by heart than by mind in what officials later aptly dubbed "an act of faith and courage." That their dream even survived, and eventually flourished, is a tribute to both the noble vision and the good fortune of the founders.

The birth of what came to be known as Memorial Health System took place in a period of rapid growth and dramatic change for American medi-

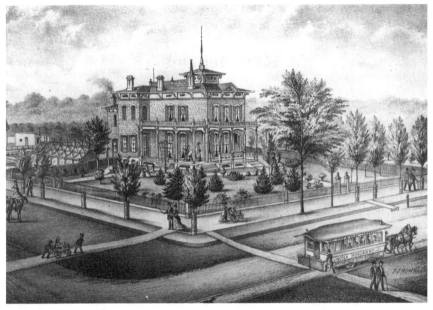

The original site of Springfield Hospital and Training School—the home of Dr. William Langdon at the corner of Fifth Street and North Grand Avenue, East

cine, nursing and hospitals. Partly the product of these broad cultural and technological developments, it also was intimately connected to the more prosaic history of its local religious sponsors and of the capital city of Springfield. To fully understand the distinctive patterns of Springfield Hospital's early years, it is necessary to appreciate the professional, institutional, religious and civic context that spawned and shaped it. One historian of American hospitals has described them as "adaptive, pragmatic organizations" that interact constantly with their political, technological, and socioeconomic environments. The birth and early years of Springfield Hospital and Training School illustrate this assertion.

Medical Milestones

The closing years of the 19th century were a time of scientific break-throughs and professional ferment for American medicine and its practitioners. In the brief span of several decades there were dramatic advances in the diagnosis and treatment of disease, the practice and success of surgery, and the professional development of physicians. For the general public this meant the rise of a startling new dream: that medical science had the potential to conquer disease and injury, ensuring a full lifespan to all.

The popular heroes of the age were neither statesmen nor warriors, but medical scientists. Citizens avidly read press accounts of the path-breaking discoveries of Joseph Lister, Pierre and Marie Curie, Robert Koch, and Louis Pasteur. Their laboratory and clinical exploits elicited admiration, hope, and visions of longevity. After much early skepticism and controversy, the germ theory of disease won acceptance, leading to revolutionary advances in medical diagnosis and treatment, surgery, and hospital practice. The miraculous power of the x-ray, developed in the 1890s, generated as much excitement with the public as among physicians.

Dread diseases like yellow fever, tuberculosis, smallpox, malaria, and cancer showed no abatement, but doctors and their patients for the first time could entertain some realistic hope for their cure or even prevention. Rare but well-publicized incidents of successful cancer surgery, plus the novel idea of radium treatment, gave some early hope of victory over this mysterious disease that annually killed 65 of 100,000 Americans. Three times as fatal was tuberculosis, the "white plague," yet the discovery of its bacillus raised prospects for a cure. The virtual eradication of yellow fever and malaria in Havana, Cuba and later Panama vividly demonstrated how rigorous public health efforts could contain disease.

There also were modest but nevertheless promising developments in pharmaceutical therapy. While most available drugs were either folk remedies or commercial nostrums aimed at a gullible public, a few scientifically validated medications like aspirin and quinine came into use. Unfortunately, the extensive advertising and merchandising of unregulated patent medicines and miracle devices captured more public favor than the bonafide drugs.

Surgical procedures dramatically transformed from a grim and seldom successful last resort to a viable medical option. New concepts of antiseptic and aseptic surgery vastly improved a patient's prospects for at least recovery if not cure. There also were primitive but promising refinements in anesthesia, reducing the specter of surgery as a form of voluntary torture. Consequently, there was increased pressure within the medical profession for surgery to be performed only by specialists with added training and experience, and in controlled, sterile environments. Both of these concerns spurred the growth of hospitals, where it was easier than in private homes to control both the eligibility to operate and the sanitary conditions. Hospitals also enjoyed increasing respect with physician-surgeons who appreciated the value of a full-time and fully equipped surgical arena for their own training and development.

American medicine's scientific and technical improvements were accompanied by similar advances in the education, certification, and professionalization of physicians. Through most of the 19th century, doctors had little professional authority or stature. Their ranks included many lay practitioners with no formal training. State licensing requirements were at best lax, and medical education was notoriously uneven. The typical small-town physician needed a second livelihood to make a living, earned (and too often deserved) a pittance from local patients, enjoyed no higher status than the undertaker or barber, and had neither the opportunity nor the motivation, for professional interaction with peers.

During the century's final quarter this bleak picture began to change, as physicians sensed the first stirrings of professional regulation and enhancement. The American Medical Association (AMA), founded in the 1840s, finally gained the collective purpose and influence to promote its reform agenda. One key gain was its success in pressuring various splinter factions (homeopaths, herbalists, eclectics and others) to either embrace conventional medicine or perform as outsiders. Its campaign for uniform and heightened state licensing standards made some progress. For example, an Illinois statute of 1877 empowered state examiners to deny licenses to graduates of disreputable medical schools. The AMA also made inroads in its effort to create a vertical federation of local and state medical societies that would reinforce its determination to be the powerful organized voice of American medical practice.

An interesting example of this latter trend was the founding, in 1874, of the District Medical Society of Central Illinois. Inspired by the 1873 AMA convention in St. Louis, 82 progressive physicians from more than a dozen mid-Illinois communities held an inaugural meeting in Pana, 40 miles southeast of Springfield. Their day-long gathering included a business session and election of officers, discussion of pending state legislation, and an afternoon devoted to technical papers and clinical reports. Thus began a lively model of continuing education and regional fellowship that thrived for 70 years. Through its well-attended semiannual meetings, the society epitomized the important changes underway for the American medical profession.

Other gains occurred in the quality of medical education and the ranks of women entering the profession. Under pressure from the nation's elite colleges, the AMA and state licensing reforms, long overdue improvements began to appear in medical curricula and instruction in the late 1800s. These early steps were neither substantial nor widespread, but served as a prelude to the celebrated study and report (1910) by Abraham Flexner that led to rigorous accreditation standards.

Women comprised a small minority of physicians, but their relative presence increased sharply in the century's final decades. By the 1890s they had doubled (to 5.6 per cent) their representation in the profession. However, the leading medical schools continued to limit admission, and as marginal institutions succumbed to the reform wave, women faced diminishing opportunities for study. Thus the brief surge was destined to reverse in the 1900s, a victim of education reform and the mounting resistance of male physicians who coveted their growing status and income.

While uneven and incomplete, American medicine's progress was a notable feature of the late 19th century. Its achievements gave new authority and stature to physicians, and nourished rising popular demand for medical care by qualified professionals in modern and sanitary facilities.

District Medical Society of Central Illinois

Meticulously kept minutes detail the 70 year history of this noteworthy venture in continuing medical education for central Illinois physicians who sought the stimulus of periodic interchange with their peers. The District Medical Society filled a regional need and served the profession well during a period of dramatic medical progress.

The founding members (82 men from more than a dozen communities) could scarcely have envisioned the enduring value of their experiment when they initially met, in 1874. For the first 46 years their semiannual conclaves took place in the small town of Pana. Thereafter the meetings circulated, and Springfield was the site five times in the 1930s. By then the group numbered nearly 150 members.

Sessions covered the entire range of clinical subjects, such as gallstones, rectal cancer, infant feeding, and skull fractures. Short papers and informal clinical reports highlighted each meeting.

The earliest Springfield physician to play a leading role was George A. Kreider, who delivered many papers and served two years as president, 1896-97. Dr. Don Deal was another active Springfield participant, and later Dr. Emmet Pearson held office. During the 1920s and 1930s a dozen or more Springfield physicians regularly attended.

St. John's Hospital and the Sangamon County Medical Society played institutional hosts for the Springfield meetings during the 1930s. Several times the group adjourned for dinner and entertainment at the Sangamo Club. Members continued meeting during World War II. The minutes fail to recount or explain the group's demise after that. Perhaps the regional approach proved cumbersome and outlived its usefulness. The society nevertheless set a good example of professional dialogue during its long life.

A Radical Metamorphosis

These same years were a time of "radical … metamorphosis" for American hospitals. One change was quantitative: the number of hospitals increased 24-fold between 1873 and 1909, from 178 to 4,359. The growth in patient capacity was substantial but less dramatic (from 50,000 to 421,065 beds), reflecting the disproportionate sprouting of small community hospitals. Many of these new institutions were sectarian in purpose and sponsorship, with Catholic hospitals heading the list.

Many influences contributed to this rapid proliferation, which in one generation significantly altered the American social landscape by bringing hospital access to nearly everyone. One obvious cause was demographic: a rapidly rising industrial age population needed more hospitals just as it needed more schools, roads, and parks. More important, however, were narrower causes unique to health care. One was the example and impetus of the Civil War.

While the Union Army's treatment of diseased and wounded soldiers was primitive by today's standards, at that time it was a widely noted improvement. Thanks to such new concepts as proper ventilation and sanitation, soldiers in Union hospitals had a better-than-even chance to survive. For many men and their families, the hospital thus became for the first time in history a place to recover rather than die from injury, and to cure rather than catch a disease. Central to the war's favorable impact on the public's acceptance of hospital care were the heroic efforts of nurses led by Clara Barton, who campaigned in war and peacetime for higher standards of hospital hygiene and patient care.

Another contributor to hospital growth was the previously mentioned discoveries and reforms in medical care. The emergence of medicine as a genuine science, the new emphasis upon antiseptic surgery, reforms in medical education, and the heightened collective influence of physicians all led naturally to greater public reliance on hospitals. Shedding their traditional notoriety as "places of dreaded impurity and exiled human wreckage," they acquired new acceptance as viable institutions for the diagnosis and treatment of injury and disease.

The nation's post-Civil War industrial boom was an additional factor. Rising workplace accidents prodded both employers and labor unions to establish their own hospitals. In Springfield, for example, the Wabash Railroad established a small medical facility on South Sixth Street in the

1880s. Known variously as the Wabash Railroad or Wabash Employees' Hospital, it functioned for several decades with a small medical staff that treated company workers with job-related injuries.

One measure of the improved public image for American hospitals was the encouragement and support they received in countless cities and towns. Toward the close of the 19th century communities began for the first time to boast about their existing hospitals or to conduct civic campaigns to establish them. While county pest houses, asylums and poor farms had operated in the shadows of disgrace and neglect for many years, it suddenly became fashionable for cities to have one or more of the new charitable or voluntary institutions. Gaining a new hospital became a measure of achievement for bustling cities on the rise.

A final catalyst was the period's newly fortified spirit of religious altruism. Reacting to the industrial era's many socioeconomic ills and widening divisions of wealth was a doctrine of "pious activism." Known also as the Social Gospel, it implored American Christians and Jews to be their brothers' keepers for the common good. This religious zeal took many forms, including relief agencies for the hungry, church-sponsored orphanages, and religious hospitals.

Catholics led the way in dotting the national landscape with sectarian hospitals. The individual reasons varied, but the principal inspiration was a perceived need to serve and safeguard the faithful in an increasingly heterogeneous society where religious, ethnic, and racial prejudice often took virulent form. Catholics worried about receiving last rites in a Protestant hospital, and Jewish physicians encountered rigid barriers to medical staff membership. Lutherans and other Protestants feared the proselytizing influence of sister-nurses in Catholic hospitals. While these religious stereotypes and anxieties appealed to the basest human prejudices, they did generously feed the hospital boom. Catholic, Jewish, and Protestant denominational institutions, many also ethnic in orientation, were a major component of the multiplying hospital census late in the 19th century.

According to one estimate, approximately ten per cent of the nation's hospitals at the turn of the century had religious affiliations or sponsors. Non-denominational, not-for-profit hospitals comprised a larger share. Their label is misleading, because they were not altogether private or charitable; as privately owned institutions they relied on fee-paying patients drawn from the general public. A third type, publicly sponsored hospitals, included the large and prestigious institutions in major cities, and also county asylums for contagious and indigent patients. Finally, there was a large number of small, proprietary hospitals owned and operated by companies, labor unions, and most commonly, physicians.

A highly regarded local example of this last type was the Prince Sanitorium, which stood for many years at the southwest corner of Seventh and Capitol streets. This proprietary hospital was founded in Jacksonville, 35 miles west, by the celebrated physician David Prince, just following the Civil War. Two years following his death in 1889, his two sons, both doctors, moved the facility to Springfield. Arthur E. Prince specialized in eye, ear, nose and throat work, and John practiced general surgery. Their four-story building, later enlarged with a two-story wing on the south, included patient quarters, operating rooms, and a section devoted to Turkish and other therapeutic baths.

The hospital boom converged with other industrial and medical developments to alter the nation's health care habits and expectations. The advent of electrical and telephone services enhanced the advantage of institutional over home care, and elevators encouraged the construction of taller and more efficient buildings. Surgical advances made it feasible and even lucrative to dedicate hospital space exclusively for antiseptic operating rooms. At larger hospitals there appeared the first signs of functional differentiation, with sections and rooms set aside for pathological, obstetrical, ophthalmological, and other specialties. The rise of trained nurses, the professional strides by physicians, and the growing demand for experienced superintendents brought new expertise and the beginnings of a status hierarchy to hospitals.

By century's end, hospitals had shifted dramatically from the periphery to the center of medical education and practice. No longer mere refuges for the poor and insane, they now welcomed all kinds of patients, many of them fee-paying. Staffed by professionals and specialists, furnished with the latest diagnostic and surgical equipment, capable of maintaining hygienic and antiseptic conditions, and welcomed by civic authorities, entrepreneurs, lay boards, and religious groups alike, American hospitals were a growth industry in a time of rapid change.

The Springfield Setting

The central Illinois city of Springfield was a boisterous, polyglot, industrial boom town at the turn of the century. The 1900 census recorded 34,159 residents, a steep increase over 1890. Foreign-born whites (13.4 per cent) and African-Americans (5.7 per cent) were rapidly expanding minorities. Soot and dust from scores of factory smokestacks covered much of the city. Foundries, farm implement manufacturers, rolling mills, shoe factories, woolen mills, breweries, and boiler works—over 300 industrial firms in all—provided employment for more than ten per cent of the residents. A nearly equal number of men worked in the two dozen coal mines scattered around the city and environs, making Sangamon County the leading coal producer in the nation's leading coal state. Mining was dangerous work, leading to hundreds of injuries and many deaths every year.

Brick paving began to replace muddy streets in the 1880s, but other improvements lagged. The municipal water system depended on a large reservoir in the northeast part of town; drinking water was only marginally safe and susceptible to typhoid and other public health risks. Both rapid population growth and corrupt municipal government accounted for these problems.

Sharp ethnic and racial cleavages, accentuated by religious differences, created a checkerboard of homogeneous neighborhood enclaves throughout the city. Catering to their diverse spiritual needs were nearly 50 churches, many of them offering foreign language services. A bitter cold spell in the early winter of 1897 led to urgent appeals for donations of clothing, food, and fuel to the poor. Churches were the only source of such relief, and many responded during the crisis.

Politics always loomed large in the capital city, but particularly in the first several months of 1897. In January, newly elected Republican Governor John R. Tanner succeeded the embattled Democrat John P. Altgeld. Early in March local newspapers reported a similar party shift at the national level, when Republican William McKinley was inaugurated president. Local politics intensified in April, when a Republican sweep of city offices installed Loren E. Wheeler as mayor.

Health hazards and work-related injuries placed a strain on the community's available medical services. One measure of this need was the daily press reports of births, illnesses, and deaths, nearly all of which occurred in private homes. In addition to the two small special hospitals (Wabash

Employees and Prince Sanitorium), there was only one general facility—
St. John's Hospital—to serve the city's growing health needs. St. John's
had been established late in 1875 by 21 Franciscan nuns who emigrated
from Germany during that country's large Catholic exodus. They first
opened a small hospital-residence on South Seventh Street, then several
years later built a two-story structure with several dozen beds at Mason
and Eighth.

St. John's Hospital grew rapidly in its first quarter century, with several building additions that raised its capacity to 86 beds and reportedly
made it the state's largest outside Chicago. The pace continued, and by
1902 it could accommodate 150 patients. Although owned and operated
by the Sisters of St. Francis as a Catholic institution, it admitted anyone
regardless of creed or ability to pay, except people suffering "contagious,
syphilic, alcoholic, and mental diseases."

To house society's unfortunates who were unwelcome elsewhere, the
city opened the Isolation Hospital, a "pest house," around 1900. Located
safely outside town to the northwest, it served sufferers from smallpox,
diphtheria, and other pestilent diseases with a resident nonprofessional
staff of two. The Isolation Hospital operated for 20 years, then its land was
sold, with symbolic logic, for an addition to Oak Ridge Cemetery.

Among the city's residents needing medical care were the faculty
and students of Concordia Seminary, a Lutheran institution founded in
1875 on the near east side. Concordia replaced the ill-fated Illinois State
University, founded before the Civil War as a Lutheran school and college.
It was owned by the Missouri Synod and Springfield's Trinity Church,
founded in the 1840s. There was a close linkage between Trinity Church
and Concordia Seminary, with overlapping boards and scriptural instruction by church pastors. At this time the Missouri Synod was actively
building colleges, seminaries, orphanages, and hospitals throughout the
Middle West.

Twice late in the 1880s Concordia Seminary suffered typhus epidemics. The worst was in 1888, when an outbreak led to nine deaths and a
three-month closing of the school. A recurrence in 1889 sent several
Concordia students to St. John's Hospital for treatment and convalescence.
According to subsequent reports, some local Lutheran leaders were dis-
mayed that impressionable young men were in the care of Catholic nuns
who might or did seek to convert them. As the Seminary added new space

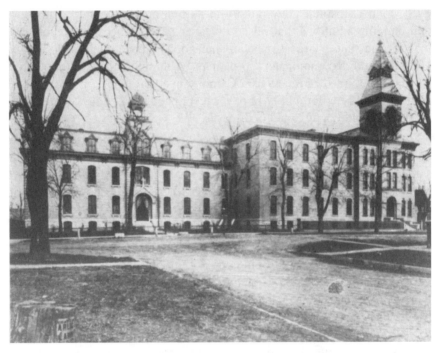

St. John's Hospital, circa 1887 (ten years before Springfield Hospital was founded). Another wing (to the left) was added in 1891. This view looks northward, from Mason and Eighth Streets. (Photo courtesy of Illinois State Historical Library, Old State Capitol Building, Springfield, IL)

and more students (reaching 280), pressure arose at both Concordia and Trinity to create a Lutheran alternative for local hospital care.

The earliest overt evidence of this initiative was a letter in 1887 from Missouri Synod officials to Dr. William O. Langdon, a Kentucky native then practicing in Houston, Texas. Langdon had studied medicine at a Lutheran school in Missouri, and seemed a good prospect to direct a new hospital in Springfield. On family business in Illinois, he met with a committee of Trinity parishioners and civic leaders. The idea died for the time, however, due to inadequate funds. Nevertheless Langdon's trip was important because he met his future wife, and in 1889 decided to transfer his medical practice to Springfield. Several years later he purchased a home on the northwest corner of Fifth and North Grand streets.

While their first effort was stillborn, Lutheran leaders continued to press for a hospital. Key figures during the 1890s were Trinity's pastor Martin H. Luecke and Concordia professors John S. Simon and Frederick Streekfuss. The "prime mover" was Luecke, who reportedly spent two years (beginning in 1895) raising interest and financial pledges. Other prominent local Lutherans evidently were also supportive.

An Ideal Retreat for the Sick

During the winter months of 1897, broad national trends, unique local circumstances, religious zeal, and a few visionaries converged to create Springfield Hospital and Training School. The first public inkling of these plans came on January 20, when the **Illinois State Journal** announced "ANOTHER HOSPITAL" in a ten paragraph story. One day earlier the Illinois Secretary of State had issued a not-for-profit corporation license, listing as incorporators Luecke and Simon, Dr. Langdon, and local businessmen Ben F. Caldwell and John Bressmer. Unnamed supporters reportedly had subscribed $20,000 toward the purchase of property and start-up costs. Numerous likely sites were under consideration, notably the Prince Sanitorium and Dr. Langdon's residence. It was optimistically anticipated that the new institution would be ready within a month.

Possibly to defuse suspicions of sectarian rivalry, sources told the newspaper that "It is not the intention of those in charge to be antagonistic to St. John's Hospital." The new facility probably would charge similar fees, and "the city is large enough to support two such establishments." Before long, however, this issue would resurface and persist, occasionally in bitter invective.

Meanwhile there was much to do. During February and early March the organizing group met at least ten times to handle myriad questions and details. Committee members and stockholders convened February 3 to narrow the choice of sites. Five days later, assembled for the first time as the board of directors, they selected Dr. Langdon's spacious two-story, brick Italianate mansion, facing North Grand Avenue on the northwest corner of Fifth Street. Situated in a quiet neighborhood, this was considered "an ideal retreat for the sick." The purchase price was $10,000 (less a $1,000 gift from Langdon), due for payment in June.

The board included Luecke, Simon, and Langdon, plus three lay leaders at Trinity: Michael Timm, John B. Maurer, and local druggist William Zapf. Mrs. Fredericka Bolte also served, and a regular attendant was Miss Mary E. "Lizette" Nagel, a nurse from St. Louis who was not a board member but was authorized to temporarily run "the household" and purchase supplies. At this inaugural board meeting on February 8, Simon was elected chairman, Luecke president, Langdon treasurer, and Zapf was named "English secretary" (reflecting the fact that German was the language of choice).

One week later the board considered a draft of hospital bylaws, ordered necessary equipment and utensils to be acquired in St. Louis, and discussed remodeling the Langdon home. On the 17th they agreed on the institution's name: Springfield Hospital and Training School, and sought help with the bylaws from local lawyers John S. Schnepp and John G. Friedmeyer, both active at Trinity.

Rapid progress continued the next week, when Miss Helena Hanser of St. Louis was named hospital matron and nursing instructor, at a salary of $25 per month plus free room, board and laundry. The daughter of a prominent St. Louis Lutheran pastor, she was a graduate of St. Louis City Hospital nursing school. Soon her sister Selma would join the hospital first as cook, then as a nursing student and later as nurse and assistant matron.

On March 1 the board approved bids for carpentry ($155) and hospital beds ($5.90 each, including springs). Attorney Schnepp was added to the board, and Dr. Langdon was named hospital superintendent. Suggestive of the fast pace of decision-making, there was some confusion over job titles and also a new election of officers that switched Langdon to vice president, eliminated the chairman's post, and reassigned Simon as secretary and Zapf as treasurer.

Periodic reports during early March of the new hospital's imminent opening proved unrealistic, as board members juggled remodeling decisions with financial, personnel, and purchasing transactions. March 9 brought an announcement of the newly formed medical staff of twelve physicians, including "some of the best known medical men (and one woman, Elizabeth Matthews) of this city." Among them were surgeons John A. Prince and John N. Dixon, obstetrician Langdon, and general physicians George F. Stericker and Ralph C. Matheny.

Opening day actually occurred Monday, April 19, just three months following the first public announcement. Neither board records nor contemporary newspapers reported any formalities or even data about patient admittances; the sole notice was of Dr. Langdon's experimental use of x-rays (discovered only two years earlier) to locate the bullet fragments in Joseph Yowell's knee. The next day was somewhat livelier, as Dr. Dixon, with two assisting physicians, performed a laparotomy (abdominal incision) to remove more than one gallon of "pus" from a seriously ill ten-year old girl. This procedure was regarded as a desperate last resort for the girl, and the "chances of recovery are against her."

The hospital that greeted patients and visitors in 1897 was as unremarkable as the public notice of its inception. The first floor of the former Langdon residence had been hastily converted into a small reception area and office at the entrance, a kitchen, dining room, and two patient rooms. On the second floor, former bedrooms had been remodeled into three rooms for patients and a combination x-ray and operating room. In mild weather another patient or two could be accommodated in an unheated hallway. Lavatory facilities were limited to a toilet on the first floor and a large sink on the second. A brick barn in the backyard was destined for conversion to quarters for staff and nursing students.

The patient capacity of this modest facility was twelve beds. A board resolution assured that "persons of all creeds and no creed are admitted and receive the same quality of nursing and care." However, those "suffering from contagious or infectious disease or mental aberration or alcoholic mania are not eligible." The last exclusion evidently did not always apply, because one early nursing student recalled her struggle to control a state legislator who had been admitted, suffering from delirium tremens. Without any male orderlies to help them, the nurses on duty had

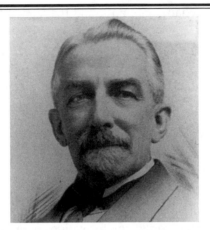

Springfield Hospital's principal founder;
Pastor Martin Luecke.

Martin Luecke, Founding Father

Martin H. Luecke deserves credit as the principal founder, or "prime mover," of Springfield Hospital and Training School. While notable by itself, this achievement was but one in his busy and illustrious career.

Luecke was born in Sheboygan, Wisconsin, in 1859. Educated at Concordia College in Fort Wayne, Indiana and then Concordia Seminary in St. Louis, he held pastorates in Bethalto and Troy, Illinois before moving to Springfield in 1892. There he had dual responsibilities as pastor of Trinity Lutheran Church and president (as well as an instructor) at Concordia Seminary. Considered one of Trinity's "ablest and most gifted pastors," he significantly reduced the church's debt and organized several charitable and relief efforts for the poor His most enduring accomplishment in Springfield was to spearhead the drive for a Lutheran hospital.

In 1903 Luecke moved back to his alma mater in Fort Wayne, serving a long term as president, until his death in 1926. Always interested in Springfield Hospital's welfare, he regularly returned to attend its annual membership meetings.

no alternative but to lock him in a basement supply room. This was an extreme example of the local adage that citizens were not safe when the legislature was in session.

Hospital staffing was commensurately small. Matron Helena Hanser was typical of hospital superintendents of that era, who generally were women with nursing experience who lived on the premises. She oversaw three nurses (including Lizette Nagel), a housekeeper (paid $1 per day), a janitor ($12 per month), and a part-time cook ($6 per month plus room and board).

Financing even such a limited establishment was a pressing board concern at every meeting. Like other voluntary community hospitals of its time, Springfield Hospital functioned awkwardly in a "middle ground between government and commerce," providing a community health service but without reliance upon tax resources. While some charitable cases were admitted, the hospital was expected to operate largely from fee income. During the spring of 1897 the board tinkered with the rate schedule for patients, eventually settling on $3.50 per week in the two wards, and $7-10 for a private room. Negotiation with the sheriff led to a $3 per week rate for county relief cases. Occasionally a special long-term need or opportunity arose, as in the board's June decision to accept the large sum of $850 "to allow the 73 year old Irish person" to remain indefinitely. Room rates did not include laundry service, special nursing care, or use of the surgical room; the latter cost "$5 to $10 extra." All charges were to be payable in advance.

Like its many proliferating peers around the country, Springfield Hospital faced chronic financial difficulty. The board's first fiscal report, late in May, revealed total income of $6,864 and expenses of $6,005, leaving some unpaid remodeling bills and a precarious cash balance of $859. The nation's new hospitals scrambled to raise funds and reduce costs. One vital recourse was the use of nursing students as staff; for a small monthly stipend they performed most of a hospital's necessary labor. Church and other charitable donations of cash, foodstuffs, and supplies were another approach. One promising source of fee income was surgery, so hospitals invested all available funds in the necessary space and equipment.

Board minutes are filled with references to cost cutting and revenue raising schemes. Late in April Dr. Langdon announced his success in persuading funeral homes to remove corpses at no cost to the hospital, and the board selected a favored undertaker after he offered free ambulance service. Contributions were solicited, with but limited success, from Lutheran churches and their congregations throughout central Illinois. Despite these and other efforts, by October the board decided that its "weak hospital fund" would permit only partial payment of the matron's $25 monthly salary. Year-end figures were no better, and also revealed the enterprise's primary reliance upon patient fees. Total receipts for 1897 were $9,253 and expenditures were $9,113, leaving a cash surplus of only $140. The bulk of receipts (81 per cent) came from sale of $7,500 in stock; fee income provided 15 per cent ($1,426), and donations (a paltry $327) less than four per cent. However altruistic and dedicated the founders and sponsors may have been, these figures were at best inauspicious omens of the fragile hospital's future.

People And Piety

One promising development in an otherwise difficult first year was the early and emphatic decision that nursing education would be integral to the hospital's operation. Indicative of this firm commitment were the words "and Training School" in Springfield Hospital's legal and formal name. Matron Hanser and board members knew that low-paid nursing apprentices were essential to controlling hospital costs, so they moved quickly to establish a curriculum and recruit students.

Nationally, nursing schools spread as rapidly as hospitals in the late 19th century. Clara Barton and others had demonstrated the value of professionally trained nurses in medical care. Like a career in teaching, nursing was a respectable occupation for millions of young unmarried women who needed to support themselves or wanted to leave home. Many of the newly founded hospitals needed their own nursing students for cheap labor and staff recruitment. Consequently, the number of nursing schools rose sharply, from three in 1873 to 432 in 1900 and 1,129 in 1910.

New standards of medical hygiene, sanitation, and antiseptic surgery largely shaped the workload of hospital nurses. Particularly among the student nurses, but also generally true for all nurses, the work was menial, monotonous, and technically unchallenging. Nurses spent much of their long work days scrubbing floors, walls, and furniture, bathing patients, making gauze bandages, emptying bedpans, and sterilizing instruments. They were not authorized to conduct even the simplest technical procedures, like measuring a patient's temperature or blood pressure. By modern

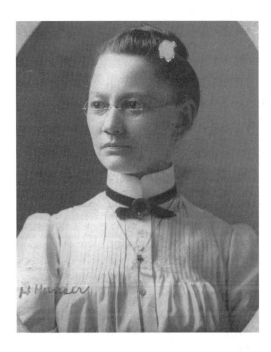

Helena Hanser, the first matron of Springfield Hospital and Training School.

Selma Hanser, sister of Helena Hanser and one of four charter students of Springfield Training School.

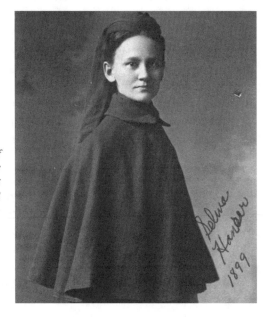

standards they resembled housekeepers, but the appeal of gainful employment in a nurturing career open to virtuous women was strong.

Under Helena Hanser's leadership, plans took shape to launch the nursing school within six months of the hospital's opening. Area Lutheran churches were invited to encourage young women over 18 to apply. The inaugural class of 1899 began its two-year program on October 15, 1897. There were four charter students: Irene Kestler, Ida Vasconcelles, Mary Rentschler, and Selma Hanser, the matron's younger sister. With two weekly lectures by physicians and one by Helena Hanser, the curriculum heavily emphasized practical subjects. Only later did science courses appear, as a means of enriching what students learned.

Nursing students were required to "assist with patient care" as part of their education. The combination of instruction and work left almost no free time. Students lived in the Training School dormitory. By 7:00 every morning they had dressed, eaten breakfast, and attended chapel. At roll call they were rigorously inspected for cleanliness and neatness. This meant no makeup or nail polish, hair in nets, shoes brightly polished, and heavily starched clean uniforms. Workdays covered 12 to 16 hours, plus lectures, and nearly consumed the entire week. A half day on Saturday or Sunday was the only available leisure time, and even then students were expected to attend church or study.

For this demanding regimen student nurses received free tuition, room and board, plus $3 a month for sundry expenses. In its early years the Training School had to recruit vigorously for its small enrollment, as each year's class never rose above six. By 1906, eight successive classes had produced 40 graduates, among them Selma Hanser, Kathryn Matthews (who became a surgical nurse at the hospital), and Anna Tittman, who became probably the most illustrious alumna of the Training School.

The regular nursing staff worked just as hard and long. Their twelve hour days ran all week, except for Sunday afternoon and one free evening "for courting purposes." Nurses were prohibited from smoking, drinking alcohol, visiting dance halls, or getting their hair styled at a "beauty shop." Out of their modest $20 monthly salary (plus free room and board), they were expected to save a sizable share so as not to be a burden in their "declining years." One potential source of additional income was an occasional outside nursing assignment. Early in 1898 the board approved such arrangements, provided the client paid the hospital $1 per day and $1 per night, to be split equally with the nurse.

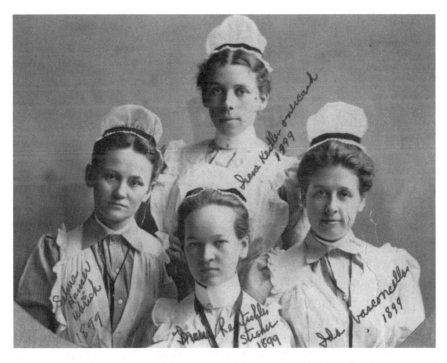

The charter graduating class (1899) of Springfield Training School—Selma Hanser Ubrich, Mary Rentschler Stisher, Ida Vasconcelles and Irene Kestler Overcash.

The anomalous relationship between a hospital and its medical staff was a unique American development of this era. Physicians were not hospital employees, but instead had a symbiotic relationship that also led easily to tension and even conflict. Doctors on the staff could care for their patients at no personal expense for overhead and equipment. In return, their referrals were the institution's lifeblood. Consequently hospitals eagerly sought the good will and confidence of a community's most active physicians, most notably its surgeons who produced lucrative fees for the operating room(s).

Springfield in 1898 listed 67 physicians. The hospital's charter staff consisted of John Prince and John N. Dixon (surgery); Elizabeth Matthews, Langdon, and Addison C. James (gynecology); George F. Stericker, A. Douglas Taylor, Ralph C. Matheny, and Riland O. Berry (general medicine); Wilber P. Armstrong (homeopathy); Ninus S. Penick (eye, ear); and E. Foster Hazell (dental surgery). Joining them early in 1898 was William A. Young, who when he died in 1943 was the last surviving member of the original group. Conspicuously absent was the city's most prominent physician of that time, George N. Kreider, who was a leader of the District Medical Society of Central Illinois and founder (in 1899) of the Springfield Medical Club. Apparently his relationship with St. John's Hospital was too strong to warrant affiliation with its Protestant rival.

Reflecting a previously noted national trend, women held a fair share of staff appointments. In addition to Matthews, Helen A. Babb served beginning in 1899, and Estelle Paullin joined in 1900, as "Ladies Physician."

It took nearly two years for Springfield Hospital's medical staff to formally organize themselves. Their first official meeting occurred January 22, 1899, "to perfect a permanent organization." In addition to drafting bylaws and rules for membership, they elected Dr. Taylor as the first president. The staff minutes reveal only one other meeting that year, and for several years thereafter they met only once annually, to elect new members and officers. At the January 1900 meeting they elected Dr. Dixon to succeed Taylor, and approved a resolution of thanks to board member William Zapf for supplying a box of cigars. By then the staff had grown slightly, to 15.

Elizabeth Matthews, M.D.

Noteworthy as a charter member of Springfield Hospital's medical staff, Dr. Elizabeth Matthews was a pioneer in other respects as well. Born near Detroit, Michigan in 1861, she graduated from the University of Michigan and then taught school, one of the few respectable occupations for women at that time. Restless for a new career; she enrolled at the Women's Medical College of Chicago in 1888. This pathbreaking school resisted male domination of the medical profession by graduating 400 women during its brief and beleaguered history.

In 1891 Matthews was licensed to practice in Illinois, and she moved to Springfield, opening an office at Fifth and Monroe streets. Six years later she was among the coterie of twelve physicians who joined the fledgling Lutheran hospital. Like most women doctors of that era, she practiced gynecology, which was considered the only specialty that justified their membership in an otherwise male profession.

Always adventuresome, Matthews was absent for extended periods traveling in the United States and overseas, usually to gather information and experience at noted clinics. During World War I she was a Red Cross physician and surgeon in France. After that she stayed in Europe, settling in Italy as the personal physician to an exiled Russian nobleman. In 1933, at age 72, she returned to Springfield, where she died two years later. Gender and lengthy absences prevented her from leaving a major mark in Springfield, but her career and habitual independence are worthy of note.

Among the hospital's physicians several individuals stood out for their steadfast commitment and active participation. Drs. Dixon, Langdon, Stericker, Young, and Taylor often attended board meetings to report on developments or request the purchase of new equipment. Their loyalty during these perilous early years was vital to the hospital's viability.

While open to people of all faiths, Springfield Hospital retained and promoted its close relationship with Trinity Lutheran Church and the Missouri Synod. It was generally believed and never denied that the hospital was founded as "an infirmary for Concordia Seminary." Press reports often called it "Springfield Lutheran Hospital," and its own publications added "Under Lutheran Auspices" to its official name. Board meetings often began and ended with a prayer.

Another measure of Lutheran influence was the composition of Springfield Hospital's board and even the nursing staff. As noted previously, every member of the original board was either a pastor or lay leader at Trinity or Concordia, except for Dr. Langdon, whose membership (and appointment as superintendent) undoubtedly owed to his generosity in providing his residence as the hospital's first building. Both the matron and the cook (Helena and Selma Hanser) came from a prominent St. Louis Lutheran family, and the German surnames of most other staff and charter nurses at least suggest Lutheran affiliation. For its remodeling and the construction of an annex in 1899, the board selected local contractor Henry Bettinghaus & Son, a family that was active in Trinity Church affairs. George Bettinghaus also served on the board at Concordia Seminary.

From the outset hospital board minutes were written in German, which was consistent with practice at Trinity and Concordia. The original stock certificates also were German, and it is nearly certain that board meetings were conducted in the language that members knew and used regularly. A curious exception occurred in 1898, evidently precipitating a board crisis that had serious community repercussions and nearly destroyed the embryonic institution.

For reasons unstated, during the twelve months beginning in February, 1898 board minutes were recorded in English rather than German. This may have stemmed from a board decision in 1897 to drop "Lutheran Auspices" from the hospital's name. Then, at a special meeting on January 18, 1899, Pastor Luecke (who served as vice president during 1898) was restored to the presidency and made an important statement:

Anna Tittman, Notable Nurse

One of the Training School's early graduates, Anna Tittman, parlayed her education and early experience into a long and distinguished career in nursing and public health. Born in Springfield to a poor family in 1884, she had to work for room and board to attend Springfield High School, where she graduated third in her class. She entered nurse's training in 1904, spending two years living and working in the original hospital building and its two annexes.

After six years of private duty experience, Miss Tittman was named the Springfield school system's first nurse, in 1912. That same year, displaying a bent for public health work, she opened the city's first dental dispensary. Major recognition and opportunity came in 1914, when Governor Edward F. Dunne named her to head the State Board of Nurse Examiners. Her frequent inspections and critiques of Springfield Hospital made her a familiar and controversial figure in hospital board deliberations.

During World War I Anna Tittman served in the American Red Cross, and was its chief nurse for the U.S. Army expedition to Siberia in 1919. Advanced study at Johns Hopkins and Columbia universities led to a degree in public health nursing, and new work of national scope. For nearly 20 years she was an executive with the National Organization for Public Health Nursing.

In 1936, on the 30th anniversary of her graduation, Miss Tittman returned to Springfield Hospital to address nursing graduates. After retiring she moved back to her native city, where she was named to the Springfield High School Hall of Fame in 1975. She died in 1977, at age 93.

As this institution is to become the property of our Lutheran congregations, as has been resolved by the delegates during last session of synod, and as the business meetings shall be conducted by means of the German language, I have been charged by the stockholders to cast the votes as I have done. All rules and regulations therefore contrary to this are null and void henceforth.

Cementing this change was the removal of Dr. Langdon from the board, though he remained as superintendent of the hospital. Immediately (and continuing for the next 20 years) board minutes reverted to German, except for occasional financial reports in English.

Reportedly the synod had acted to establish the "Evangelical Lutheran Hospital Association of Central Illinois," in order to consolidate its hospital activities and to ensure strict adherence "to Lutheran principles." Earlier claims that Springfield Hospital and Training School would be "strictly non-sectarian" came under doubt with this series of steps.

Tension mounted all year, bursting to a bitter public dispute in 1900. Officials at St. John's Hospital issued a seven-page tract entitled "Selfdefense vs. The Springfield Hospital," accusing their rival institution of conducting a covert and malicious campaign against it and "its managers, the Sisters of St. Francis." The pamphlet merits detailed summary even though it presents but one side, because it illustrates the sectarian hostility that had developed.

Author of the tract was Rev. Louis Hinssen, director at St. John's, who addressed his message to the citizens of Springfield. He claimed that officials at Springfield Hospital had issued two different annual reports for the year 1899, one in English and the other in German. Ostensibly covering the same subject, they in fact (according to Hinssen) had different titles and very different contents. The English version, called simply "Report of the Springfield Hospital," reiterated the institution's non-sectarian mission, described the nursing school, and provided readers with a summary of hospital rules and other general information. The report was factual and inoffensive: "nobody could find any fault with it."

Hinssen proceeded to describe the German version, which officials at St. John's had obtained with some difficulty. Its longer title was "Report of the Springfield Hospital of the Evangelical Lutheran Society of Central Illinois." Both its contents and the tone amounted to a diatribe "of dishonest means and slanders" against "an honest competitor" and "the noble Sisters." To prove his point, Hinssen included lengthy excerpts from the "false charges" in the report.

The alleged document's preamble complained that, before 1897, "Rome ruled ... with absolute power" over central Illinoisans needing hospital care. Citing the two typhoid epidemics ten years earlier, it claimed that "fanatical nuns" had attempted to convert some Concordia students who convalesced at St. John's. Protesting these "false charges" and the "despicable means" that Lutheran leaders had employed to spread them, Hinssen branded his adversaries as the real fanatics. Going further, he accused them of shielding their real intent with a benign, non-sectarian face in order to attract broad public support for the new hospital. Now, he concluded, Springfield Hospital "has thrown off its mask," confirming the original fears of local Catholics when they learned that "the professors of Concordia" had spearheaded the movement for a new hospital.

Among the early records of Springfield Hospital there is no mention of this dispute, or record of the different reports for 1899. However, there is evidence in the board minutes, as previously noted, of the synod's action early in 1898 to reassert complete Lutheran control and restore the hospital to "Lutheran principles" under Pastor Luecke. Also, the board did authorize issuance of annual reports and other publications in both German and English. Therefore, while the record is incomplete and highly partisan, evidence from the two antagonistic institutions is in general agreement.

Clearly there was a bitter rivalry and war of words underway between the larger and more established St. John's and the struggling upstart several blocks north. Worse, the feud had reached public attention, with ugly undertones of religious bigotry. Whatever its causes and course, it damaged the public face of both hospitals, and inevitably exacerbated their natural rivalry for staff physicians, patients and civic support.

In its third year of operation, Springfield Hospital and Training School therefore faced new and prickly challenges in addition to the familiar issues of space, staffing, credibility, and finances. Never fully secure or established during its infancy, it now had the added burden of an internal struggle over control that had spread externally, to a public fight and a public relations disaster. Founded by citizens and medical professionals who were dedicated to curing ills and alleviating pain, Springfield Hospital ironically was in danger of becoming more a problem than a solution to the citizens of Springfield. Nevertheless, its birth had been opportune, because a rapidly growing populace needed more and better medical service, and Americans by the millions were turning to hospitals over home care.

As the nation welcomed a new century, Springfield Hospital faced an array of problems and challenges. Time would tell whether its earnest board, its able physicians, its dedicated nurses, and its loyal managers could repair the damage, tap the growing market, and achieve financial stability.

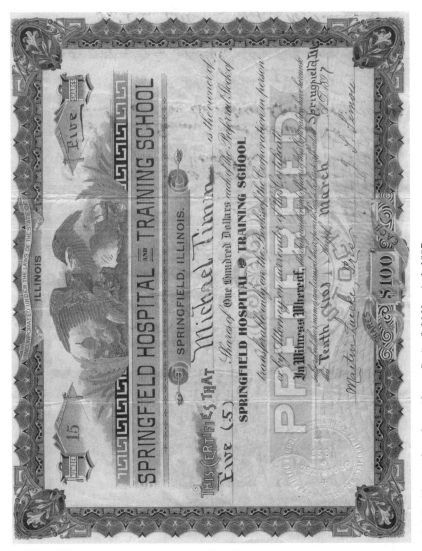

Original hospital stock certificate. Springfield Hospital, 1897.

Memorial Milestones

1900   Smallpox epidemic

        Martin Luecke leaves Springfield

        Construction of south wing

        Dr. Charles Patton joins medical staff

        Typhoid outbreak

        Ira Gerding and John Hoffmann appointed

1910   AMA Flexner report

        Palmer Tuberculosis Sanitorium opens

        "Springfield Survey"

        Matron Rosa Waltke (1913-17)

1915   Three story addition opens

        U.S. enters Great War

        Spanish Influenza epidemic

        Board minutes in English

1920   Pastor Paul Schulz joins board

        Frederick Streckfuss leaves board

        Frank Siebert and Louise Lindemann resign

1923   Debt crisis

Chapter Two

Innocuous Desuetude

The dawn of a new century brought social and political reforms, resurgent public optimism, and bold visions of inevitable progress for most Americans. The nation's medical industry participated in this burst of energy and confidence, as physicians, scientists, nurses and many hospitals built on the substantial gains and numerous discoveries of the previous several decades. Scientific breakthroughs in the prevention of dread diseases, a continuing boom in hospital construction, and rising standards for medical schools were just some of the signs that American medicine was in tune with the spirit of the "progressive era."

Such, unfortunately, was not the case with Springfield Hospital and Training School. Following soon upon the fervor of its founding was a long, slow period of institutional struggle and decline, punctuated by periodic crises. For the next 25 years board members and a tiny staff bravely worked to keep pace with changing technology, recruit physicians and nursing students to the staff, earn public confidence, and pay both operating expenses and the interest on a mounting debt. Of course there were some bright moments and solid achievements, and no dearth of heroic supporters, but in general Springfield Hospital during the first quarter of the 20th century suffered a withering of the energy and resources that had launched it and were vital to sustaining it. Looking back on this bleak era in the hospital's history, a consultant in the 1930s aptly labeled it a time of "innocuous desuetude."

Growing Pains

The shrill sectarian invective that marked Springfield Hospital's feud with St. John's Hospital in 1899 receded thereafter, at least in its public expression. A bitter and mutually suspecting rivalry persisted, but officials of both institutions at least managed to avoid any further public embarrassments. Lutheran control and orientation continued, and most of the founding directors stayed in charge. Joining Pastor Luecke, Professor Simon and Messrs. Schnepp and Zapf on the board in 1900 was Herr Boye, pastor of a Lutheran church outside Springfield. The next year Professor Frederick Streckfuss of Concordia Seminary began a lengthy board tenure that lasted until his death, in 1924. Pastor Luecke resigned his position as officer in 1903, when he left Trinity to serve as president of Concordia College in Fort Wayne.

As long as the Evangelical Lutheran Association of Central Illinois owned and controlled the hospital, its member churches had a stake in the institution's welfare. Their interest was conspicuous at the annual meetings, which ministers and laity from a dozen or more central Illinois cities attended. In 1901, for example, there were Lutheran church representatives from Lincoln, New Berlin, Beardstown, Decatur, Petersburg, Pekin, Chandlerville, Havana, Manito, Chestnut and Mt. Pulaski, in addition to Springfield. Thus was established, albeit in a narrow fashion, the regional scope that would much later distinguish Memorial Hospital's expanding market and reputation.

Control also meant responsibility and stewardship, so churches and their congregations in the association were expected to serve the hospital in various ways. Not only did they supply board members and officers, but they also were supposed to steer patients to the hospital. In addition, there were periodic calls for them to encourage young women in their congregations to enroll in the nursing school. Finally, of course, they were subject to constant appeals for monetary and in-kind donations. In order to renovate the hospital's third floor, directors in 1901 pledged to raise $500 from each of their respective congregations. That same year the board expressed "heartfelt thanks" to New Berlin Lutherans for a gift of 45 dozen eggs. Affiliated pastors occasionally were asked to devote their sermons to an appeal for gifts.

Hospital Hyperbole

*Striving to win civic stature and a steady influx of patients, Springfield Hospital's leaders did their best to advertise the new institution. One conspicuous example was the space they purchased in a 1903 promotional booklet, **State Topics: Springfield in the Twentieth Century**. Both text and illustration rendered the hospital in highly flattering terms. The artists' drawing, for example, portrayed a much larger and grander complex than contemporary photographs reveal.*

The accompanying description resorted to dubious superlatives ("highest ... first class ... best") and inflated prose. Springfield Hospital's north side neighborhood was dubbed "salubrious and pleasant," and patients reportedly appreciated its expansive and beautiful lawn. Inside the facility were "spacious wards and splendidly furnished private rooms," plus an "operating room (that) is a model of beauty." Skilled nurses and nursing students worked under "the best medical and surgical staff obtainable in Central Illinois."

The authors mixed pride with prayer in forecasting "a bright future for our young and efficient institution."

Additional money was one way to attack the hospital's chronic financial peril; another was curbing costs. In 1901 the board agreed that the annual budget for building repairs could not exceed a miserly $100. That same year, after some discussion, it authorized paying a housekeeper $8 per month "on the condition that she would not break so many dishes any longer." In 1902 a maid was offered $10 per month provided she also helped with the laundry. When she complained about this salary, the board voted to dismiss her.

Added to the original mortgage debt were the expenses of adding a north wing (1899) and a south wing (1904). These facilities were necessary to raise the hospital's capacity and thus generate more income. The 1899 wing more than tripled capacity to 40 beds, and the south wing doubled that, to 80. Local architect Murray Hanes designed both structures, and the Bettinghaus firm was contractor. The earlier construction was budgeted at approximately $10,000, and the latter at $15,000. Contributing to the south wing's greater expense was a $2,000 elevator. When completed, the total cost actually exceeded $22,000. Nearly every board meeting during these years dealt with construction decisions and the negotiation of loans to cover costs.

Hospital debt correspondingly rose at a steep rate, reaching $43,000 in the early 1900s. Board members frequently wrestled with the challenge of allocating a slender cash balance between the twin demands of current obligations and debt payments. One brief bright moment occurred in 1906, when rising income enabled the board to reduce debt by ten per cent, to $39,000.

One curious measure of this period's financial strains was the occasional discussion at board and stockholder meetings of proposals to sell the hospital. Even in the midst of major construction projects there were calls to unburden the Evangelical Lutheran Association of its costly young hospital. The first such discussion came in 1900, and was promptly dismissed by a renewed commitment to raise construction costs from area Lutherans. The issue surfaced again in 1906, when board members agreed that a minimum selling price would be $85,000. The next year they were more interested and less demanding. Mr. Zapf was instructed to inform an unidentified prospective buyer that the hospital was available for $60,000, and that negotiations were welcome. Nothing, however, came of these overtures.

Financial results were on the agenda at nearly every early board meeting. The annual report for 1898, the hospital's first full year, revealed total income of only $2,842 and nearly equal expenditures, $2,821. Patient fees comprised 96 per cent of the revenue, with donations of only $105. Income jumped to nearly $5,000 the next year, due to the expansion completed that year. To save on food costs, hospital employees tended a vegetable garden behind the building, solicited donations of canned goods and jellies, and sometimes accepted meat and poultry in lieu of cash from patients. An annual fundraising event, the "Hospital Fest," generated some cash donations. Staged in the summertime on the seminary campus or at the state fairgrounds, this event drew volunteer help from Trinity Church and netted modest returns; for example $125 in 1899.

Monthly operating income and expenses naturally grew as additional beds became available. In the hospital's first few years monthly income was in the mid-hundreds range, but by 1902 it began exceeding $1,000. Total operating income in the 1903-04 year was over $12,000, sufficient to meet periodic debt payments of $500. With more space and beds, the hospital payroll also rose. Three nurses were added in 1904, bringing the nursing staff to ten plus 38 students. Other employees (the matron, housekeepers, receptionist, kitchen staff, janitor) totaled ten.

There was corresponding growth of the medical staff, which reached 27 by 1904. Much of the expansion took the form of new specialists. Assignment of space and personnel for pathological work began early but modestly; in 1900 the board approved providing a small room "behind the wood house" for post-mortem examinations. At a cost of $100 this 14 x 18 foot space was converted to a mortuary in 1904. Dr. Samuel E. Munson joined the staff as pathologist in 1907, and was succeeded by Dr. Harrison C. Blankmeyer two years later. A pediatrician, Dr. George T. Palmer, also served beginning in 1909.

Among the new medical staff recruits was Charles L. Patton, who returned to his hometown in 1906 after training and a residency in obstetrics-gynecology at the University of Michigan. Dr. Patton was in the vanguard of Springfield physicians to boast advanced training in a specialty, and thus to signal a major medical trend of the 20th century. He quickly gained stature as one of the city's most capable and progressive physicians, serving his first of three terms as president of the hospital's medical staff in 1913. He (and later his son Robert L. Patton) worked hard to enhance the quality and reputation of Springfield Hospital's medical services.

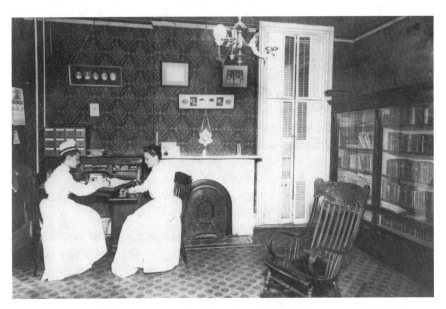

Nursing personnel in the hospital's central structure, Dr. William Langdon's former residence. The year is 1905.

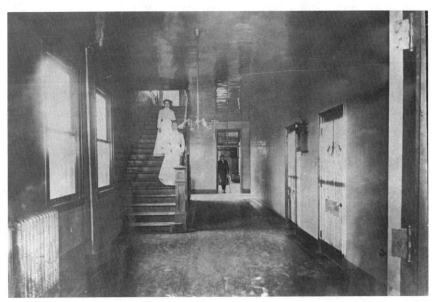

An interior hallway at Springfield Hospital, 1903.

The demand for X-ray services grew steadily during those years. Dr. Fred S. O'Hara specialized in this work, and generated valuable income from it for the hospital. By 1914 his cramped quarters were inadequate, so the board reluctantly authorized him to use its meeting room to store supplies, inspect X-rays, and confer with patients.

Reform and organized action were hallmarks of the American medical profession in the new century's first decade. During those ten years, membership in the American Medical Association swelled from 8,400 to 70,000, giving physicians for the first time a powerful national voice. Organized medicine's agenda echoed the Progressive Era's reform themes: efficiency, the application of knowledge to solve society's ills, a reliance upon experts, and faith in a better future. Two notable developments illustrated this trend. One was the AMA's success in welding state and local medical societies into a potent alliance that pushed to upgrade the qualifications and performance of doctors, particularly in their hospital service. The second was AMA's drive for improved medical education, which began with an inspection program in 1905 and culminated in the famous 1910 report by Abraham Flexner, calling for close integration of hospital care with medical science and medical education.

A central tenet of this reform surge was the emphasis upon detailed and timely medical records as a requisite of good patient care. Hospitals and their medical staffs were the fulcrum for accomplishing this progressive advance. Thus was inaugurated a chronic contest between hospital administrators and physicians over the maintenance of satisfactory medical records. Hospital officials and medical staff officers periodically pleaded and even threatened doctors to comply and thereby satisfy a crucial accreditation standard. One final tendency of this period was the growing influence of staff physicians in the governance and management of hospitals.

Springfield Hospital's medical staff gradually began adopting these ideas and practices in its own collective actions. In 1907 it successfully petitioned the board to dismiss an incompetent member from practice in the hospital. Shifting from pro forma annual meetings to monthly meetings, staff physicians frequently transmitted requests and recommendations to the board. One major appeal that failed was its 1912 suggestion that the religious institution convert to "a general hospital," and add a new pediatric wing. In this and other actions it was demonstrating a fresh concern for the hospital's general standing, not simply medical concerns. On more technical matters, like hiring a nurse anesthetist to assist in surgery, the physicians were more successful.

Relations between the board and the medical staff reached a peak of interaction during 1913-14. At several joint meetings doctors raised such disparate issues as the need for land acquisitions to accommodate future expansion and a concern for cleaner and safer milk supplies. Participants in a joint dinner gathering noted with satisfaction the "good will existing between the Board and the Staff." This cordial spirit was interrupted in 1916, when the two groups feuded over Dr. Blankmeyer's election as a medical staff officer. As physicians gained greater community stature and technical proficiency, their parallel quest for more influence in hospital decision making confronted a lay board equally determined to maintain its hegemony. This was the outset of a natural contest over hospital governance that would affect Springfield Hospital and its peers nationwide throughout the new century.

New Leaders, New Challenges

The profession of hospital administration was in its infancy during these early years at Springfield Hospital. A national Association of Hospital Superintendents was organized in 1899, and in 1908 changed its name to the American Hospital Association. Compared to private business, hospitals were slow in developing corporate models of efficiency and organizational hierarchy. Dubbed a "peculiar bureaucracy" by one historian, they took decades to devise administrative structures, professional training, or a systematic approach to capital development, pooled purchasing, and fee collection.

At Springfield Hospital, even administrative titles and roles seemed fluid. Helena Hanser began in 1897 as matron, but two years later, with no change in duties, she was called superintendent. By 1901 she again had the title of matron. There was no clear delineation between her executive responsibilities and those of the hospital's other appointed head, Dr. Langdon. In all likelihood their respective duties were a reflection of their differential professions and genders. As a woman and a nurse, Hanser fit the conventional role then prevailing for a hospital's day-to-day operations manager. She lived at the hospital, supervised the nurses and other staff, directed the nursing school, and generally oversaw patient care. In 1905 her salary was $40 per month. By then her duties were sufficiently burdensome for the board to recruit a nurse to relieve her of one task: chloroforming surgical patients.

Because he regularly attended his own patients at the hospital, Dr. Langdon was accessible for key decisions, and he routinely represented the institution at board meetings. Sometimes he also was referred to as superintendent. Evidently this vague division of labor (and confusion of titles) worked reasonably well; at least there is no evidence to the contrary in the records.

By 1900 Selma Hanser was serving her sister as assistant superintendent, after successive stints as cook, nursing student, and nurse. Helena became ill in the summer of 1905, and took a lengthy vacation "for rest and recuperation." That fall she resigned, reportedly due to a "situation that required her presence elsewhere." Whatever her health at the time, Helena Hanser lived to the ripe age of 86, and before her death in 1954 offered reminiscences about the hospital's early years. Her departure triggered an interregnum of several months in which three women were offered the position, followed by successive resignations and appointments that reflected administrative confusion for the next several years.

First was Kathryn Matthews, a surgical nurse at the hospital, who apparently declined. In December the board approached a St. Louis nurse named Amies, promising her a nursing job and the prospect of being named matron. She accepted the first but never received the latter appointment, and resigned later to get married. The next month, January 1906, Ira Gerding was appointed. After eight months illness forced her to resign, so the board prevailed upon Miss Matthews to serve as acting superintendent.

Within a month, and "overwhelmed by work," Matthews also resigned, leading the board to reappoint Miss Gerding, whose health evidently had improved. She remained in the position from 1907 to 1913, but again there was confusion in administrative titles. In July of 1907 the board negotiated with John A. Hoffmann to serve as superintendent, though clearly he was succeeding Dr. Langdon as the hospital's chief executive. Hoffmann was offered $65 per month, but managed to obtain $68 plus a telephone connection at his residence. He held the office for nearly seven years.

Like other hospital boards of the day, the directors of Springfield Hospital made decisions on even the pettiest issues and transactions. In a habit that survived to the 1960s, board members frequently visited the facility, walked the corridors, and conferred with staff and patients alike. Meeting formally once a month, they discussed and decided all personnel matters, and purchases as small as several dollars.

Reporting the News

Beginning soon after it was established, and continuing fitfully in its early decades, Springfield Hospital publicized its services and reported its news through various publications. One early item, "Pages from the Hospital" (1901), was a promotional pamphlet with text by Pastor Martin Luecke and photographs of staff physicians. Its cost was borne with advertisements by friendly businesses.

A monthly newsletter, "Hospital News Sheet," first appeared late in 1900. This modest two page publication began as a promotional piece rather than a house organ, and was available for an annual subscription of 25 cents. Within a few years it was renamed the "Hospital Journal," offering lists of the medical and hospital staffs and nursing students, and also reporting monthly expenses and income.

Hard times and more pressing concerns occasionally interrupted publication, but the newsletter continued its irregular run. By the 1920s it had another new name, "Springfield Hospital News," and a more realistic quarterly schedule. During these years it remained something of a hybrid, partly house organ and partly external promotion. Not until the hospital's reorganization and financial recovery did its publications diversify into separate intramural and extramural periodicals. Such were the modest origins of the numerous glossy publications that today report on Memorial Medical Center to employees and various interested publics.

During the hospital's early years the board included various physicians, all drawn from the medical staff. In 1898 the board voted to add Dr. William A. Young, providing he either made a gift or purchased stock. Also serving that year were Drs. Lewis C. Taylor, Addison James, and Wilber Armstrong. After the hospital's transfer to strict Lutheran control in 1899, physicians ceased representation on the board (for over eighty years).

As previously noted, Miss Lizette Nagel had an anomalous role that combined administrative and governing activities. She regularly attended board meetings and was authorized to make routine purchases of supplies. Apparently she was the institution's chief financial officer, because the ledger and account books were her responsibility. When treasurer William Schnepp resigned due to illness in 1901, Miss Nagel was named to succeed him. In this capacity she was an officer of the corporation while also an agent of board governance. Her death late in 1903 led to the appointment of Selma Hanser to succeed her.

Rarely if ever was Springfield Hospital filled to capacity. The bed census for January, 1902 was typical. There were 29 patients when the month began, and 34 when it ended, comprising approximately 75 per cent of the 40-bed capacity. During January 39 patients were admitted, 30 were released, and four died. Five years later, with capacity doubled to 80, the hospital still had fewer than 30 patients on most days. During August of 1907, for example, patient care days totaled 799, for a daily average of less than 27.

While the hospital generally operated well below capacity, its directors still believed that it must grow in order to survive. Considerably smaller than its local Catholic rival, and housed in an inefficient cluster of small buildings, Springfield Hospital might yet find success through construction. Accordingly, the board decided in 1914 to build a three-story addition with 40 beds, bringing the total capacity to 120. Current debt was to be consolidated with construction costs in a new $50,000 mortgage at five per cent, payable over ten years. Whether born of optimism or desperation, this additional debt burden proved troublesome and nearly fatal in the early 1920s. Speaking prophetically, a local banker warned the board in 1914, "You'll never see the end of that debt."

The new facility opened in 1915, as Europe was settling into war. With it the original property at Fifth Street and North Grand Avenue became a Hydra of separate buildings, cumbersomely connected. Dr. Robert Patton remembered visiting the facility often as a young boy, while his father made rounds. Its principal entrance still looked like the residential entryway that it had once been. The hospital's lobby bore unmistakable traces of its original function as the Langdon family's front hall and parlor. The overall appearance was "rather dark and gloomy." By then the second floor space for surgery had grown, with one minor and two main operating rooms. Nearby was the X-ray department, with "ancient equipment" and a tiny darkroom.

In those years the average hospital stay, nationally, was 25 days. Three out of four patients paid the full rate, another ten per cent made partial payment, and 15 per cent were charity cases. These general factors placed a heavy strain upon Springfield Hospital's operating finances. Faced with excess capacity and substantial debt, the board frequently implored staff physicians and Lutheran pastors to refer ill and injured patients to its empty beds.

Bequests were a welcome but rare source of financial relief. Two generous bequests totaling nearly $5,000 came in 1915. By then the expanded hospital's operating income had grown considerably, but still barely covered expenses. At year's end total income was $38,804, only $28 above total expenses. Debt exceeded $49,000.

One key to maintaining financial viability lay in the nursing school, which supplied cheap student labor and graduates to replenish a regular staff subject to frequent turnover. By the early 1900s the hospital's Training School accepted 12 or more new students every year, and had an average total enrollment of 30. For nursing students it was clear that "Your work came first, not your books." Classes were canceled whenever students were needed to help overworked nurses. Dr. Langdon regularly lectured on obstetrics and Dr. Dixon on surgery, while Helena Hanser covered all aspects of practical nursing. Gradually and grudgingly the board raised the monthly stipend from $2 to $5, and also offered advanced students a modest increase. Beginning in 1914, the hospital rented a North Fifth Street residence to house nursing students.

As the nursing profession organized itself nationally, it also began promoting educational reforms. The most serious deficiency in nursing education was instruction in the basic sciences. In 1912, following the national trend, Springfield Hospital stretched its program from two to three years, and added science instruction to the curriculum. The next year, signaling the school's coming-of-age, an alumnae association was founded to provide a social outlet for more than 100 graduates. The association continued to operate, even after the nursing school closed in the 1970s.

In addition to administrative, financial, and staffing challenges, Springfield Hospital confronted serious public health problems in its host city. A landmark social survey of Springfield, conducted in 1913 under the auspices of the Russell Sage Foundation, documented grave inadequacies in housing, education, charitable care, public health, and the treatment of mental illness. At least by implication, the city's medical institutions shared in the responsibility to address the litany of problems.

The "Springfield Survey" was notable as one of the first in a wave of community studies during the Progressive Era. By combining the survey research skills of social scientists with the volunteer assistance of local citizens, reformers hoped to supply factual ammunition and grass roots enthusiasm for civic uplift. Under the guidance of Russell Sage Foundation officials, an army of 600 Springfield citizens conducted a massive door-to-door survey. The findings were published in a three-volume, 1,600 page report and also publicized in an elaborate ten day public exhibition of charts, lectures, motion pictures, posters, and tableaux at the State Armory.

The documentary and statistical findings were sobering for parents, educators, employers, public officials and doctors, for they revealed a city with serious socioeconomic and health problems. In a public school system of 7,000 students, there was only one nurse and no physician to monitor contagious diseases and other problems. Systematic inoculation was "neglected," as three-fourths of all schoolchildren lacked vaccination. Community care of "mental defectives" and alcoholics was seriously deficient. The report noted that Springfield Hospital "has refused all mental cases," and St. John's only admitted some, consigning most of the troubled patients to either the county jail annex or the Sangamon County Farm (almshouse).

Scattered throughout the city, but especially on the east side, were numerous wretched neighborhoods with ramshackle houses, open sewage ditches, and dangerous drinking water. Springfield's public health rested precariously on an unregulated surfeit of 7,500 wells and an equal number of privies. Contagious diseases and even occasional epidemics were the inevitable result of such conditions.

Mortality statistics confirmed this troubling picture. During a six year period, 1908-13, there were 490 reported deaths from tuberculosis, 227 from pneumonia, 84 from typhoid, 61 from diphtheria, 44 from whooping cough, 31 from measles, and 23 from scarlet fever. Infant deaths from all causes totaled 727. Experts estimated that at least one quarter of all deaths (1,687) were preventable with good public health practices. The yearly average of 121 infant deaths struck observers as "appalling," particularly because at least one third were preventable.

Not surprisingly, the toll was disproportionately heavy among poor, ill-educated, and non-white families. For example, the tuberculosis death rate was more than four times higher for non-whites. This imbalance was in part a reflection of the uneven and generally poor quality of charitable medical care. In the absence of a free city medical dispensary, indigent patients generally headed either to the county poor farm, some 15 miles outside Springfield, or (if suffering from a contagious disease) to the city-county isolation hospital, just north of town.

Neither St. John's nor Springfield Hospital readily offered free beds for indigent adult patients, though both accepted county-subsidized referrals at the minimum rate of $4 per week. In 1913, for example, Springfield Hospital admitted only eight charity cases. It also notified authorities at the Washington Street Mission that ill or injured persons in their custody were not welcome. The hospital's policy for children was more liberal; it maintained a small free ward for them. With scant resources and a limited financial base, it could not afford to operate as a charitable institution. Realistically, Springfield Hospital officials had little choice but to discourage indigent patients.

Pestilence and War

Most of the hospital's problems during these years of struggle were self-imposed, or at least the products of its own nature: an inefficient physical plant, slender financial support, a sharply sectarian identity, and high administrative turnover. However, certain other challenges and one acute crisis during the 1910s stemmed from malevolent forces that were national or even global in scope, and insidious in their local impact. They further taxed Springfield Hospital's human and fiscal resources.

Not unlike most cities of its size and era, Springfield periodically endured outbreaks of virulent and often fatal disease. Cholera struck with devastating results several times in the 19th century. Typhoid fever, a direct result of poor sanitation and drinking water, killed between five and thirty-five people annually early in the new century. The city "suffered severely" from it in 1907, when the mortality rate jumped to 82 per 100,000 population.

Because it could have been prevented or at least mitigated through modern public health practices, the 1907 typhoid outbreak prodded Springfield officials to upgrade the city's small and inactive health department. In 1907 they filled the superintendent's position for the first time with a physician, and a very capable one as well. Dr. George T. Palmer came from a well known area family, earned recognition as a dedicated pediatrician, and was an early member of Springfield Hospital's medical staff. City health inspectors under his supervision became more diligent in enforcing public health ordinances. The new commission form of municipal government that commenced in 1911 supported Dr. Palmer's efforts to address health concerns raised in the Springfield Survey. Illegal privies and unsafe wells shrank in number, and consequently so did the incidence of typhoid. When Palmer left office in 1918, the city's public health office had transformed into a modern and vigilant agency under a full-time medical doctor.

Smallpox was another preventable disease, through vaccination. Efforts to enact compulsory vaccination were thwarted by court rulings, and an epidemic in 1901 produced over 500 cases, with 335 the next year. This outbreak in turn led to establishment of the previously mentioned isolation hospital, or "pest house."

The most intractable and chronic scourge of this era was tuberculosis, which killed an average of over 80 Springfield citizens annually in the early years of the 20th century. The Springfield Survey reported that both of the city's general hospitals were "averse to accepting tuberculosis patients." This was certainly true at Springfield Hospital, which limited its admissions to space available in a small backyard tent on its property at Fifth and North Grand. City health superintendent George Palmer spearheaded a civic solution by opening a clinic in 1911 and then persuading donors to underwrite construction of a sanitorium. Located in a converted farmhouse at the end of West Lawrence Avenue, the Palmer Tuberculosis Sanitorium

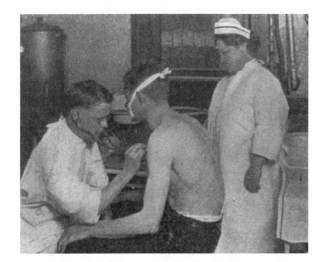

*The Springfield
Tuberculosis Association
operated a community
dispensary, circa 1916.*

*Sangamon County and
the City of Springfield
jointly maintained the
Contagious Disease
Hospital located north
of Oak Ridge Cemetery,
circa 1918.*

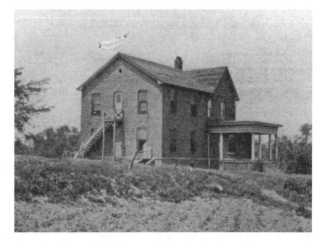

operated for 40 years under the dedicated leadership of its founder and namesake. Later the expanded facility and its 26 acres were sold to the Presbyterian Synod for use (still today) as a home for the elderly. A second facility opened in 1919, when St. John's Hospital established its tuberculosis sanitorium near Riverton, northeast of Springfield. This initiative, when first proposed, aroused suspicion and resistance among the Lutheran leaders at Springfield Hospital. Board members resolved to monitor "these machinations of Rome," and protest if city funds were solicited.

Springfield Hospital's record in response to the community's public health needs and especially its contagious diseases was spotty and meager, but not surprising or unusual for its circumstances and the times. As already noted, it could not afford to operate as a charitable institution. Moreover, its compact facilities would have made admitting contagious cases an unacceptable risk to other patients. Walking a narrow pathway between prudent management on one side and compassionate care on the other was not easy, but it became an uncomfortable fact of life for directors and staff.

This ambivalence was put to its ultimate test when Springfield and the nation suffered through the great influenza epidemic of 1918. Worldwide in scope and staggeringly deadly in its toll, the strain known as "Spanish Influenza" made its American appearance at an eastern seaboard army base early in September, then quickly spread west. Successive waves struck for nearly six months, then the plague disappeared as swiftly as it had first occurred. One out of four Americans suffered, and at least 675,000 died. Estimates of the global toll range from 20 to 40 million.

One reason for the pandemic's catastrophic impact was the tendency among its victims to also catch pneumonia, which commonly led to death in those pre-penicillin days. Another unusual trait was that its target population was predominantly young adults rather than more vulnerable age groups such as infants or the aged. Ironically, wartime U.S. servicemen were principal carriers and victims, because they were concentrated at crowded military bases, and their constant movement between bases effectively transmitted the disease. It is therefore no surprise that the epidemic quickly surfaced in the Middle West at Great Lakes Naval Training Station, north of Chicago (which eventually counted over 14,000 deaths). Alarming news reports prompted Springfield public health director Dr. Albert E. Campbell to take emergency steps on October 15, when he arranged to close public schools and ban public gatherings. The next day

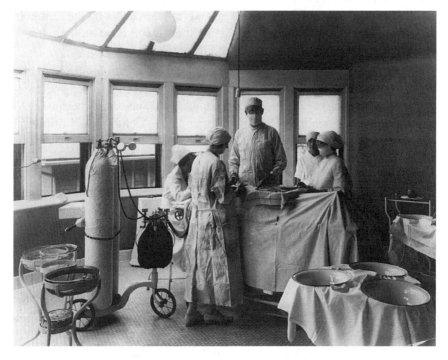

The irregularly shaped, top floor surgery room provided natural light and fresh air for Dr. Charles Patton and his team in this 1920 view.

the onslaught reached its first peak, with 127 new cases reported, plus a sharp increase of pneumonia. During that terrible week more than 100 new cases occurred daily. City authorities closed churches, theaters and billiard halls, and eventually banned any meeting of more than three people. Court was recessed and funeral homes were asked to limit the escalating number of services to immediate families only. One last desperate measure was a city-wide house quarantine. Still, by October 22 the tally was 2,500 reported cases and hundreds of deaths.

City physicians, nurses and hospitals strained to the breaking point in addressing the crisis. Early in the deadliest week the local press reported that Springfield and St. John's hospitals were "taxed to their capacity." The Red Cross opened a makeshift facility at the state fairgrounds, but most victims had no choice but to suffer in their homes. This in turn placed even heavier demands on those doctors and nurses who were well enough to help. Endangering their own lives, they made house calls around the clock for ten exhausting days. One nursing student at Springfield Hospital later recalled, "It was just terrible." Another student, Hallie Kinter, remembered "a very difficult time … we had so many sick patients."

An aura of manageable bedlam prevailed at the hospital, where all staff physicians, nurses and students toiled with scarcely a break. There was no effective medication to use, only bed rest and careful monitoring. Fresh air was the prevailing regimen, so hospital windows were kept open, making the rooms "awfully cold at night" because of the early fall chill. As a makeshift isolation gesture, nurses draped sheets around the beds of flu patients. Most of the staff, including Kinter, caught the virus, and at least one student later died from related tuberculosis.

By early November the number of new cases dropped sharply, permitting schools and stores to reopen. Then a second wave occurred, but by December the crisis ended. Nevertheless both hospitals remained crammed with pneumonia patients for many months. There is no exact record of area deaths, but among Springfield citizens alone the toll from flu and related pneumonia was nearly 400. Even so, the city's suffering was relatively moderate in comparison with larger urban and transportation centers. For Springfield Hospital the experience was traumatic and memorable, the most dramatic of its numerous challenges during these difficult years.

Hospital Discipline

Recruiting adolescent women from area Lutheran families to become nursing students placed heavy in loco parentis responsibilities upon the board and matron at Springfield Hospital and Training School. Strict rules governed the appearance, schedules and behavior of student nurses at all times. Infractions were a serious business, as three students learned in 1915. Board minutes reported the episode:

Hazel Jones, Minta Merry and Bessie Kirk have violated the rules of the institution, the former two in that they returned at a very late hour of the night and then used the fire escape to get to their rooms on the third floor, and the latter in that she fell asleep at her post. All three have already had a ten day suspension as punishment. Bessie Kirk showed herself to be repentant, and with the warning that a repeat offense will necessitate her immediate discharge, she was let off by the mercy of the Board of Directors. Hazel Jones and Minta Merry had not voluntarily admitted the offense to the matron at first, but were about to do it, when they were made to explain themselves by her. They both appeared before the Board of Directors and recognized their fault and expressed their regret about it. On that they were let off.

The next year another nurse was immediately dismissed for "running around with a married man" and using "very improper and unchaste expressions in the hospital."

One other vexing issue, a form of cultural or political epidemic, arose during the nation's involvement in the Great War, 1917-18. The hospital's close ties with German Lutherans subjected it and its directors to suspicion during the wartime hysteria directed against the treacherous Hun enemy. Actually, nativist prejudice began resurging before the war, but it reached a peak of virulence once American soldiers entered battle. Ad hoc patriotic societies in cities like Springfield sought to ban the performance of Wagner's music and German language instruction in public schools. A mood of "100 per cent Americanism" led to extremes, including violence.

Trinity Lutheran Church, the hospital's original patron and longtime advocate, was among the most vulnerable local institutions. Bowing to patriotic pressure, it converted to English language services during the war, and even refrained from celebrating the 400th anniversary of the Reformation, owing to the Springfield populace's "fanatical frame of mind." The exact impact at Springfield Hospital is unknown, but its directors also succumbed to the prejudice against German language in its board proceedings and minutes. For the first time since its earliest years, the board began recording its minutes and committee reports in English, a practice that continued intermittently after the war, until the final switch to English later in the 1920s.

Sparse records for this period make it unclear whether Springfield Hospital, its Lutheran directors, and its predominantly German Lutheran staff suffered in other ways from the overzealous patriotism of the war years. Given the experience of countless other Germanic organizations and institutions throughout the country, they probably did. Community ostracism may readily have tarnished the hospital's reputation and undermined its effort to attract more patients. Board minutes in 1917 did note a serious attrition in patient admissions, and directors voted in mid 1918 to print the hospital's newsletter in English.

Therefore, contagions of both disease and discrimination posed yet another unwelcome burden for the struggling hospital during the war years. While in general the nation's hospitals continued to grow in size, stature and public acceptance, Springfield Hospital was beset by problems of both its own making and unhappy circumstance.

Wretched Money

With the end of the Great War and the influenza plague that accompanied it, Americans embarked upon a decade marked by great (but uneven) prosperity, the advent of mass consumerism, and a retreat from foreign adventures. Dubbed by President Warren Harding a "return to normalcy," the times were anything but that. The nation's health care institutions and practitioners continued to expand rapidly, introduce new drugs and techniques, and acquire wider public acceptance. Springfield Hospital, on the other hand, continued to face its all-too-familiar challenges, enjoying neither prosperity nor stature. Approaching the hospital's 25th anniversary, directors and staff had little to celebrate except survival.

Ratification of the 18th Amendment and passage by Congress of the Volstead Act embarked the nation on its 12 year "noble experiment" with Prohibition. Hospitals generally were unaffected by this controversial reform effort, except for their singular eligibility to acquire alcoholic products for antiseptic and medicinal purposes. Rising consumer demand led to extralegal and criminal efforts to obtain alcohol, so hospitals had to carefully manage their supplies. Springfield Hospital officials learned this lesson quickly, when Matron Lindemann reported in 1921 the theft of 40 gallons of alcohol from the hospital's storeroom.

American hospitals generally entered the new decade on the crest of a sustained boom. A 1923 census counted nearly 5,000 institutions, a spectacular (nearly 30 fold) jump from the 178 of fifty years earlier. The largest and most progressive hospitals began exhibiting characteristics that would become the standard for others to emulate. They were governed by lay boards and managed by professional administrators or physicians. They boasted state-of-the-art technology in radiology and surgery equipment. Their high standards and regional or even national reputations rested largely on the presence of an affiliated medical school which gave them added stature as educational and research institutions.

Such were the hallmarks of the successful urban hospital of the 1920s, but they were well beyond the reach of Springfield Hospital and Training School. The evidence was all too clear. In 1918 the American College of Surgeons promulgated voluntary criteria of hospital management, staffing and record keeping, and began sending teams to evaluate the nation's health institutions. These were the initial steps in a program of "standardization" that would evolve into accreditation under the American Hospital Association. Springfield Hospital first confronted this in the summer of

The Nursing School

Among the hospital's myriad problems during the postwar years was its constant struggle to recruit and retain nursing students. Stable enrollment at the Training School was vital both as a means of low cost nursing help and as a supply of future employees.

At one point, in 1920, the challenge became a crisis. Far too few matriculants and too many dropouts forced the hospital to hire 22 regular nurses. Paying each of them $100 per month instead of using student nurses ($10 a month) imposed a massive burden on the hospital's straitened finances. Matron Lindemann and board members urgently asked area pastors to encourage young Lutheran women to enroll. They also inquired if state authorities would waive the existing requirement that applicants have at least one year of high school education.

By 1921 the picture had brightened somewhat. Lindemann reported 17 students in that fall's entering class. Four came from Springfield, ten from other central Illinois towns, and three from out of state. The struggle persisted, however, with an average of one dropout reported every month. Nearly every board meeting included a report of names dropped and added on the school roster. Dismissals on disciplinary grounds aggravated the problem. An underlying factor, duly noted in board minutes, was the low morale and turnover among regular hospital employees. It was difficult to attract students to an institution beset with other problems.

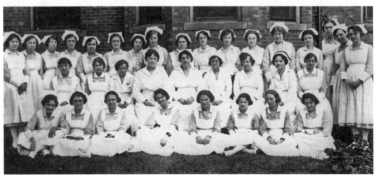

Nursing students (1921) were a vital source of inexpensive labor.

1920, when the board received a critical report from the Illinois Hospital Association, questioning its admissions criteria for student nurses and its lack of provision for legal liability of doctors on staff. Rebuke from one's peers was scarcely an auspicious omen as the new decade began.

Once again there was talk, prompted by medical staff complaints, of converting the hospital to a secular institution. Financial woes, staff turnover and a deteriorating physical plant led many area citizens to conclude that "things are very sad for the hospital." With a major new building program underway at St. John's, physicians warned that Springfield Hospital was on the verge of failure. Board members insisted that most of the criticism came from hostile sources, but they would consider offers to sell the hospital to a non-sectarian entity.

Meanwhile, the hospital remained under "Lutheran auspices," and all corporation members, directors and officers were required to be members of congregations in the Evangelical Lutheran Synodical Conference. Officers at the decade's start were Pastor W. Heyne from Decatur (president), Pastor Kuppler (vice president) from Jacksonville, Pastor Weiss (secretary) from Petersburg, and the venerable Professor Frederick Streckfuss (treasurer), who taught at Concordia in Springfield. Rounding out the board through most of the decade were active parishioners at Trinity Church: newly installed Pastor Paul Schulz, William Schnepp, Frederick Van Horn, Frank Siebert, and Harry Koopman. After years of devoted service in nearly every possible capacity, Streckfuss was forced by illness in 1920 to take an extended leave of absence. In 1922 he was named honorary director, and he died a few years later. Schulz came to Trinity in 1921, and quickly rose to a position of leadership on the board. Tireless, dogged and dedicated, he bore many of the hospital's mounting burdens through these difficult years.

Rumors and inquiries continued to surface about terminating the hospital's Lutheran affiliation. In mid-1921 a special board committee reiterated the standard argument that "our people should first be given the opportunity to help," and if that failed, "then we are prepared to make it a public one." The issue persisted for several years, but the board held firm. If anything, the religious hold strengthened. A Synod committee in 1922 urged every effort "to make the hospital a Lutheran one in every respect." This meant limiting the institution's charity to needy Lutheran pastors, teachers, students and laity. The Synod in return would try to allocate an annual $5,000 subsidy. New bylaws in 1924 officially added the phrase "Under

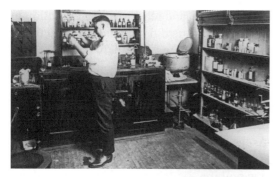

The old hospital dispensary was Spartan, but serviceable.

Springfield Hospital's central office on the ground floor was crowded, as seen in this 1921 photograph.

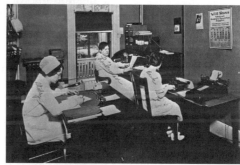

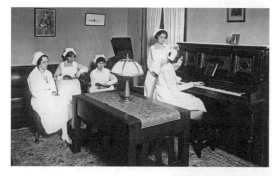

The student nurses' residence included a common room (1921), where the young women could gather during their precious free time.

The austere pediatrics facility, circa 1921. Evidently this was a special occasion, the presence of Springfield Hospital's first triplets.

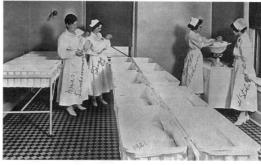

Lutheran Auspices" to the hospital's name, and reasserted the affiliation in strong language. Curiously, the patient profile did not reflect this sectarian identity. Among the 2,307 patients admitted in 1919, only 215 (less than ten per cent) declared themselves Lutheran. Unmoved by this incongruence, the board persisted with the hospital's Lutheran identity.

At the annual summer meeting of corporation members in 1921, President Heyne succinctly declared their gravest problem: "we are always missing the 'nervus rerum,' the wretched money." A debt burden of more than $60,000 cost the hospital $3,000 in interest annually. Operating income barely covered expenses, leaving nothing for debt reduction. Almost plaintively he added, "We have done what we could," but the financial dilemma seemed intractable.

At board meetings there was discussion of every possible way to reduce expenses, raise income, and stall creditors. This last tactic, a sign of desperation, took various forms. For example, it was noted that one creditor's $5,950 note would soon be due; "The opinion was that we should wait quietly until Mr. Jannsen announces himself." Two months later, to the board's likely consternation, Jannsen demanded payment. Similarly, there were periodic appeals that Lutheran parishes either forgive or at least extend their loans to the hospital. The pressure was relentless, as nearly every month one or more note holders demanded payment.

Another recourse was to pare operating expenses, which became a standard refrain at board meetings. Cost-cutting measures ran the gamut. When patients complained about being served oleomargarine, the board reluctantly decided to provide them with butter, but instructed the superintendent to continue using oleomargarine for nurses and students. It indefinitely deferred action on a $2,708 bid for "necessary" plumbing repairs, dismissed a housekeeper ($50 per month) in hopes that some ladies aid society would perform the work, and after discharging a male cook decided to "hire a woman ... in lieu of a man for economy." When superintendent Frank Siebert resigned in 1922, the board was in no hurry to replace him, because the lapsed salary was more valuable at that time than executive leadership. Although a Synod survey had revealed that Springfield Hospital salaries were below average, every request for a raise was denied.

Fundraising was a third approach. Invoked frequently, it seldom made any headway. Appeals to the Synod and to area pastors yielded meager results if anything, because churches had their own pressing needs.

Medical Staff, 1923

After operating for a quarter century, Springfield Hospital had nearly twice as many physicians (23) on its medical staff as when it opened (12). Three of the men listed in 1923 had been in the original group: Drs. Hazel, Stericker and Young. The entire group, arranged by practice, follows:

General Medicine: Frank N. Evans, Samuel Munson, George F. Stericker, Lewis C. Taylor

Surgery: Don W. Deal, Daniel M. Ottis, Charles L. Patton, William A. Young;

  Assistants: Robert E. Smith, Harry H. Southwick

Ear-Nose-Throat: Robert I. Bullard, Charles P. Colby, John F. Deal, Arthur E. Walters

Obstetrics: Harry Otten

Gynecology: James A. Day

Dental Surgery: E. Foster Hazel

X-Ray: Frederick S. O'Hara

Urology: Herbert B. Henkel

Sanitation: George T. Palmer

Orthopedics: George W. Staben

Tubercular: Herman H. Cole

Pediatrics: Harrison C. Blankmeyer

These 23 staff members comprised less than one quarter of Springfield's listed physicians at the time, and numbered far fewer than the staff at St. John's Hospital. Interestingly, the 11 specialties represented on the staff were more than double the corresponding variety in 1897. This reflects the powerful trend toward specialization that American medicine was experiencing even early in the 20th century.

Recognizing that concerted effort by a paid specialist might work better, the board engaged an area Lutheran pastor to serve as a combination debt collector and fundraiser. In four months he managed to raise $1,567, but his salary consumed one-third of this, and he had exhausted all realistic sources. In 1923 this tactic again received consideration, when the representative of a New York firm offered its services for a fee. Uneasy about such a radical solution, the board decided to stick with local volunteers.

If fundraising could not substantially raise income, perhaps higher patient receipts would. Pastor Paul Schulz believed that advertising the hospital might generate more referrals and admissions, thereby increasing revenue. Accordingly, he arranged publication of a promotional brochure. Illustrated with photographs of the facility and a group of nurses, this 1922 flyer touted the hospital's "atmosphere of sincere, earnest devotion" in a "beautiful, quiet, home-like setting." Staff physicians were "men of the very highest standings." Schulz also advised the board that he would install an exhibit about Springfield Hospital at the Illinois State Fair. These gestures may have been useful, but not enough to appreciably increase operating income or avert the financial deterioration.

A day of reckoning loomed, with the 1924 deadline on the hospital's $48,000 bond issue. It weighed heavily on Pastor Heyne as he delivered his presidential address at the July, 1923 annual meeting. In a largely religious message he interspersed thanks to God with bitter regret that the hospital had no endowment fund or any "large donation ... from rich patrons." The board's cost-cutting "efficiency committee" had realized every possible economy. Nevertheless, Springfield Hospital was losing between $3,000 and $5,000 annually, a disastrous trend that foretold insolvency. Funds were insufficient for the institution to own or equip its own laboratory and laundry. One year later the hemorrhage had worsened; total receipts for 1923-24 were $94,463 against expenses of more than $100,000, for a deficit of $5,552. Stubbornly hopeful, and still dedicated to the hospital's cause, corporation members approved a board recommendation to issue new bonds at the increased level of $50,000. The picture was bleak, but, maybe faith and hope could save charity.

Administrative turnover was another ominous sign of the hospital's precarious status. After the awkwardness of 1905-07, when four women successively served as matron and nursing director, Rosa Waltke managed to retain the position for five years, 1913 to 1917. She generally earned high marks, but recurrent health problems and a nagging dispute with one staff physician led to her departure. Then the revolving door began spinning again. Sophie Sherpeltz succeeded Waltke in 1917, but staff turmoil led to her abrupt replacement by Regina Hackman and Laura Turner, who also left almost immediately. Mary Shields held the job for one year, followed by Louise Lindemann, who served from 1920 to 1922.

Board minutes from 1917 to 1920 revealed nearly constant turmoil among hospital employees and administrators. At various times the matron, superintendent, surgical nurse, certain physicians and groups of nurses presented separate grievances and implored the board to take swift action. Directors frequently met in special sessions to conduct informal hearings over personnel disputes. Charges and countercharges touched nearly everyone working at the embattled hospital. One dispute was over allegations of "gross indecencies" between a physician and the surgical nurse. Board members lurched from one crisis to another, reprimanding some parties, firing others, supporting still others, and occasionally reversing their decisions in response to pressure or new evidence. The only consistent theme through these troubled times was agreement that the hospital's occupancy and reputation were suffering as a result.

Lindemann's tenure was clouded by controversy that eventually led to her departure. During the fall of 1922 the board received complaints about her from several staff nurses and one student, whom Lindemann had expelled. After meeting with her, the board reported that "peace was established," but several weeks later it accepted her resignation, after which the secretary noted with either relief or fervent hope: "peace, harmony and cooperation are very much in evidence."

The superintendent's position proved only somewhat more secure. John A. Hoffman served for six years, resigning in late 1913. Pastor Charles Gross, who moved to Springfield that year, held the job for five difficult years. His performance initially pleased the board, which in 1915 raised his monthly salary from $80 to $125. Later, however, he quarreled with successive matrons and resigned under board pressure. He was followed in 1919 by local shoe store proprietor Frank Siebert, who served until 1922. By then board members seem to have finally settled on executive titles. Siebert's position was called hospital "manager," with the superintendent's mantle finally resting with the unmarried female nursing directors who lived at the hospital.

The abrupt and nearly simultaneous resignations of manager Siebert and superintendent Lindemann came in Springfield Hospital's 25th year, an anniversary that passed without ceremony or even notice. Moreover, there was symbolic meaning in their joint departure. It capped two demoralizing decades of struggle, decline, and executive instability. Moreover, the hospital's severe financial straits were starkly evident when the board decided to postpone filling either vacancy for reasons of economy. It was a reflection of Springfield Hospital's near-paralysis and bleak prospects that in 1923 its board sought financial relief by leaving its two management positions unfilled. Saving nearly $200 a month in payroll costs may have suited a hard-pressed board, but it also was a melancholy measure of the hospital's desperate situation. How much longer, observers might have wondered, could the dreams and prayers of its founders and valiant supporters survive in a losing cause?

Memorial Milestones

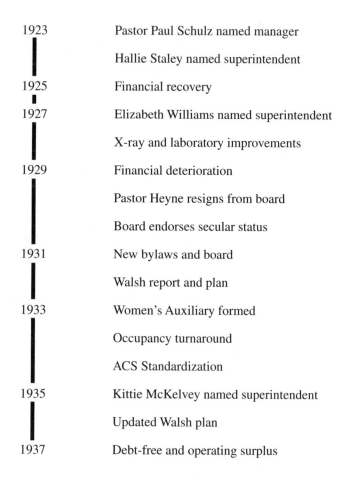

1923	Pastor Paul Schulz named manager
	Hallie Staley named superintendent
1925	Financial recovery
1927	Elizabeth Williams named superintendent
	X-ray and laboratory improvements
1929	Financial deterioration
	Pastor Heyne resigns from board
	Board endorses secular status
1931	New bylaws and board
	Walsh report and plan
1933	Women's Auxiliary formed
	Occupancy turnaround
	ACS Standardization
1935	Kittie McKelvey named superintendent
	Updated Walsh plan
1937	Debt-free and operating surplus

Chapter Three

An End And A Beginning

During the late 1920s and 1930s, Springfield Hospital experienced both a fatal crisis and a timely rebirth, mimicking on a very small scale the entire nation's roller coaster ride from boundless optimism through the despair of the Great Depression and then renewal under the New Deal banner. In both instances the changes were convulsive and far-reaching. Superficially the aging hospital at Fifth and North Grand looked in 1939 much as it had in 1925, but in fundamental ways it was an entirely different institution. Sectarian control had given way to secular governance by community leaders of many beliefs and both genders. A dramatically improving financial picture for the first time in the hospital's history enabled it to emulate national trends in progressive health care. Released from the fundraising constraints of its original Lutheran identity, the institution soon drew sufficient community support to plan a modern new facility at a carefully selected site.

After decades of struggle and near-paralysis, Springfield Hospital emerged from the ashes of its founding vision as a transformed and revitalized institution. Devout and compassionate Lutheran leaders had struggled and sacrificed for more than thirty years to offer a Protestant alternative in health care for area citizens. That their singular dream died was a reflection of their own self-imposed limits, but the strength and structure of its successor owed much to the steadfast commitment of the founding pastors and laity.

Two Generations in Medicine

During the 1930s there were many prominent names on the hospital's medical roster. Two stand out, both for long service and for the advent of a second generation to maintain the family tradition of medical leadership.

Dr. Charles Patton joined the medical staff in 1906, and was a key figure for the remainder of his long and distinguished career. He served as president in 1913, and again during two critical years, 1932-34. He was instrumental in every constructive step taken during that fateful decade. His son Robert later entered practice, spending 40 years as one of the area's most respected surgeons. Like his father, Bob Patton worked hard for Memorial Hospital's success, and served as staff president, 1953-54. Widely admired among peers and in the community, he retired in 1981, ending 41 years of service.

The Stericker name also stood out in hospital annals. George F. Stericker was a charter staff physician who held office as president from 1903 to 1907. Equally active in medical and civic affairs, he headed the county's tuberculosis association for a term. His death in 1935 ended 46 years of practice. At that time his son George B. already was an established physician. The younger Stericker was in practice for 48 years, led Memorial's medical staff in 1946, and served as president of the county medical society in 1953. He died in 1976.

We Have Done What We Could

After years of deteriorating finances, deferred maintenance and administrative turnover, Springfield Hospital enjoyed a brief Indian Summer of solvency at mid-decade. The financial results for 1925 were heartening, as a sharp increase in receipts enabled the board to finally pay the remaining balance of a $5,800 note to Ridgely-Farmers Bank. Bonded debt dropped from a high of $50,000 early in the decade to $36,000, prompting the venerable board member Martin Luecke to declare that 1925 brought the "greatest success ... in the history of the hospital." This in turn made it possible to raise Superintendent Hallie Staley's monthly salary to $150, and also to perform some long overdue physical improvements. Among the major projects were an overhauled heating plant, some new wiring, the construction of a sleeping porch for nurses, a new roof on the south wing, and fresh paint in patient rooms. The financial respite continued through 1926, when debt was reduced another several thousand dollars.

Composition of the board of directors scarcely changed during most of the decade. Rev. William Heyne of Decatur served as president, William H. Schnepp as vice president, and Robert O. Gaudlitz as secretary. Other familiar names—Siebert, Koopman, Luedke and Horn—remained on the board. The most active new voice was that of Rev. Paul Schulz, Pastor of Trinity Church. Named hospital manager in 1923, he added the board title of treasurer the next year.

Schulz naturally and rapidly rose to a position of board leadership, by virtue of his dual responsibilities, his stature as Trinity pastor, and his dedication to the hospital's welfare. Minutes reveal that his was the dominant voice in shaping the agenda and making decisions. The venue for these deliberations ordinarily was a cramped basement classroom, but at times the board met in "the green operating room."

Schulz's lengthy tenure helped stabilize management of the hospital. Joining him as in-house superintendent in 1923 was Hallie Staley, whose "highly satisfactory" performance in an acting capacity led to a permanent appointment. Ill health forced her to take a two month leave of absence during the summer of 1926, followed by her resignation in October. Kittie McKelvey served for six months as acting superintendent, while the board advertised for a successor. Early in 1927 Elizabeth Williams of Baltimore began a seven year tenure, while McKelvey stayed as director of nursing until resigning later that year. She would return as superintendent in the mid 1930s.

Superintendent Williams got off to a shaky start, evidently due to an ambitious agenda for improvements. Within two months the board received complaints that she was moving too quickly with operational changes, and it reacted cautiously to her expensive wish list for new equipment. She gradually gained the board's confidence, however, and in 1928 she prevailed in a dispute over staffing the x-ray facility. That summer there were resignations of key hospital personnel in the laboratory, x-ray room, kitchen, and anesthesiology.

Managing, staffing and equipping both the laboratory and the x-ray facility were nearly chronic board concerns through much of the 1920s. At mid-decade Dr. Fred S. O'Hara was approved to oversee both departments, but this arrangement fell victim to his extended sojourns in Florida and his eroding support on the medical staff. Hospital directors conducted a careful review of the problem in 1927, calculating that a properly equipped x-ray department would cost $12,000, plus perhaps $5,000 annually in personnel expenses. A survey of other hospitals in central Illinois revealed that such a facility could yield up to $15,000 income per year, and that most area hospitals earned a net profit on their x-ray services. This information persuaded the board to proceed, and also to replace Dr. O'Hara. After a New York City physician declined the offer, Dr. Jerry S. Bell of Fort Wayne, Indiana accepted, at a monthly salary of $250. Bell soon lost favor with the board, and was succeeded in 1929 by Dr. Lawrence Hilt, who divided his time between the hospital (for $225 per month) and the Patton Clinic. Before long he too was at odds with directors over staffing and other issues, but the board sidestepped these differences in order to protect its investment in a profitable unit. The application of x-ray technology for diagnostic and therapeutic purposes had become one of the medical marvels of the age, and also a catalyst for growing public dependence on hospitals in place of home care.

The hospital's laboratory also was growing in importance. For example, blood transfusion was evolving from an exceptional to a routine component of surgery, sometimes (critics charged) more to impress the patient and relatives than out of necessity. In these early years there was no community blood bank, so physicians personally had to arrange as well as perform blood donations for their patients. One Springfield surgeon recalled much time devoted to finding donors, drawing blood in the hospi-

The Palmer Legacy

Mentioned occasionally throughout this history is Dr. George T. Palmer, a physician of considerable ability and broad interests. Moreover, members of at least three generations of his family dedicated themselves in diverse ways to distinguished service, making the Palmer legacy a remarkable record.

George was the grandson of John M. Palmer, long a resident of Carlinville and then Springfield. The elder Palmer was one of Illinois' notable public figures, serving as both Governor and U.S. Senator, and also a third party candidate for the presidency in 1896. Palmer's wife cofounded the local YWCA, and he was pivotal in persuading fellow Springfield school board members in 1874 to adopt equal educational access for African-American children.

John Palmer's daughter (George's aunt) was Jessie Palmer Weber, who devoted a singularly productive career to promoting Illinois history. She was a founder of the Illinois State Historical Society, librarian of its distinguished historical collection, and charter editor of its prestigious journal.

Born in 1875, George began medical practice in Chicago, but returned home in 1903 as assistant secretary of the state health board. A pediatrician, he was an early member of Springfield Hospital's medical staff. His appointment to head the city health department led to its reform as a model of professional service. He founded and directed the Palmer Tuberculosis Sanitorium, which served area patients for 40 years. As noted elsewhere in this chapter, his wife helped found the Springfield Maternal Health Center.

Dr. Palmer also found time to write a highly regarded biography of his statesman grandfather. Ever the thoughtful citizen, he established a $150,000 trust that was given to Memorial Hospital in 1967, years following his death.

tal laboratory, and then personally administering transfusions. In 1927 the board borrowed $14,000 to upgrade and re-equip both the x-ray room and the laboratory, and to add a second operating room. All of these improvements reflected the technological advances in medicine and surgery that underscored the new primacy of hospitals in American health care.

Specialization was another sign of the times. In 1927 the hospital added its first staff physician (part-time at $100 per month) with formal training in anesthesiology. Several years later it appointed a half-time pathologist, Dr. Perry J. Melnick, who also worked in a Decatur hospital. Also in the 1930s the board considered establishing a pediatrics department in affiliation with Children's Memorial Hospital in Chicago, but the plan was deferred.

Medical science was making significant strides, but many procedures remained primitive by modern standards. For example, nurses providing steam treatment for pneumonia patients lacked a steam machine, and therefore resorted to using a hot plate, tea kettle, funnel-shaped roll of newspaper, and a suspended bed sheet canopy. "We did a lot of improvising," recalled one nurse, who also reported that delirious pneumonia patients had to be shackled with two leather straps (a leg to one side rail, the opposite arm to the other rail), to keep them safely in bed. Victims of lip cancer were treated with radium needles, held in place with wax. The radium inventory was maintained by a physician, who brought doses to the hospital as needed.

Patient admittance levels were a continuing board concern, because empty beds jeopardized the hospital's solvency. Annual reports from the late 1920s indicated that Springfield Hospital operated at 75 per cent of capacity or lower. The per capita daily cost of patient care hovered between $3 and $4, depending directly on occupancy figures. One recourse was to negotiate agreements with major local employers that also were hospital vendors. Thus in 1927 the board persuaded its coal supplier, Peabody Coal Co., to refer all mine accident victims to the hospital. Conversely, when the hospital's dairy vendor balked at such an arrangement, the board switched suppliers.

If patient admittance was a problem, at least the hospital could expect lengthy stays. The typical obstetrical patient was hospitalized for ten days, and recovery from hernia surgery consumed two weeks. A demographic picture of Springfield Hospital's clientele emerges in detailed figures for 1926. Surgical patients outnumbered medical patients, 56 to 44 per cent, and women were nearly twice as numerous as men. A slight majority of patients came from towns outside Springfield (e.g., Petersburg, Girard, Lincoln, Morrisonville, Gillespie), reflecting in part the steady influx of accident victims from area coal mines.

The hospital's medical staff of more than two dozen physicians struggled over several problems during the 1920s. In the previous decade the staff had convened nearly monthly, kept detailed minutes, and occasionally met jointly with the board. These healthy steps abruptly changed after the war. Medical staff minutes indicate only one meeting in 1920, two in 1921, none in 1922, and one annually through 1926. Formal interaction with the board also virtually ceased. Whatever the cause, this was a troubling trend that was bound to undermine any hospital bid for accreditation ("standardization"), a growing movement now under the auspices of the American College of Surgeons (ACS).

Concerned physicians took steps beginning in 1926 to reinvigorate their collective voice. They elected Dr. Harry Otten, one of the city's busiest physicians, as president of the medical staff. In turn he opened an informal dialogue with hospital directors, leading to a joint meeting early in 1927 at which 18 physicians registered concern over a deteriorating physical plant. Later that year, led by Dr. Charles Patton, they formulated new operating room regulations and also agreed to prepare a new staff constitution and bylaws, probably in alignment with ACS standards. One other initiative was to persuade the board to add at least one physician as a voting member, in order to improve communication and to add a medical perspective to its deliberations. Under Pastor Schulz, however, the board firmly resisted any such change. It would be more than fifty years before doctors gained voting membership on the hospital board.

One other vexing issue did by necessity engage both the medical staff and the directors. Reports began circulating in 1927 that several physicians with staff privileges at both hospitals were actively counseling their patients against using Springfield Hospital. One doctor in particular, Robert Bullard, openly declared that he could get "better service" at St. John's Hospital. Staff physicians argued that the solution was for Springfield Hospital to upgrade its equipment and plant, but board members reacted that disloyal behavior warranted dismissal from the staff. It was Dr. Otten's delicate task to mollify the board without losing the support of his colleagues. This issue dragged on for several years and contributed to the crisis and transformation of 1931.

Crisis and Change

After several comfortable years, Springfield Hospital once again slid into financial jeopardy in 1927. This began a long, slow slide that anticipated the nation's economic crisis, and had comparably convulsive repercussions, leading in 1931 to the hospital's rebirth as a secular community institution.

Treasurer Schulz informed the board in the spring of 1927 that the hospital was unable to pay over $2,000 in overdue bills, due to inadequate operating income. To reduce expenses he laid off a hospital painter and the telephone operator. Superintendent Elizabeth Williams reported that room rates were relatively low, so the board raised them 20 per cent. More discouraging news came in July, when the Lutheran Synod announced it would soon discontinue its annual subsidy in excess of $1,000. Pastor Schulz noted that such action was unwise, because in return the hospital was providing free care to Lutheran pastors, seminary students and professors, but the Synod's decision was irreversible.

Lutheran affiliation had always been considered a hospital asset, but now the equation was changing. That fall, for example, the board held a prolonged discussion over accepting donations from other Protestant churches, but Schulz reminded his fellow pastors on the board that help from non-Lutheran organizations would violate the hospital's distinctive mission. Gradually the directors were discovering that their sectarian status was constrictive and possibly destructive.

The financial plight steadily worsened, prompting the board, Schulz and Williams to pursue three by now familiar steps: reduced expenses, increased operating revenue, and outside donations. Bids were sought for lower utility rates and laundry charges. Early in 1928 Schulz curtailed all buying in order to meet an interest payment of $800. Still, the accounts payable rose ominously, to nearly $9,000. One cost-saving measure, recycling rubber surgical gloves, consumed much nurses' time. They cut gloves that were beyond repair into patches, used an oxygen tank to inflate others in order to locate holes and tears, then glued the patches. The recycled gloves were too bulky for surgical use, but found a second life in the emergency room.

Fred W. Wanless

Fred and Charles Wanless were Springfield's leading real estate developers during the depression and war years. Born in 1881, Fred had many civic interests and responsibilities as well. He was an active Mason and director of First National Bank. Politics and public service were a lifelong activity. He served on the county board and also one term in the state legislature. For 20 years he was chairman of the Sangamon County Republican Committee.

Recruiting him to the reorganized hospital board in 1932 was an act of wisdom and good fortune. In nine years as president he steered the hospital from near death, through spectacular recovery, and to final planning for the newly constructed and newly named Memorial Hospital. More than any single individual he was responsible for the institution's second birth and bright future. He died in 1949.

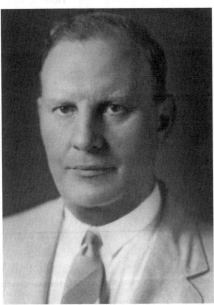

Fred W. Wanless

By early 1929 trouble was brewing on other fronts as well. Key staff resignations the previous year were evidence of low morale, and it was no secret that several physicians were steering their patients to St. John's. The purchase of medical equipment was effectively stalled, as were repair and maintenance requests. A routine Fire Department inspection reported the alarming news that the hospital's extinguishers were inoperable. There was mounting nationwide pressure for hospitals this size to be standardized, but Springfield Hospital was deficient in too many areas even to apply.

In March a group of concerned physicians told Schulz they needed to meet with directors to discuss the grave situation. At the April board meeting they declared their belief that it had become "necessary to change this hospital to a general Protestant institution." Further, there was a chance that doctors might be able to organize and purchase it. This prompted the board to call a special meeting in May of the members (stockholders) of the Springfield Hospital Association. There it was announced that hospital physicians and others "are clamoring for a more up-to-date and larger hospital ... which can successfully compete with the large and well-equipped Catholic St. John's Hospital." Stockholders responded with a resolution authorizing the board to sell the hospital if they deemed that in the best interest of members. Several days later the **Illinois State Journal** reported this fateful development, adding the rumor that "some influential men of means" were ready to buy and then replace the facility with a new, larger building.

Discussions and negotiations dragged on for the remainder of 1929. That fall Pastor Heyne resigned as president, because he was scheduled to leave his Decatur church for a new assignment. Fellow directors wanted to salute him for several decades of faithful service, but a board resolution to purchase a farewell gift was "tabled indefinitely owing to the financial condition of the hospital." Such was the institution's perilous condition.

Early in 1930 the board heard presentations by two hospital consulting firms offering their services to raise nearly $750,000 to build a new 125-bed facility and nurses' home, provided the charter was changed to "include other Protestants" and the word "Memorial" became part of its name. The prospect of abandoning their Lutheran mission was a devastating disappointment to many veteran directors, and led to a dramatic August board meeting at which Vice President Siebert, Secretary Gaudlitz and Treasurer Schulz submitted their resignations. Several days later, responding to appeals, they agreed to remain until the October annual meeting.

Meanwhile rumors circulated that potential buyers included Springfield's Protestant churches, or either the city or county governments.

At the 1930 annual meeting Pastor Schulz warned stockholders that the hospital could not function much longer as a Lutheran institution and in its dilapidated quarters. Members present approved a resolution "that the Springfield Hospital, now under Lutheran auspices, be changed to a General Nondenominational Hospital." Schulz now had the cruel task of approaching civic leaders to save the institution he had vigorously and faithfully served for nearly ten years.

There were rumors early in 1931 that "a wealthy coal mine operator" had pledged one-half the cost of constructing a $1 million new building on property adjoining the existing hospital. Like previous overtures, this idea died, as did any lingering hopes to actually sell the rapidly depreciating asset. The most that Schulz and others could expect was a direct transfer of ownership, including the hospital's existing debt.

During the spring Schulz conferred with Dr. Charles Patton and prominent attorneys Bayard L. Catron and R. Allan Stephens. They in turn developed a list of nearly two dozen individuals with the collective influence and resources to assume the debt and manage the hospital. By May of 1931 Patton, Catron and Stephens had recruited businessmen Pascal Hatch, George W. Bunn, Jr. and Robert C. Lanphier, plus attorney Logan Hay. This group met in Stephens' office with Schulz and board president William H. Schnepp, and agreed "that the citizens of Springfield should assist the Hospital Association in working out its problem" by organizing a new board and making the institution non-sectarian.

Further discussions led to drastically altered bylaws that both the hospital board and the stockholders (meeting June 5) duly adopted. Henceforth Springfield Hospital would be "a general non-denominational" institution, governed by a 27-member board. The group had to be this large to include many new faces plus (temporarily) the nine Lutheran incumbents. Significantly, the bylaws stipulated that nine board members (one-third) would be women, a break with board precedent nearly as radical as the secular composition. Joining the board would be prominent businessmen Fred Wanless, Herbert Bartholf and Thomas Rees, plus a slate of women comprising a "Who's Who" of Springfield society: Elizabeth (Mrs. Frank) Ide, Alice Bunn, Mildred (Mrs. Jacob) Bunn, Niana (Mrs. Henry) Davis, Frances (Mrs. George) Keys, Mrs. John Cook, Jeanette (Mrs. Joseph) Hammerslough, Emma (Mrs. Fleetwood) Connelly, and Jane Brown.

Mildred Bunn

Mildred (Mrs. Jacob) Bunn served on the hospital's board of directors during 16 crucial years, helping lead it through the Great Depression, its transformation to secular standing, the building campaign, World War II and postwar adjustment. Her tenure included stints in several offices, including board president, and a record of extraordinary commitment, leadership and generosity.

Mrs. Bunn became a young widow when her husband died in the mid 1920s. For the next 30 years she devoted herself to raising their three children and serving the community. She was a director of Sangamo Electric Company, which her husband had cofounded, and she served on numerous civic boards, but none as long or as productively as Memorial Hospital's.

A faithful and active participant at hospital board meetings, Mrs. Bunn deserves primary credit (along with Fred Wanless) for steering the institution through its near-miraculous recovery from insolvency and stagnation to robust health and respectability. One admirer described her as "a real kingpin" of Memorial's ascent.

The hospital benefitted from her philanthropy as well. An early and generous donor to the building campaign, she also gave funds to construct the Henry Bunn Chapel, in memory of a son who died in military service during World War II.

Mildred Bunn resigned from the board in 1947, at age 60, so that "a younger person might be appointed." Fittingly, her son Jacob Jr. succeeded her, and sustained a family tradition by later donating funds for the installation of an organ in the chapel. Mrs. Bunn died in 1958.

In addition, the hospital would have an Advisory Committee consisting of the early recruits (Hatch, Lanphier, Hay, Catron, Bunn, Stephens) and Robert E. Miller. There also was to be a 27-member "Board of Women," with representatives from every temple and Protestant church in Springfield, the Temple Sisterhood, and various civic organizations like the YWCA, Springfield Women's Club and the American Association of University Women. This group's purposes were to oversee volunteer and other affiliated groups, improve hospital efficiency, and win "increased public understanding and support" for the troubled institution.

The new bylaws were a veritable revolution from the top down. Overnight Springfield Hospital and Training School was to be a secular community institution governed, advised and supported by the city's wealthiest and most powerful leaders, both male and female. For a hospital on its death bed, this was a massive transfusion of fresh blood, fresh ideas, and fresh money. The most notable feature of the new governance structure was the prominent and vital role assigned to women, both on the board of directors and their own support board. Not since the founding year (over 30 years earlier) had there been a woman director at Springfield Hospital. This statutory quota of at least one-third female representation remained in effect for another thirty years, until new bylaws in 1960 ended it, ushering in another (briefer) era of an exclusively male board.

Another important bylaw change was to limit board meetings to a quarterly calendar, with the annual meeting slated for January. Clearly the 27-member board was expected to exercise broad oversight rather than detailed management, another sharp departure from tradition. A seven member executive committee, consisting of the four officers and three other directors, would meet as needed between board meetings to monitor hospital operations and approve personnel and financial transactions. With a massive job awaiting it, this executive committee would quickly emerge as the fulcrum of hospital governance, with its members convening frequently and for long hours. For the remainder of 1931 it was a transitional group, with the four holdover officers (William Schnepp, Pastor Edwin Summer, John Horn, and Schulz) joined by new board members Fred Wanless, Michael Eckstein (law) and Edward E. Staley (manufacturing). Another element of continuity was the retention of Pastor Schulz as manager of the hospital, though on a part-time ($20 per month) basis. He loyally remained in this capacity until 1933, when he resigned for personal reasons.

A New Deal

The timing of Springfield Hospital's rebirth could not have been less auspicious. Both the city and the entire nation were mired in an economic and social crisis of unprecedented magnitude. Industrial production and employment plummeted in the wake of Wall Street's 1929 crash. Building construction virtually ceased. Thousands of banks failed, including the once proud Ridgely Farmer's Bank of Springfield. Commodity prices dropped too low for farmers to make a profit. Coal mining, long a staple of Sangamon and neighboring counties, shrank drastically, due to meager industrial demand. Despite efforts by President Herbert Hoover and Congress, unemployment steadily rose to reach 15 million workers, or 25 per cent of the labor force. Those bankers and financiers who were still solvent had been discredited by the stock market's steep descent. A dangerous mood of despair and social unraveling hung over the country during the 1932 election year, as many troubled Americans questioned capitalism's resilience under such stress.

The nation's hospitals were not immune from these alarming developments. In 1930 average receipts per patient plunged 75 per cent, from $236 to $59, and bed occupancy drifted down to 62 per cent. The combination of drastically lower per capita receipts and fewer patients put even the healthiest institutions in serious trouble. At voluntary hospitals the percentage of indigent and partial payment cases rose sharply. Compounding these ills was a steep decline (over 50 per cent) in the nationwide level of charitable support for hospitals. While all types, sizes and regions suffered, the hardest hit were the nation's 1,600 proprietary hospitals, which shrank by 25 per cent (to 1,200) by decade's end.

Desperate circumstances led to desperate measures for survival. Hospitals found it necessary to cut wages and salaries, delay improvements, defer maintenance, and cancel new construction. At Springfield Hospital, sadly, such measures were already commonplace long before the 1929 crash, leaving scant opportunity for further economies. Another recourse among voluntary hospitals was to seek local government assistance for the swelling ranks of charity patients. However, struggling municipalities like Springfield were in no position or mood to help.

With private charity and local state relief efforts inadequate, desperate citizens (including hospital officials) then turned to the federal government for help. Franklin D. Roosevelt in 1932 promised Americans a "New

Deal" that would provide emergency relief, restore confidence, correct the ills and abuses that had triggered the depression, and get people back to work. The resulting plethora of statutes, programs and agencies was a double-edge sword to hospital officials, who saw both opportunity and peril in a larger, more active central government. Consequently, the American Hospital Association (AHA) and likeminded organizations divided their time between promoting their pet ideas and resisting unwelcome ones.

For example, AHA lobbyists began urging Congress to enact some form of federal reimbursement for medical care of indigent patients, and also to subsidize new hospital construction. It would eventually take nearly 20 years for these programs to materialize, but the seeds were sown in the 1930s. As will be noted later in this chapter, a parallel drive in the private sector to establish prepaid hospital and medical insurance won earlier acceptance, with the rapid spread of Blue Cross.

Just as energetic were the efforts to protect hospitals from federal laws viewed as intrusive or costly. One such threat was the National Industrial Recovery Act of 1933, which among other things ensured collective bargaining for many American workers. The AHA and the newly formed American College of Hospital Administrators successfully petitioned to exempt hospital workers from this potentially costly leverage. Similarly, they won exemption from coverage under the Social Security Act of 1935, on the grounds that hospitals were charities in partnership with government. Not until the 1950s would hospital employees become eligible for Social Security coverage.

Entering this vortex of crises and competing nostrums were the newly named stewards of Springfield Hospital. Naive about the particulars of hospital management, they nevertheless had the wit and determination (not to mention the necessity) to learn quickly. In the space of five years they managed to save the institution, reverse its deficit tradition, elevate staff morale, launch a major planning process, rehabilitate the physical plant, acquire needed equipment, earn accreditation, raise patient usage, and build community goodwill. The turnaround for Springfield Hospital was faster and more comprehensive than was the nation's own recovery from depression. In a manner and with a dedication resembling their institutional forebears, the Lutheran founders of 1897, this new generation of loyal supporters achieved a near-miracle in the midst of national despair.

At the first annual meeting under new bylaws, in mid-January of 1932, directors named their officers for the year. Elected president was Fred

Wanless, a prominent realtor, who would retain the post for nine years, steering the hospital from its death rattle to vigorous health. One keen observer recalled that Wanless and Dr. Oscar Zelle deserved principal credit for keeping "the hospital afloat during the worst years." Joining him as vice president was a respected lay holdover, William Schnepp. Elizabeth Ide was named secretary, and realtor Milton Hay Brown treasurer. Three other directors joined them on the executive committee: grocer Leon Fisher, Mildred Bunn (widow of Jacob), and Niana Davis (widow of Colonel Henry).

Next to Wanless, the most active and influential executive committee member during these critical years was Mildred Bunn. She rarely missed the weekly meetings, participated fully in discussions and typically offered successful motions on the most fateful issues. For example, she exerted leadership to seek ACS standardization and also to produce a comprehensive long range plan. Within two years she joined Elizabeth Ide as a hospital officer, serving next to Wanless as vice president.

For the remainder of the decade, meeting weekly and later less frequently, the executive committee effectively managed Springfield Hospital, because Pastor Schulz's managerial position went unfilled following his departure in 1933. Its agenda and deliberations quickly settled into a businesslike routine. As recorded crisply by secretary Ide, each session began with a hospital report by the superintendent, then turned to finances and the approval of bills for payment. Any special topics would then conclude the meeting.

The executive committee faced a formidable array of pressing issues and problems. The principal tension in its agenda was between long-range strategic concerns like standardization and a new physical plant, and more immediate challenges such as rising deficits and a disgruntled medical staff. Urgent matters necessarily took precedence, but directors also sought to address the future whenever possible. For example, the full board held a special open meeting late in 1931 to hear the concerns of staff doctors, citizens and others. Dr. Charles Patton was among those declaring the critical need for a new facility. In response, board members personally pledged $900 as a down payment to underwrite the cost of commissioning a comprehensive survey and report on Springfield Hospital's future.

Meeting again early in January of 1932, the board decided to approach Dr. William H. Walsh, a nationally recognized hospital consultant with the American College of Surgeons. Walsh visited with the executive commit-

Mitzvah For Memorial

As long as Springfield Hospital was a sectarian Lutheran entity it failed to tap the volunteerism and generosity of area Jews, who in Springfield had a longstanding record of success and good deeds, or "mitzvah." That limitation ended abruptly in 1931, when the newly non-denominational institution sought broad community support.

Among the new directors that year was Michael Eckstein, a prominent lawyer and leading member of Temple B'rith Sholom, one of Springfield's three Jewish congregations. This break-through inaugurated a tradition of Jewish representation on the hospital's governing board. In addition to serving the hospital, Eckstein earned distinction on the local and state bars, helped found the Springfield Urban League, headed the area B'nai B'rith chapter, and was chairman of the city's Human Relations Commission. He died in 1960.

Also named a director in 1931 was Jeanette (Mrs. Joseph) Hammerslough, one of the coterie of prominent women who invigorated the board during that decade. Mrs. Hammerslough was a member of B'rith Sholom and the Temple Sisterhood, and a volunteer on several other civic boards. In addition, each of the Jewish temples was represented on the hospital's new Board of Women.

In later years many Jewish civic leaders served as director, including Albert Myers, Jr., William Gingold and Alvin Becker.

With its welcoming hand extended, Springfield Hospital won active and generous support from the Jewish community. That tradition has continued to the present, and has been an important factor in the hospital's growth and success.

tee in February, and again with both the board of directors and the newly formed advisory board in March. For a $1,000 fee, he and another experienced consultant, Dr. Malcom T. MacEachern, would conduct a survey of community needs and then offer a detailed plan for Springfield Hospital. The board agreed, and Walsh promised to submit his report in time for the quarterly board meeting in May.

With this emphatic commitment to a better future, the executive committee necessarily turned to messier concerns over its troubled present. As always, finances were the central worry; throughout the winter months of 1932 the hospital continued to struggle with operating deficits. The symptom was a rising level of accounts payable, but the cause lay in accounts receivable. Worsening unemployment left one of every three patient bills uncollectible. The problem was systemic, but the only viable solutions were piecemeal. President Wanless lent his automobile to an office assistant for afternoon collection forays. The executive committee wrote off unrecoverable debts. It accepted in-kind payments: a contractor widened the hospital driveway for $44 credit on his bill, and another offered to paint the third floor washrooms. To stem the financial hemorrhage, officials decided to require a credit application upon admission, and to request early payments while a patient was in the hospital.

Eventually these steps, and a slowly improving economy, would solve the problem, but in the late spring of 1933 it spiraled into another cash flow crisis. The immediate solution, common among employers during the depression, was to slash payroll costs by 25-30 per cent. Vacancies among janitors and in the laundry went unfilled, and salaries for the 33 hospital employees were temporarily reduced by as much as 30 per cent. These and other cost-cutting steps made it possible to begin reducing the $16,000 in accounts payable by at least five percent a month. The results were prompt and welcome; by the end of the year accounts payable had fallen to $10,000, and for the first time in years the trend was favorable.

A longer term answer to chronic financial woes was fundraising, specifically the establishment of an endowment. Late in 1932 Mildred Bunn and Leon Fisher consented to form a committee for this purpose. Either to treat all five of Springfield's banks equally or to diversify the hospital's risk in an age of bank failures, they opened five identical trust accounts under the name, "Springfield Hospital Endowment Fund." R. Allan Stephens symbolically launched the campaign with $5 deposits to each account. Bunn and Fisher immediately began soliciting with a seasonal campaign, "Putting Your Christmas Present Where it Counts."

Increased patient use, at least for paying patients, was another urgent concern. During the early depression years, when the hospital's stature and future were shakiest, occupancy levels also slid disastrously. After hovering in the low 70 per cent range during the 1920s, the rate slipped to 65 per cent in 1931 and to the mid 40s in 1932 and 1933. In June of 1933, for example, 41 patients were admitted, 47 were discharged, four babies were born, and there were five deaths. The average daily occupancy for that month was 46 per cent of the hospital's capacity.

The turnaround in occupancy and finances was rapid and substantial. Early in 1934, after two years under the new regime, Superintendent Williams reported an apparent increase in patient admissions. This was confirmed the next month, which boasted "the largest number of patients and the best collections for a long period of time." Later that year directors had no difficulty meeting the semiannual deadline for paying interest on its bonded debt. At the October quarterly board meeting it was announced that current debt had fallen (from $16,000) to under $3,000, and bonded debt was down to $23,500.

One key to the hospital's reversal of fortune in the 1930s was the nationwide spread of voluntary group medical and hospital insurance. Patient fees, which were a hospital's lifeblood, plunged during the depression but recovered just as quickly, thanks in part to Blue Cross and other insurance programs. Blue Cross was founded in Texas in 1929, as a non-profit cooperative venture between doctors and hospitals. Designed as a voluntary alternative to the specter of compulsory government insurance, it proved immensely popular during the troubled depression years. By 1940 Blue Cross had enrolled six million subscribers, providing an enormous boost to hospital revenues. It created a new and potentially powerful third party in the complex financial relationship between patients, doctors and health care institutions.

The improved fiscal picture made it possible to tackle the lengthening list of repair and equipment needs. New wiring and plumbing were installed, the aged heating system received a new boiler and smokestack, and in July of 1934 air conditioning was installed in the operating rooms. Medical staff president Dr. Zelle named a committee of physicians to advise the superintendent and executive committee on priorities for new medical equipment. Among the items acquired were anesthetics equipment, sterilizers, a pneumonia treatment tent, an electric cardiograph, and a diathermy machine.

By mid-decade, Springfield Hospital was beginning to enjoy a healthy cash flow, renewed staff loyalty, enhanced community stature and a confidence about the future that had eluded it for most of the previous 35 years. At the February 1935 annual board meeting, Fred Wanless announced a sharp upturn in patient occupancy, many physical improvements, and a "materially reduced" hospital debt. One year later the news was even better. Results for 1935 were a "splendid showing" in all areas. The hospital had no current debt, and its bonded debt was steadily shrinking. Admissions had doubled over the level of 1933, elevating occupancy to 87 per cent and occasionally exceeding capacity. There had been sufficient funds to buy and furnish a neighboring house for additional nursing quarters and also to purchase $63,000 of new equipment. Clinical advances included a well equipped x-ray facility and safeguards in surgical work that had produced only four infections among 171 clean operations.

A Hospital of the First Class

Two other announcements at the 1936 annual meeting offered additional evidence of the hospital's dramatic recovery and its brightening future. President Wanless noted with understandable satisfaction that Springfield Hospital now boasted both a plan for replacing its antiquated facility and the status of ACS approval. While coping with urgent operational problems at every meeting for four years, the executive committee also had devoted effort and funds to long range needs for institutional self-study and self-improvement. The Walsh Report and standardization were hospital milestones that warrant special attention.

In assembling data for their May 1932 report to the hospital board, Drs. Walsh and MacEachern carefully inspected the aging facility on North Grand Avenue. What they discovered was an "old, dilapidated institution" that posed an extremely dangerous fire risk. Even the younger wings were "quite out of date and no longer suitable for the conduct of a hospital." Walking the dark, narrow hallways on all three floors of the original structure, the two wings and the 1914 addition was enough to prove their point. To the left (north) of the entrance and offices was the ten person men's ward, nicknamed the "miner's ward" for its most common patients. Crank-operated iron beds comprised the principal furnishing here as in the other wards and private rooms. The entire facility's "antiquated" plumbing meant that there were no private or even ward bathrooms; one utility room in each wing was available to empty and clean bed pans. Patients were given a bowl of water, soap and dish cloth to wash face and hands before breakfast.

To get to the second or third floor, one could use the stairs or a "rickety elevator." On the second level there were two operating rooms with "old-fashioned" equipment, a ceramic tile floor, and a bay window often left open to admit fresh air. Two small emergency rooms adjoined the operating suite, and they often were used for minor surgery (tonsillectomies, circumcisions) and transfusions. The remaining clinical space on the upper two floors housed wards and private rooms, a small obstetrical unit, and a pediatrics section. Back on level one was a cramped kitchen and staff dining area.

Walsh quickly concluded that, whatever its fate, Springfield Hospital could not maintain or even rehabilitate its existing facility. The deeper questions were over long term medical needs in central Illinois and the existing resources in Springfield. To answer them the consultants gauged the area market, spoke to civic leaders, visited St. John's Hospital, inspected potential building sites, and compared their findings to national data and standards. Their 60-page report was ready for board consideration at its May 1932 meeting. A foreword paid tribute to the "generous sacrifice, patient persistence, and never failing faith" of the Lutheran founders. Times and needs had substantially changed, however, so that the hospital now faced a critical decision to either "press forward to a fuller realization of its aims," or "relapse into a condition of innocuous desuetude."

It was clear to Walsh that Springfield and environs, while temporarily hobbled by the depression, constituted a viable market for modern, high quality medical care. Within a 50 mile radius there was a shortage of beds and not a single accredited hospital. To satisfactorily meet the need, a hospital must be (1) governed by an active and diligent board, (2) staffed by competent and progressive physicians, (3) constructed and equipped according to modem standards, and (4) sanctioned by the American College of Surgeons. Both of the local hospitals fell short of these goals, but they had the potential to achieve them.

Springfield Hospital, the consultants continued, had made progress through its new bylaws and broadened base of support. In order to become a "community hospital of the first class," it needed, most of all, to build a new 150-bed facility on a suitable site, at an estimated cost of $931,000. The ideal location would be a residential neighborhood not far from downtown, easily accessible to streetcar lines and highways, away from factory noise and fumes, and capable of expansion. Walsh mentioned four possible sites (one of which was eventually selected), noting their pros and cons. Finally, Walsh argued that the board should plan to raise an endowment of $250,000 in addition to the construction cost, in order to provide an adequate financial cushion.

For an institution that at the time could not even pay its current bills, this was a daunting challenge that required a broad leap of faith by the new board. Even their consultant acknowledged that current economic conditions were "not an opportune time" for such ambitious plans, but with a blueprint the directors would be ready when the time came. With no dissent or hesitation, Wanless and his colleagues approved the plan. Local newspapers duly reported this lonely bit of good news to depression-weary citizens. There would be many steps and hurdles along the way, but the board's boldness in 1932 initiated a process that would culminate 11 years later, hard times and war notwithstanding, in the new Memorial Hospital.

For the remainder of the decade the executive committee and board methodically pursued their dream. As early as 1932 a special committee began scouting possible sites. In 1936 the board named a building committee headed by businessman Robert C. Lanphier. The next year he and Wanless met with Walsh to update and amplify the plans. Walsh's nine-page memorandum recommended raising the capacity from 150 to 175-200, creating an isolation ward for communicable disease patients, including a "children's pavilion," and providing for possible expansion. Such a structure would require seven floors, plus a separate building for the heating plant, laundry and work shops. To build and furnish this facility and a nurse's home would cost $961,000, a modest increase over the original estimate. It was this amended plan that set in motion the architectural design and fundraising for the new hospital.

Integrally related to any massive investment in the future was action on the long deferred issue of standardization. Both the American Hospital Association and the American College of Surgeons had been prodding the nations's hospitals for 15 years to establish internal procedures and regulations consistent with modern medical practice. After a slow start in 1918, the movement gained momentum, and by 1941, 93 per cent of all hospitals with more than 100 beds met the standards.

An ACS pamphlet specified the criteria and offered sample forms and bylaws to applicants. To be approved, a hospital needed (1) a medical staff with eligibility requirements, regular meetings, bylaws and rules of behavior, (2) a system of complete, timely and accurate patient records, and (3) a reasonable level of diagnostic and therapeutic services, including a fully functioning laboratory and x-ray facility.

One of the new executive committee's earliest acts in 1932 was to instruct superintendent Elizabeth Williams to contact Dr. MacEachern of ACS about qualifying for standardization. The subject recurred at weekly meetings, and the committee met with MacEachern that August. In November the medical staff reorganized under stricter new bylaws, and elected Dr. Charles Patton its chief. Patton, a respected local surgeon and a longtime champion of standardization, was the ideal leader for this effort. He successfully urged fellow physicians to keep better records and remove a few incompetent staff members.

Throughout 1933 Miss Williams regularly reported to the executive committee on her progress in bringing the hospital in compliance with ACS standards. Many of these steps were modest but essential; for example she adopted new patient admission and medical history forms according to models in the ACS standardization brochure. She also announced equipment purchases intended to upgrade the laboratory. By consulting periodically with Walsh and MacEachern she was able to identify weak areas needing further attention.

The application process continued in 1934, with superintendent Williams managing the effort and reporting to the medical staff and the executive committee. That summer her work bore fruit. In June an official from the American Hospital Association conducted an inspection that left him "much pleased with the hospital," and confident that it would receive AHA approval. The next month Dr. MacEachern wrote the board that Springfield Hospital now enjoyed "full credit" for having achieved ACS standardization.

Reaching this second institutional milestone in two years was a culminating achievement of Elizabeth Williams' tenure, as she resigned several months later, in October 1934. Originally appointed in 1927, she had loyally served during the hospital's darkest hours, and now could enjoy its better times. She had been a solitary figure of continuity during the crisis years, when there was substantial turnover in the ranks of directors, hospital employees and medical staff. The board regretfully accepted her resignation and paid tribute to her faithful service. After interviewing several candidates and conferring with Dr. Zelle and others on the medical

staff, directors named Prudence Appleman to the superintendent's position, at a monthly salary of $150.

Appleman's tenure was briefer and more troubled than her predecessor's.
Within months of starting she was under attack by Dr. Hilt and other physicians for taking control of the laboratory and x-ray facility. Unlike Williams,
she only rarely attended executive committee meetings, which undoubtedly
weakened her standing there. Trouble surfaced again in mid-1936, over her
expulsion of a student nurse, but once again she was not present to defend
her actions before the executive committee. Whether these absences were
her or the board's responsibility cannot be determined, but the outcome was
her resignation in July to accept a job in New Jersey.

Appleman's successor proved a happier and more successful choice.
Kittie McKelvey had briefly served as acting superintendent and then
director of nursing, 1926-27, and in 1936 was assistant superintendent at
Jewish Hospital in St. Louis. Fred Wanless and his board colleagues inter-
viewed and promptly hired her effective October 1, for $200 per month, a
substantial increase in the superintendent's salary.

McKelvey enjoyed excellent relations with the board and hospital staff
from the outset, and served capably until 1942. She regularly attended
executive committee and board meetings to report on hospital operations
and answer questions. In addition to a one third higher salary, the board
awarded her a larger office than Appleman's. One veteran hospital worker
recalled her fondly, adding that "We called her pussyfoot" owing to a habit
of moving quietly and quickly to monitor staff performance.

With the Walsh Plan, standardization and Kittie McKelvey's appointment, Springfield Hospital's directors could look back on a five year
period of intense activity and remarkable progress. Fred Wanless, Mildred
Bunn and their colleagues, cordially allied with a medical staff led by Drs.
Zelle and Patton, had performed a near-miracle in resuscitating a deeply
troubled institution. The most difficult challenges were behind them, but
new demands and opportunities lay ahead.

A Progressive Social Agency

One vivid measure of Springfield Hospital's dramatic recovery was the
changing frequency of board and executive committee meetings. During
the crisis years directors had met quarterly and delegated active manage-

ment to their seven-member executive committee, which met nearly every week for several years. By 1935 the committee felt comfortable convening biweekly, and two years later it changed to monthly meetings. That year, moreover, the board altered its bylaws to provide for a single annual meeting in place of the quarterly calendar then in place. Deliberations were still lengthy and fateful, but an air of routine oversight had replaced the original sense of urgency.

Through most of the 1930s the board's membership changed only slightly. Fred Wanless and Mildred Bunn retained their leadership positions, and were joined on the executive committee by Herbert Bartholf (treasurer), Bertha (Mrs. Robert C.) Lanphier (secretary), Donald Funk, Louis W. Southard, and Ellen (Mrs. Pascal) Hatch. Incumbent board members typically were re-elected for another three-year term. A clear pattern had been established of tapping civic leaders from Springfield's major businesses, banks and industries, plus prominent women with records of active community service. The board and its allied advisory groups consisted of the city's wealthiest and most influential Protestant and Jewish citizens, giving the hospital both stature and access that were of inestimable value.

Following the early and damaging effects of the depression, the nation's hospitals quickly rebounded by mid-decade. Occupancy rates soared as hospitals achieved standing as the centerpiece of American medical care. Between 1935 and 1940 annual admissions jumped 33 per cent, leading in many areas to chronic overcrowding. Springfield Hospital followed this trend; its annual patient census increased nearly 75 per cent between 1930 and 1940. Every winter season brought many pneumonia cases, pushing the occupancy beyond its 100-patient capacity. In March of 1938, for example, superintendent McKelvey reported a brief peak of 120 patients. One nurse recalled having to place two patients in each hallway of each floor wing. Another nurse's father was assigned to a cramped file storage room where staff members ordinarily enjoyed their coffee and cigarette breaks.

Hospital fees had not changed markedly over the years. Daily rates in the 1930s ranged between $1.50 and $6.00, depending on room type and location. Reduced rates were assigned to personnel of certain cooperating companies, and various discounts were available to hospital employees, staff physicians and area ministers.

Both the increased demand and the income it generated led to growing equipment purchases. In 1937 hospital officials spent $15,000 on new beds and room furniture, operating room equipment, a portable electric inhalator, new sterilizers, and replacement items for the kitchen and laundry.

Hospital finances reflected the boom. Operating close to capacity brought the daily per patient cost of care sharply down; in 1938 alone it shrank by 36 per cent, from $4.77 to $3.08. A fiscal milestone occurred early in 1937, with final payment on the bonded debt. Several months later the executive committee confronted an unfamiliar but welcome task: how to invest surplus operating funds. Additional cushion came in the form of gifts that were a direct result of the hospital's broadened community identity. Robert Lanphier donated $5,000 for new x-ray equipment in 1938, and board members proudly noted a $15,000 bequest the next year.

Like hospitals, American physicians enjoyed rising influence and income during these years. With improved controls over eligibility, the trend toward specialization, and a powerful collective voice (the American Medical Association), doctors were reaching a privileged position in the public eye and sovereign status in the nation's hospitals.

Not many years earlier Springfield Hospital's medical staff had been ill-organized, uneven in quality, and demoralized. These problems began disappearing with the institution's reorganization. The staff met regularly, kept detailed minutes, and took disciplinary action as required. One constant concern was each doctor's obligation to maintain timely patient records. In 1935 staff members voted to reduce delinquent members from active to associate status, and to set rigorous standards for surgical privileges.

The hospital's most active physicians also were among the city's medical elite. Drs. Charles Patton and Oscar Zelle led a staff of highly regarded practitioners, notably brothers Don and John Deal, H. Street Dickerman, Frank Evans, Herbert B. Henkel, Sr., Richard Herndon, David Lewis, Thomas Masters, Harry Otten, Kenneth Schnepp, George Staben, and George Stericker (father and son). Don Deal was regarded as "an excellent surgeon" who was "way ahead of his time" in such pioneering procedures as the 'button hole' incision that led to faster recovery and less pain for appendectomy patients. Otten, who began his career in 1914, had a prodigious general practice that drew him into many fields and keen competition with his peers.

Group practice, long discouraged by the AMA and state authorities, proliferated in the interwar years. Inspired by the Mayo and Menninger clinics, doctors throughout the country but especially in the Middle West began forming their own groups. Springfield's first such effort was launched by Charles Patton and included other Springfield Hospital leaders: Dickerman, Evans, Herndon, Lewis and Masters. Later (1939) the Springfield Clinic was established, principally by doctors more closely associated with St. John's Hospital. Its original partners included Drs. Richard F. Herndon, James Graham, Harold Ennis and Raymond Eveloff. In these years an office appointment typically cost $3, an appendectomy or hernia surgery $50-$75, and the most complex operation as much as $250.

The 1930s also brought the dawn of federally sponsored medical research. Congress established the National Institute of Health in 1930, and then in 1937 the National Cancer Institute under NIH auspices. Both the Public Health Service and the office of the Surgeon-General also expanded their programs and research activities. Government patronage had its own ripple effect, prompting doctors and hospitals throughout the country to undertake clinical research.

At Springfield Hospital the consequences were noticeable. Thomas Masters obtained basement space and modest support for his ongoing diabetes research, a dynamic field owing to the discovery of insulin in the 1920s. The introduction of sulfa drugs revolutionized the treatment and recovery rate for pneumonia, resulting in a sharp drop in mortality. Perversely, the incidence of cancer was rising as Americans lived longer. By the 1930s, cancer had replaced tuberculosis as our "dread disease," causing 140,000 deaths in 1937. This alarming trend prompted physicians and hospitals around the country to open cancer clinics and departments.

Responding to this new concern, physicians at Springfield Hospital inaugurated their own weekly tumor clinic. Specialists took turns presenting papers, followed by discussion of diagnosis and alternative treatments. Occasionally a cancer patient was brought in to illustrate clinical issues. The clinic was open to the entire medical staff, and attracted much interest.

Other specialties were experiencing growth as well. Several area physicians who had treated World War I soldiers with venereal diseases parlayed that experience into careers in genital-urinary work. Drs. Henkel and Evans conducted much of their specialized practice at Springfield Hospital. One new interest, birth control, proved too controversial locally to attract hospital support. Prominent area women founded the Springfield Maternal Health Center (a forerunner to Planned Parenthood) late in the decade. Operating out of a second floor downtown office, the clinic offered birth control examinations, devices and counseling. Its first president was Mrs.

George Thomas Palmer, wife of the versatile physician. Strong resistance from Springfield religious leaders discouraged physicians and either hospital from cooperating with this pioneering initiative.

The hospital's laboratory and x-ray units continued to grow. By this time the demand was sufficient to assign a full-time physician to manage the x-ray department and a part-time pathologist for the laboratory. Late in the 1930s Dr. Aloysius Vass, a heavy-accented Hungarian, began a lengthy tenure as head of the laboratory.

The depression had meant hard times for nurses as well as other groups. Up to 10,000 nursing graduates were out of work in the early 1930s. The labor surplus fueled a campaign to close hospital diploma programs in favor of collegiate nursing education. Many training schools did cease operation, but soon accelerating hospital growth transformed the surfeit into an acute shortage. For example, Springfield Hospital's training school grew to record levels late in the decade; in 1937 it boasted a total enrollment of 63, more than double its size a few years earlier. That June's graduating class was 15, the largest ever. Most of the hospital's staff of several dozen nurses were alumnae of its school, demonstrating the practical value of offering an in-house diploma program.

Other than slightly higher monthly pay ($12), little had changed for students at the training school. Helen Shull, who matriculated in 1936, remembered the dormitory rooms crowded with eight students each, the "very dark and dingy" basement classroom, the exhausting 12-hour work shifts interspersed with classes, and the heavily starched special uniforms assigned to all "probies," or entering students. Occasionally rabbits kept in the basement laboratory for pregnancy testing would escape, creating pandemonium among students in the adjoining classroom.

Strict rules and supervision prevailed. The half day of free time every week permitted a streetcar ride downtown, a walk through nearby Lincoln Park, or socializing at the corner drugstore, a favorite haunt for nursing students and orderlies, who typically were young men enrolled at Concordia Seminary. Trainees could anticipate only three full days off every year: Thanksgiving, Christmas and New Year's. During any night shift lull students would be assigned to make gauze bandages, compresses and swabs, clean syringes, and patch surgical gloves.

The nursing supervisor and her instructional associates inspired fears of discipline or expulsion. Frequently one or more students would be expelled for "not cooperating," being secretly married, or conducting themselves "improperly." Shull's class consisted of 24 students at the outset, but shrank by a third before finishing. The minority of kindly and compassionate supervisors were remembered with affection. Alumnae displayed remarkable loyalty and nostalgia for a program that more closely resembled army boot camp than a school. Founded in 1912, the Alumnae Association held programs for its members and performed various services; by 1937 (the school's 40th year) it boasted over 300 graduates.

Consultant William Walsh had envisioned Springfield Hospital's brighter future as "a progressive social agency." In the decade's final years the board of directors and its allied organizations took various steps to fulfill this dream. One key outreach medium was the advisory board, consisting (like the board itself) of prominent civic leaders. Its meetings were infrequent, but it provided invaluable public credibility for the resurgent hospital.

Other affiliated groups, old and new, also worked to enhance the hospital's reputation. The Springfield Hospital Club began in 1909 as a small group of women volunteers and fundraisers. By 1937 its 25 members remained active supporters and could note with pride their countless gestures and projects. One circle of the King's Daughters dedicated itself to weekly volunteer assistance. The 1931 bylaws had created a new body, the 27 member Women's Board, representing Springfield's Protestant and Jewish religious institutions as well as other community organizations. It developed an ambitious agenda of volunteer services.

The next year yet another group appeared, the Women's Auxiliary. In 1933 the two new organizations merged as the Women's Auxiliary of Springfield Hospital. Its 74 person charter membership mushroomed to more than 1,000 members by 1940. Both dedicated and resourceful, these women performed many services, most of them designed to raise money for the hospital. For example, they inaugurated a popular annual ice cream social, which evolved into a lucrative fund-raising event.

Yet another community medium was the hospital's occasional newsletter. Known as the **Bulletin,** this four-page publication reached many Springfield homes with news of the nursing school, equipment purchases and noteworthy gifts. One issue, for example, acknowledged donations of tomato preserves, dresser scarves, boxes of candy, apple butter and three geese. Gradually its contents grew more reader-oriented, offering homilies and gentle humor, poetry, religious messages and general advice on family health.

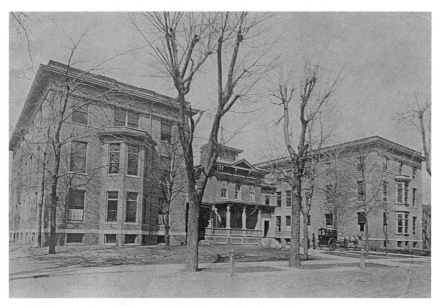

This 1903 view of the hospital's central building and two wings remained relatively unchanged in the 1930s.

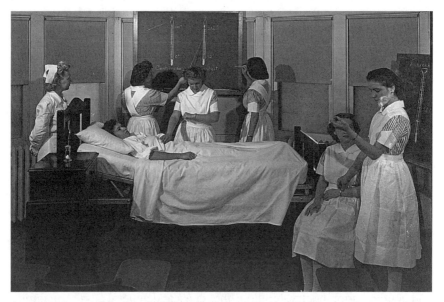

An obviously staged portrayal of clinical nursing education, in this case the comparison of centigrade and Fahrenheit temperature scales.

Mindful of the hospital's opportunity and responsibility as a broad-based community institution, board members frequently sought ways to build goodwill and community recognition. One approach was to encourage Women's Auxiliary members to address church groups about the hospital's progress. Another was to meet with civic clubs. In 1934 directors hosted a dinner meeting with the local Rotary Club, later reporting that it had been "a great success and a good advertisement for ... the hospital."

Reaching the general public was a larger challenge that hospital officials met with a popular annual event, "Hospital Day." Inaugurated nationally in 1921, Hospital Day occurred every May 12, the anniversary of Florence Nightingale's birth. By the late 1930s this had become a highly success-ful local event, with 1,000 and more visitors. The Women's Auxiliary planned and staffed the various programs: an open house, tours, exhib-its and refreshments. The 1937 celebration, widely reported in the city's press, stressed healthy babies. The hospital proudly displayed photographs of every baby born during the past year. Visitors could get advice and free literature on infant care.

As the decade ended, Springfield Hospital showed every sign of robust health at age 40. Operating at full capacity and with modest but heartening annual surpluses, its directors, doctors and employees could look back on ten years of remarkable achievement. A condition of grave peril had given way to a healthy and reenergized institution that finally had achieved the community standing its founders had envisioned. Now it was poised with confidence for a future of new opportunities and challenges.

Memorial Milestones

1938	New hospital construction announced
1941	Capital campaign
1942	Royal E. Raper hired, executive director
1943	New hospital dedicated
	Renamed Memorial Hospital of Springfield
	Participation in U.S. Cadet Nurse Corps
1944	Victor S. Lindberg replaces Raper
1949	Local polio epidemic peaks
1951	Lindberg dies, Frank R. Shank is hired
	Baby boom, overcrowding
1953	Nurses granted 5-day work week

Chapter Four

Building A Future

On National Hospital Day, May 12, 1938, the **Illinois State Journal** announced that Springfield Hospital would construct a new $1 million facility on the historic property at Miller Street, bounded by First and Rutledge. It had been six years since hospital directors had hired Dr. William H. Walsh, at the height of the Depression, to assist them in charting a course for the future. The board reactivated the plan in the spring of 1937 and, by the time of the announcement in the local press, the hospital was debt-free and able to purchase the site with surplus funds. Walsh had based his original recommendations in part on an analysis that the region's existing bed capacity was inadequate. Yet five months after the announced construction, officials at rival St. John's Hospital laid the cornerstone on a $1,250,000 addition which would make it, as described in the **Journal,** "the largest private hospital in the United States." Undaunted, the Springfield Hospital board proceeded not only to build its new facility but also to double the bed capacity from the originally recommended 150. The story of the struggling hospital's successful completion of ambitious building and fundraising efforts is one of the most significant in its history. Without a modern physical plant the hospital could not have survived. Thus the story, rich in detail, dominates a decade of general development.

Walsh had urged the board to create a first class hospital and, under the leadership of president Fred Wanless, it boldly moved to achieve that goal. The timing could have seemed ill-fated; the effort began at the ebb of the Great Depression and culminated at the height of a world war, events which claimed the preponderant resources and attention of communities across the United States. To understand how the board achieved this feat it is useful to review the American hospital environment as well as the spirit of Springfield in the pre-war years.

Springfield emerged from the Depression with a frenzy of building activity. When the new hospital was announced in 1938, the project joined many others. In addition to the St. John's Hospital addition, the Illinois State Archives building was dedicated, scout camps were opened, construction began on the John Hay Homes public housing project and a major addition to Lanphier High School was completed. While some projects benefited from New Deal recovery programs designed to put Americans back to work, voluntary hospitals would not realize federal assistance for construction until the 1941 Community Facilities Act, known popularly as the Lanham Act. Even then, the attack on Pearl Harbor led to strict restrictions on the use of those funds.

In the United States there was no simple division of hospitals into "public" and "private." Voluntary hospitals were a hybrid, with characteristics of both. Nonprofit, voluntary hospitals were looked upon as symbols of the American ideal of community spirit and were, as one historian described them, "beacons of hope, science, faith and caring." Thousands of Americans served without pay on hospital boards and contributed their time as hospital volunteers. In the uniquely American approach to health care, nonprofit hospitals in the 1930s had labeled themselves "public," by which they meant voluntary. Hospital associations representing the voluntaries used this attractive rubric to separate themselves from both for-profit and government hospitals, to claim that they deserved to receive federal funds and to maintain tax exempt status without government interference. Then in 1934 the American Medical Association classified hospitals into three categories: government, proprietary and nonprofit (voluntary). Among these types, voluntary hospitals represented the largest segment, with two-thirds of all hospital admissions. Hospital associations were quick to take advantage, pressing their message that the voluntaries ensured access to health care via the new insurance plans. As Springfield Hospital laid its plans for a new building, somewhat more than 600,000 Americans were covered by Blue Cross hospital insurance plans, soon to become a national movement that would cover 4.4 million Americans by 1940.

Another trend emerged in the late 1930s which affected not only Springfield but hospitals throughout the country. Federal support for biomedical research began in earnest with the 1937 federal act supporting cancer research and, by 1949, had grown to include mental, dental and heart diseases. Medical research, fueled by the second world war, led to new wonder drugs, including penicillin and other antibiotics. The burgeoning new medical and surgical techniques increased hospitalization 32 per cent from 1941 to 1946.

Despite the rapid advances in medical knowledge, hospital stays remained quite long in the late 1930s in order to carry out the tedious and prolonged patient care techniques of the day. There were no specific therapies for most conditions until 1937 when sulfanilamide was developed. This drug eventually led to a 40 per cent drop in the pneumonia death rate by 1945. But most care remained unsophisticated. As late as a decade after the development of this drug, one veteran nurse recalled that every evening nurses placed all flowers on the hallway floors outside patient rooms in order "to improve the oxygen supply." Nevertheless, the technique and technology of the modern hospital was such that by the mid-1930s there was "no alternative to hospitalization." By 1940 nearly one-quarter of physicians were full-time specialists whose services required the equipment available at hospitals. The 1940s saw a rapid growth in specialties and subspecialties, as physicians who returned from the war used the GI Bill of Rights to acquire specialty training, then returned from large, urban teaching hospitals eager to bring the latest techniques to their hometown community hospitals. The demand for hospital services was poised for takeoff and Springfield Hospital was on the cusp of the best vehicle for success, the modern hospital building.

Make No Little Plans

Hospital construction during this period was generally viewed as a social benefit, because new buildings promoted an image of success and financial recovery. Dr. Malcolm T. MacEachern, who had directed the American College of Surgeons' hospital standardization program since 1921, reviewed and concurred with Dr. Walsh's report. By consulting these two notable physicians, both known to be champions of the modern hospital, Springfield Hospital officials were emphatically making big plans. In 1935 MacEachern published a widely consulted textbook on hospital administration in which he depicted hospitals as "shining, scientific citadels." Illinoisans who were shopping for new citadels in the 1930s could find them in Chicago, already an international leader in modern architecture.

The 1938 construction announcement reported that definite plans were incomplete, but the hospital was to "be of the skyscraper type." At a special meeting on December 10, 1938, directors approved contracts with Dr. Walsh for additional planning assistance and with the Chicago firm of Burnham and Hammond, architects, for design of the new building. In its selection of this venerable firm, the board made a direct connection to the skyscraper. Hubert Burnham, whose signature adorns the original architectural drawings, was the son of the legendary Daniel H. Burnham, known as the father of the skyscraper and a principal designer of the 1893 World's Columbian Exposition. One historian has noted that hospital architects of the time were "tapping into the American dream." So, too, were the hospital directors.

The announced construction and subsequent capital campaign generated phenomenal attention in the local press, which continued almost daily for more than three years. Large feature stories discussed the site, the plans, the fundraising campaign and the construction. No detail was too trivial to receive coverage. The press even ran a large photograph of construction workers digging the sewer line. In the process of funding, building, and promoting a new hospital, Springfield citizens were quintessential examples of community boosterism.

Board president Fred Wanless appointed a special committee to review Walsh's four suggested sites. Members included George W. Bunn, Jr., Henry Merrium, Robert Lanphier, Herbert B. Bartholf, and Reverend Paul Schulz. They chose the Coleman property, which Walsh had originally described as "too distant but acceptable." The site consisted of two parcels, comprising four square blocks. The litany of names over three generations and two branches of the same family makes description of these properties difficult. One of the parcels, at First and Miller Streets, was donated to the hospital by Logan Hay, a member of the hospital's advisory committee, a partner in the law firm of Brown, Hay and Stephens, and a two-term State Senator. Hay also happened to be the keynote speaker and organizer for the dedication of St. John's Hospital's new addition. The Hay property had once been the site of the well-known and historic Littler home, which had been razed several years earlier. During the Depression, Lucy (Mrs. Logan) Hay had permitted several dozen needy families to raise vegetables on the lot.

Link to a Legend

Architect Hubert Burnham was the third of Daniel H. Burnham's five children. He was a 1905 graduate of the U.S. Naval Academy, appointed through President McKinley, who "believed in the boy from the bottom of his heart." Hubert resigned his commission to study architecture at the École des Beaux Arts in Paris. He entered the family firm as a junior associate in 1910 and thus was a seasoned professional by the time he designed Memorial. His partner then was Illinois State Architect, C. Herrick Hammond, a designer of Springfield's 1938 Illinois State Archives building. Daniel H. Burnham's name is among the 24 engraved on that edifice.

Memorial officials aimed high with their selection of a nationally recognized architectural firm. Founder Daniel H. Burnham was a major contributor to the early "Chicago School" of architecture and a nationally recognized city planner. Frank Lloyd Wright described him as an "enthusiastic promoter of great construction enterprises." Among the firm's notable designs are Chicago's Field Museum and the Rookery as well as the Lincoln Memorial in Washington, D.C. Burnham is also credited with an enduring Chicago motto: "Make no little plans. They have no magic to stir men's blood." Memorial officials shared that vision.

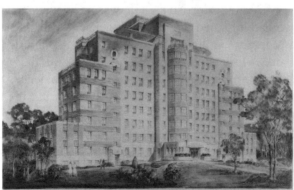

An artist's rendering of Burnham and Hammond's proposal for "The New Memorial Hospital of Springfield."

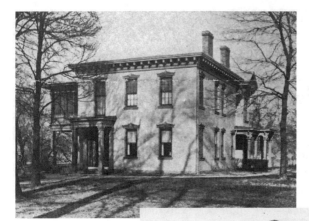

The Logan home

The Littler home

Dr. Hugh Morrison sold the adjoining property, his home, to the hospital in May 1938 for $23,000. Morrison's wife was a Coleman and the Littler descendant who had inherited the property; hence Walsh's description of the "Coleman property" in his report. The Morrison's historic home was razed on October 31, 1938, a few days after Women's Auxiliary volunteers conducted "last opportunity" tours of the 18-room residence. Several of its antique furnishings were donated to the hospital for use in the Nurses' Home on North Grand Avenue.

Though the purchase of the site left the board with a surplus of $67,000, members expressed concern about their ability to raise the required construction funds. In the 1930s nonprofit, voluntary hospitals were often built with local capital but, as hospital historian Rosemary Stevens noted, by 1941 hospital construction was generally too costly for local support. Springfield, Illinois was a striking exception.

A $1.1 million campaign was announced in May 1941, along with the board's intention to change the hospital's name to Memorial Hospital of Springfield. The name change was to be concurrent with the move to the new facility, and was selected as part of the capital campaign promoting the hospital as a memorial to all donors. It also served, perhaps intentionally, to distance the new, modern institution from the old, overcrowded, and dilapidated structure on North Grand Avenue. Whatever the board's reasoning, renaming the 46-year old institution was both beneficial and fateful. Lingering sectarian connotations were bound to die faster as were memories of the jerrybuilt north side structure. The word "Memorial" underscored the hospital's enlarged base and community mission. Other name changes would come in the 1970s and 1980s, but "Memorial" would remain the hospital's distinguishing moniker.

The building campaign was officially launched in June 1941 under the guidance of board treasurer Herbert B. Bartholf, president of the Illinois National Casualty Company and the St. Nicholas Hotel. Bartholf was general chairman of the building fund while director Edward S. Perry chaired the vitally important memorial gifts committee. In less than one month the campaign raised slightly more than half its goal. In fact, nearly half the goal was reached within the first 24 hours by four public-spirited donors: Alice Bunn, Mildred Bunn, Bertha Lanphier, and Susan Bartholf. Their generosity ensured the campaign's ultimate success and dramatized the vital role women were playing in the hospital's renaissance.

A second important funding source included central Illinois Masonic lodges and Shrine Consistory. According to one longtime board member, these were among the "known anti-Catholic organizations" that campaign organizers pointedly solicited. Thus began a cordial and lasting relationship. Aggregate Masonic contributions to the building drive exceeded $100,000, and subsequent support matched that level.

When the capital campaign passed the $1 million mark, the press reported that the effort "establishes a new high water mark for public subscription to hospital building funds since the onset of the depression." The press had based this claim on a nationwide review of records and labeled the campaign the nation's largest and most successful in over ten years. Edward S. Perry won the 1941 Distinguished Service Award from the Cosmopolitan Club for his work on the campaign. Perry was president of the Perry-Rigby Company, which operated the Leland Hotel. His was the first distinguished citizen medal awarded since 1928. The rapid fulfillment of the original

Masonic Support

Characterized by a mingling of religion, science, and ritual, modern freemasonry dates from early 18th century England. Numerous spin-offs and subgroups (Odd Fellows, Fraternal Order of Eagles, Shriners, etc.) have emerged, and these organizations took firm hold in the United States, a nation of joiners.

On June 22, 1942 the Masonic fraternity of Springfield laid the cornerstone of the new hospital. Board members Herbert B. Bartholf, Edward S. Perry, Fred W. Wanless, and Leon E. Fisher were all Masons. Newspaper editor Vincent Y. Dallman acted as Grand Orator in the absence of Governor Dwight H. Green, also a Mason. More than 600 master Masons in white aprons participated in the ceremony, witnessed by several hundred citizens. Sealed within the stone, laid in the "custom and usage of ancient craft masonry," was a copper box containing a list of the hospital directors, a description of the building, and issues of the local newspaper and the **Springfield Scottish Rite Magazine.** In an "eloquent oration," Dallman praised the role of the Masons in building a "house of mercy."

The cornerstone was removed in 1969 as part of a laboratory expansion project. The box was entrusted to hospital administrator George Hendrix until the Masons could formally lay the stone in a new location. Records of the period note a scheduled date but no record has been found of the ceremony nor evidence of the original cornerstone and its contents.

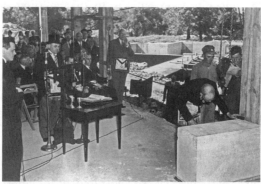

campaign by mid-September encouraged the board to expand the goal to $1.25 million.

A promotional campaign brochure, **Life and Remembrance,** outlined a community need for the hospital and cited American Medical Association statistics which described Springfield Hospital as the "most overcrowded general community hospital in the State of Illinois." The campaign strategy was to solicit memorial donations and pledges, the latter to be met in six installments payable every four months, a two-year commitment. The brochure featured floor plans and listed memorial opportunities on each. Donors could sponsor hallways, equipment, rooms, wards or floors, such as a four-bed ward on the third floor for $6,000, or the entire third floor for $141,900. Appropriately, the Masons donated the foundation and ground floor as a "Masonic memorial." The Women's Auxiliary funded the solarium and a three-bed ward on the second floor for $9,000.

The highly successful memorial fund drive was bolstered by special events, largely organized by women and held at the Orpheum Theater. Echoing their successful 1940 Jeanette MacDonald song recital, the Women's Auxiliary and the **Illinois State Journal** co-sponsored a Nelson Eddy concert in 1942. One year later they treated Springfield residents to a concert by leading Metropolitan Opera soprano, Lily Pons. The program for her recital featured advertisements from local businesses and solicitations to purchase war bonds. The hospital was also able to use its voluntary status as a fundraising tool. It released a booklet, **Out of the Shadow of Charity,** which addressed its responsibility to serve indigent patients. The booklet explained the obligation of community hospitals to serve all citizens regardless of their ability to pay and noted that with half its patients paying less than the cost of service, Memorial would have to raise rates 60 per cent if it were a private business. Its "special financial structure" meant that it could not borrow funds or raise fees to underwrite a new building, but must instead rely upon donations.

Despite this rhetoric, hospital officials did borrow money for the project. Contractors were compelled by wartime shortages to order construction materials well in advance. Bills for materials were flowing in by late 1942 although pledges were not due until 1943. A year before the new hospital opened the board agreed to borrow up to $200,000 for the building fund, to be repaid from subscriptions. Similar actions were taken in June and November 1943. Upon completion of the new building, the hospital owed three Springfield banks a total of $300,000. In less than four years this was

reduced to $120,000, with $50,000 of the debt paid from income on operations. In 1945 and 1946 the hospital "operated in the black."

Shining Citadel

Nearly three years after the construction was announced, the board
authorized architect Burnham to proceed with detailed plans, which
were finally approved in January 1942. John Felmley and Company of
Bloomington were awarded the construction contract.

Burnham's design for Memorial was described as "neither pretentious
nor elaborate." Simple lines incorporated three wings in Bedford limestone
and brick, with approximately 300 windows. The Art Deco style entrance
featured "The Memorial Hospital of Springfield" etched in stone above
the door. Glass brick above the stone admitted light to the second floor
nursery. Art Deco featured colorful finishes and the new hospital was no
exception. Walls were shades of green, peach, tan, yellow, and blue, and
furniture had light finishes of maple, walnut, and mahogany. Outside, the
Springfield Civic Garden club volunteered to landscape the new grounds
and contributed $600 for the plan and plants. At a November 1943 public
ceremony the club planted ground cover at the hospital entrance.

The hospital which finally emerged following the design and fund drive
stages more than doubled Walsh's originally recommended size. Three
wings of seven stories intersected at a 10-story tower in a T-shape with the
nurses' stations located at the intersections. The eighth floor was a "roof
garden" where patients could get sun and fresh air or stay in a solarium.
Private rooms were located near wards for ward patients "who became
desperately ill." The laundry and boiler house were separated from the hospital with access via a tunnel. The 335 bed capacity included 50 bassinets
and boasted the latest modern luxury, air conditioning, in the operating
rooms, obstetrics, and nursery. All corridors and walls were "sound proof"
and all floors had rubber tile. There were three elevators, two for the public
and one for hospital staff. Telephone service was provided in all the "necessary" administrative offices, each nurses' station and in private rooms.
Reflecting a business acumen, the board elected not to install telephone
service in semi-private rooms so that these would not "impede the sale of
private rooms."

Dedicated To Service

Arrangements for the hospital dedication were as ambitious as the capital campaign. The board appointed a dedication committee which included representatives from the board, the Nurses' Alumni Association, the Women's Auxiliary and "prominent lay persons." Doctors on the committee were Don Deal, Richard F. Herndon, and Herbert B. Henkel.

*Dr. William H. Walsh, who played a key role in conceiving and planning the new hospital, had died in 1941 without seeing his plans come to fruition. Dr. Malcolm T. MacEachern, another long-term consultant, was present to speak as associate director of the American College of Surgeons. In addition to Springfield Mayor John W. Kapp, the program featured remarks by the Sangamon County Medical Society president (Dr. Herndon) and the Memorial Hospital medical staff president, Dr. Harry Otten. Among the half dozen medical notables who were included on the program were Dr. Morris Fishbein, editor of the **Journal of the American Medical Association,** and representatives of the American Hospital Association, Illinois Hospital Association, the National League for Nursing Education, and the Army and Navy Nurse Corps.*

The principal speaker was Lieutenant Colonel Charles W. Mayo, M.D. of the Mayo Clinic. He had been granted a special leave by the U.S. Surgeon General in order to attend. Thousands joined the Springfield Municipal Band in "America" and bowed their heads to the invocation offered by Reverend William Hudnut, Jr. of the First Presbyterian Church. With civic pride and hyperbole, Mayor Kapp declared the "erection of this fine structure should make Springfield the medical center of the middle west." Nevertheless, Memorial had come a long way since Dr. W. A. Young, by then the only surviving member of the original medical staff, had introduced rubber gloves to Springfield physicians.

In marked contrast to the commonplace announcement of the hospital's founding in 1897, the dedication of Memorial Hospital was an extravaganza. Accounts of the ceremonies for the new building reveal considerable pride and commitment from the community. On September 26, 1943 an open house for the public drew over 12,000 people. Tours were halted for the two-hour dedication ceremony in the afternoon, attended by an estimated 5,000. The **Illinois State Journal and Register** produced a 12-page special section on the new hospital, complete with a half-page photograph of the new Art Deco entrance, numerous stories, and large congratulatory advertisements. Springfield enjoyed perfect autumn weather for the dedication, which was also broadcast by radio. In officially accepting the keys to the hospital from architect Burnham, board president Mildred Bunn offered simple remarks that exemplified the values of voluntary hospitals of the day: "I dedicate this hospital to the service of Springfield and the surrounding communities."

The long awaited move to a modern facility occurred on October 1, and that midnight the new hospital began admitting patients. Helen Shull, Director of Nursing, recalled that nurses were instructed to select "essential" supplies and equipment for the move that day but were in a quandary about what was essential. Patients and supplies from the third floor of the old hospital were moved to the sixth floor of the new one; the seventh floor was not yet ready for patients. Staff prepared identification tags to be tied to each patient. Each tag included the patient's name, both old and new room numbers, and the doctor's name. Six local ambulances and two other automobiles were volunteered to move 57 patients to the new hospital. Each patient was accompanied by a nurse and each ambulance was escorted by police. Dietitian Eunice Scott noted the intense planning and extra staff required for the move and recalled that breakfast was served in the old hospital and lunch was the first meal served in the new building. She remembered that her only loss was a misplaced 25-pound bag of cornstarch.

The move "went quite smoothly" despite recent turnover and vacancies in the managerial staff. Until the board hired Royal E. Raper in October 1942, the hospital had functioned with only one administrator for several years. Kittie McKelvey had been de facto executive director from October 1936 until Raper was hired and the new title created. As superintendent of both the hospital and nursing school, McKelvey was the senior administrator at the time the board was undertaking its building and fundraising efforts. Born in Sparta, Illinois, McKelvey was a graduate of the U.S.

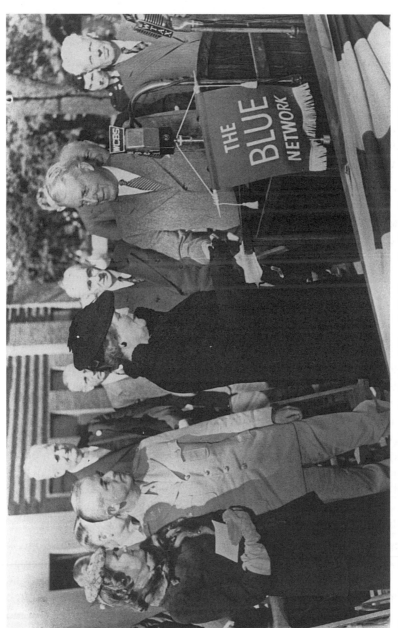

Pictured are Mildred Bunn, Hubert Burnham, Lt. Col. and Mrs. C. W. Mayo, Dr. Harry Otten and Dr. R. F. Herndon at the hospital's dedication ceremony, September 26, 1943.

Army School of Nursing, associated with Walter Reed Hospital. Her considerable experience included work at hospitals in Boston, Washington, D.C., St. Louis, and Ohio.

When Raper was hired, just one year prior to opening the new hospital, McKelvey was given the title of assistant executive director. In a telephone call to board president Mildred Bunn, McKelvey submitted her resignation just eight months later. She claimed she was unhappy and preferred to sever her connections with the hospital before the move. Bunn described the call as a surprise and accepted the resignation with regret.

McKelvey was replaced by three nurses. Harriet Sooy and Ann Tarpley were each named assistant directors and worked the evening and night shifts. Alma E. Gault became director of nursing and nursing education but resigned in 1944. Later that year, Ruth D. Riedesel was also employed as an assistant executive director. She was in charge in Raper's absence and supervised admitting, the information desk, and the elevators.

The board had discussed the matter of employing an executive director for some time before Raper was hired. He was a central Illinois native, recruited from Springfield, Ohio, who had earlier worked at Methodist Hospital, Peoria. Through Raper's efforts, the board was able to recruit Eunice Scott from Methodist to head the dietary department.

Board members suffered from an inadequate supply of qualified administrative staff to knowledgeably handle day-to-day operations. Acting as unpaid administrators, board members had to cope with the extra responsibilities involved in building and equipping a new hospital. Even McKelvey, with her considerable knowledge, was forced to handle matters which were completely outside her experience. Directors were, in modern parlance, micro managing the organization by performing duties which would later be assumed by hospital departments and myriad staff. Board members purchased typewriters, lockers, and birth certificate forms, and directly hired some professional and managerial personnel.

In the spring and summer of 1942, before Raper arrived, the board took steps to select and order supplies and furnishings for the new hospital. Board president Mildred Bunn and other committee members selected the furniture. McKelvey was charged with ordering linens and china, though directors reserved the privilege of choosing the china patterns. Fred Wanless, then vice president of the board, selected the silverware. When dietitian Scott was hired she was unable to locate any records of what supplies had been ordered. To her dismay, there were some expensive and inefficient selections already made by well-meaning board members who mimicked their own personal and household habits. Scott found ten different china patterns as well as silver-plated flatware (from Stout's, a local jeweler), including small-sized sets for pediatric patients, engraved with the hospital's name. She was forced to gradually replace lost, stolen and mismatched items with institutional china and flatware. In one particularly memorable experience, Bressmer's Department Store called to inform her that the hospital's teapots had arrived.

Raper stayed less than two years. Though Eunice Scott recalled that he was a "very nice man" with whom she enjoyed working, he apparently had some difficulty getting along with the medical staff. Quickly succeeding him was Victor S. Lindberg, appointed in June 1944. Lindberg, the son of a Lutheran minister, was recruited from Victory Memorial Hospital in Waukegan. Dr. Robert Patton remembered that Lindberg "ran the hospital by himself," with some help from Edna Huelskoetter, who "could run it herself pretty well." Lindberg was a capable and popular administrator, twice elected president of the Illinois Hospital Association. His wife, Alice, was active in the Women's Auxiliary.

Lindberg, described by Dr. Glen Wichterman as a "short, rotund, and jolly" man, suffered a heart attack at age 53 and died at Memorial on April 7, 1951. In its resolution recognizing his service, the board expressed its appreciation. "He so endeared himself to everyone connected with our institution that he has built his own imperishable memorial within its walls."

It may have been Lindberg's great popularity that caused his successor to stay only two years. Frank R. Shank, who assumed the executive director position on May 14, 1951, was recruited from Chicago Lying-in Hospital. Shank is notable as the administrator whom no one remembered. The medical staff executive committee extended a brief thank-you and letter of recommendation. Apparently, Shank did not leave to take another job but no trace of difficulties was left in the written record. He submitted his resignation in April, to be effective June 1, 1953. A former administrator alluded vaguely to "problems" with Shank and a physician explained Shank's departure with "well, it didn't work out." One veteran manager recalled that Shank was rather quiet while another was able to compliment him for painting patient rooms more vibrant colors. Eunice Scott astutely observed that the popular Lindberg had been a "tough act" to follow. Indicative of the scarcity of administrative staff, the president of the board had to spend much of his time at the hospital after Shank left,

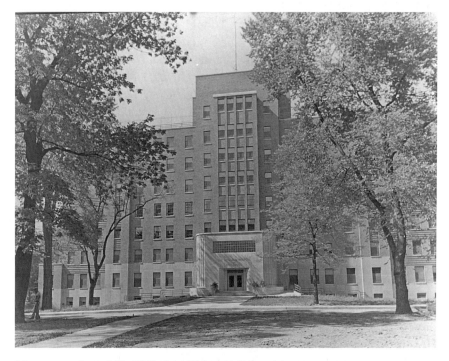

Mature trees framed this 1943 view of Memorial's art deco entrance.

working with Edna Huelskoetter on operational issues. She was granted an extra month's pay for her effort.

Wartime Paucity and Patriotism

The day after the Pearl Harbor attack the board agreed to change the hospital's name on its bank account to Memorial Hospital of Springfield. An ambitious project under normal circumstances, the construction of a new hospital during the second world war was both a challenge and a monument to hospital officials. The war marshaled an intense sense of purpose and sacrifice which carried over into the strong community commitment to the hospital. The fighting spirit, the effort required for a great cause, was echoed in the board room and the hospital hallways.

Though eleven years had elapsed between the 1932 Walsh report and the opening of the new hospital, World War II did not delay the construction. Completed in just 20 months, the project enjoyed a high priority for scarce materials. The federal Office of Production Management's "A-7" rating enabled the hospital to acquire steel and other necessary supplies. The war affected only some relatively minor features of the construction, such as the front doors. Designed for steel, they were constructed of wood until steel was more readily available after the war. By 1948, just five years alter construction, 650 "war time doors" had to be refinished or replaced, a $5,200 expense.

Hospitals had been declared "essential activities" by the federal War Production Board. Despite this priority status, the war added a considerable bureaucratic burden to the already overwhelmed staff. Hospitals were subject to rules and regulations promulgated by the War Production Board, the War Labor Board, and the War Manpower Commission, to list a few agencies. Translated to the everyday operation of a community hospital, many routine activities such as ordering supplies and hiring staff were subject to federal control and required tedious additional paperwork, record keeping and delays. New employees could not readily be hired away from other "essential activities," that is, other hospitals. Hiring had to be conducted through the local office of the United States Employment Service, and with an appropriate piece of paperwork, the certificate of availability. Late in 1944 the employment service refused to "release" a medical record librarian to accept Memorial's job offer. These were formidable obstacles to a board faced with staffing a new hospital twice as large as its present

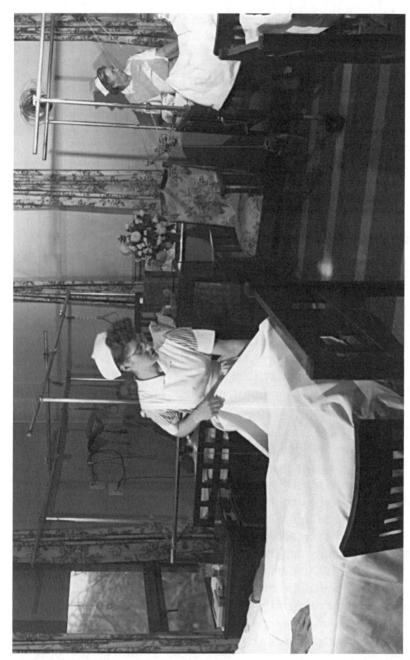

Modish draperies enlivened this ward room, which also featured orthopedic equipment for several beds.

one. Heaped further upon this burden were other government directives, such as the Surgeon General's 1943 edict to create and staff an emergency medical unit affiliated with the United States Public Health Service. The hospital was instructed to appoint a leader to the unit who would have the army rank of Lieutenant Colonel. In another instance, the Executive Director had to travel to Chicago to negotiate with the Salary Stabilization Board for the radiologist's pay increase.

Three months after the Pearl Harbor attack, Kittie McKelvey attended meetings in St. Louis on the operation of hospitals in wartime. In keeping with her recommendations, the board approved the purchase of extra sheets, blankets, and towels as part of their strategy to stockpile hospital supplies. In order to maintain a neat appearance in the new hospital, the board decided to provide uniforms for some employees, including nurses' aides, maids, laundry workers, kitchen maids, housemen, and elevator operators. The board ordered these uniforms ten months prior to the opening of the new hospital due to their concern about the wartime cotton shortage. McKelvey vehemently preached scarcity and stressed the use of one paper towel instead of two.

The rationing system added additional layers of bureaucracy. The board had long been in the habit of adjusting employee salaries in the form of meal allowances. The law now required the hospital to hold the ration books of all employees who received eight or more meals per week. The dietary department followed a government points system for scarce commodities like meat and sugar. When the local ration board granted extra sugar to the pharmacy so that certain drugs could be compounded, the board had to open an additional ration bank account in order to keep this separate from dietary sugar rations.

Many Springfield residents rode the bus to work due to gasoline rationing. Springfield manufacturers produced more than $5 million in war supplies and equipment. The community also shared the severe national shortage of physicians and nurses. At one point, 37 physicians of 127 on the attending and associate staff were in military service. Among the most challenging shortages was the 1943 loss of the hospital's only pathologist. Dr. Aloysius Vass was granted a wartime leave of absence to serve in the army. The board then hired Dr. Harry M. Steen, who worked at St. John's Hospital, and had to pay him a full-time salary for his part-time work. Raper hoped to hire a new pathologist but the medical staff refused to make a recommendation for a replacement. The board had no choice

Littler Legacy

Rooted in a rich and fascinating heritage, the site of the new Memorial Hospital was selected as the most practical and cost effective place to build a future. Though a historic home was destroyed on Halloween to make way for the hospital, the presence of the site's former owner lingers.

Both parcels had once been owned by Stephen T. Logan, a prominent early judge and law partner of Abraham Lincoln. The list of persons who had owned or visited the site's two homes constitutes a "Who's Who" of 19th century Illinois history and includes Lincoln, Jane Addams, Ulysses S. Grant, and Illinois governors Richard J. Oglesby and Joseph W. Fifer

Judge Logan built a home in 1837 at First and Miller Streets as a wedding gift for his daughter, Kate, and her husband, State Senator David Littler. The Littlers had one son, Stephen Logan Littler, who later inherited the home as well as 4,300 acres of farm land. In 1907 Stephen Littler's phobia of disease led him to cancel a trip with friends to Europe, where there was an alleged smallpox outbreak. His friends returned home to learn that he had died at home of pneumonia. Littler, who had never married, left his home to his cousin, Logan Hay, and stipulated that all his cousins equally share the income from the farm trust property. After the 26th and final cousin died in the mid-1960s, the trust's assets were destined for "a hospital." Littler had named as trustee the Sangamon Loan and Trust Company, which later became the First National Bank. In 1955 Memorial was named beneficiary and in 1967 received $770,000 from the sale of one quarter of the land. The remaining land, held in charitable trust, provides the hospital with an annual income into perpetuity. By Memorial's centennial year, proceeds from the Littler legacy had reached nearly $9 million.

Judge Logan had purchased the adjoining property in 1838 from Ninian Edwards, Illinois' third governor. Another daughter, Jenny Logan Coleman, eventually lived in the home built there.

but to await Vass's return from the war. The situation became so desperate that Dr. Don Deal and two board members traveled to meet Vass, who was serving in the United States, in a futile effort "to arrive at some satisfactory solution." A year before Vass finally returned, Dr. Deal made unsuccessful efforts to get Vass released from the army.

The nursing shortage was even worse. Local newspapers ran appeals for nurses' aides and volunteers, and the Red Cross sponsored nurses' aide classes at both hospitals. At a local Red Cross meeting the urgent plea for nurses for army, navy, and veteran's hospitals was noted with considerable alarm by Raper, who was coping with his own nurse shortage. His was no idle concern. The army and navy enrolled more than 65,000 nurses from 1944 to 1945, most from civilian hospitals. The shortage was so critical that President Roosevelt unsuccessfully recommended drafting nurses. In a 1945 letter to recent Memorial graduate Hilda Slocum Warren, the officers of the Citizens War Nursing Committee for Sangamon County congratulated her on her graduation and advised her of her opportunity to serve in the Armed Forces. "This committee is ready to do anything in the world that is reasonable, to aid you in your noble endeavors."

Hospitals with student nurses had a ready source of cheap labor. In the nation's hospitals with nursing schools, 80 per cent of the workload was carried by student nurses. Congress delivered more students in 1943 with the creation of the U.S. Cadet Nurse Corps. The Corps was a tremendously successful program which subsidized students' entire education, including maintenance and a monthly stipend, in return for a promise to work in either military or civilian nursing for the war's duration. By the time the Corps terminated in 1948 the program had trained 125,000 nurses at a cost of $160 million. A month before the new hospital was dedicated in 1943, the board approved participation in the Cadet Corps program. At the time, there were 66 students enrolled in Memorial Hospital School of Nursing. By September 1945 there were 145.

The hospital received $27,200 from the U.S. Public Health Service to inaugurate the Cadet Nurse Corps program. Most nursing students signed up as cadet nurses; all 31 students accepted into the fall 1944 term were in the Corps. These students received Cadet uniforms and adhered to the strict and detailed requirements promulgated by the U.S. Public Health Service for wearing them. Students were forbidden to wear their uniforms in taverns or other places which would "disgrace" the uniforms, and were encouraged to "harmonize" their lipstick and fingernail polish with the red epaulets.

Despite the aggravations created by the war, doctors and hospital personnel were largely uncomplaining. A 1944 issue of the **Bulletin of the Sangamon County Medical Society** listed local nurses who were serving in the military, one of whom was in Africa, and went on to editorialize about the nursing shortage:

> ...these young ladies are busy winning a war and people
> will just have to do without this luxury for the duration.
> No doubt these girls would rather be in the cool corridors
> of the hospital than the burning sands of Africa, but war is
> war. The doctors of Sangamon County salute you!

While still housed at the old hospital, the board had agreed to acquire the service flags of hospital staff and doctors in the armed services and display them in the lobby. The business office was required to maintain a list of names of those in the service. When the American Hospital Association approved a service emblem for hospital employees signifying that they were engaged in important war work, the board quickly purchased enough for all hospital employees. The war pervaded all activities, including the 1942 cornerstone dedication. In his oration, Vincent Y. Dallman, editor of the **Illinois State Register** and potentate of the Ansar temple, described the hospital as "essential to war and a contribution to peace."

Booming Business

The August 15, 1945 newspaper headline, "Springfield Goes Wild," aptly described the exuberant festivities at war's end. It also foreshadowed several decades of unbridled growth and change in the city. Springfield was perhaps too exuberant because in the postwar decade it earned a reputation for vice, gambling, and corruption. The city drifted to a white collar economy and to newly created subdivisions. Downtown buildings were demolished for parking lots while bus ridership sharply declined.

Local citizens also participated in the nationwide postwar baby boom. In 1945 there were 596 births at Memorial. The following year there were 895, a 50 per cent increase. When the annual number of births passed 1,000 in 1951, the hospital experienced severe overcrowding. Board records throughout the 1950s noted the problem infrequently but vividly. In a congratulatory tone, the board noted that 1952 was better than 1951 because the hospital had "reassembled every available bed from the Nurses' Home and in the hospital, and frequently have placed them in the

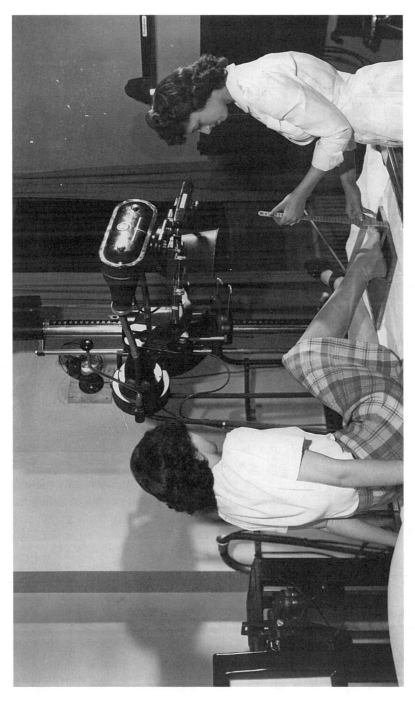

After World War II, technological advances led to x-ray equipment that was less bulky.

corridors for patients, with screens around them." Just three months later the board passed a resolution recommending to medical staff that "we try for a period of two months visiting hours that are continuous from 11 o'clock a.m. to 8 o'clock p.m. in an effort to relieve the congestion which is now prevalent during visiting hours."

Like its hometown, Memorial Hospital experienced growing pains. When the war ended the hospital had 66 inactive beds and experienced a brief postwar slowdown attributed to "higher prices" and long over-due medical staff vacations. Admissions fluctuated from about 7,000 to 7,400 annually in the late 1940s but climbed to more than 9,000 by the mid-1950s. In 1953 the seventh floor was finally opened for patients, with one four-bed room used for surgery recovery. That year the eighth floor solarium was partitioned with curtains for patient use.

Crowding had a favorable effect on the hospital's financial standing. The payroll had increased about 65 per cent with the 1943 move, but by 1945 the hospital once again operated in the black, yielding a surplus of more than $16,000. This was generally true in the postwar years, until the early 1950s. Officials were able to invest funds and in March 1950 declared "the hospital is under no indebtedness."

The tremendous postwar demand for hospital services led to the passage of the landmark Hill-Burton Act in 1946. This law provided federal funds for hospital construction and established a guideline of 4.5 general hospi-tal beds per 1,000 population. The program funded 88,000 hospital beds in its first six years. States were required to develop plans to implement the Hill-Burton standards and the concept emerged of regional medical centers affiliated with medical schools. The post-war years also produced growth in practical nursing and allied health schools as hospitals tried to handle a growing number of patients with a dwindling number of nurses. By 1947 Memorial also trained interns, residents, x-ray technicians, and medical laboratory technicians.

Critical Shortages

The dramatically increased postwar demand for hospital beds exacer-bated two nationwide problems, a shortage of beds and of trained personnel. Hill-Burton aimed to cure the former problem but hospital officials, includ-ing Memorial's, were left to struggle as best they could with the latter. After the war, financial assistance from the Cadet Corps was scaled down, preparatory to closing the program. The hospital was instructed to expect a gradual or "radical retrenchment" as the country returned to its normal supply of nurses. The return to a normal supply never materialized.

By 1950 half of American women aged 18 to 24 were married, and nurses withdrew from the workforce during the 1950s at a rate of 6.5 per cent per year in order to marry and have children. Due to nursing students' long hours and the requirement to live at the hospital, married women had generally not been eligible. Shortages and social changes inevitably forced change. Among the nurses who did return to work, many chose not to return to hospitals. Nurses who served in the armed forces could pursue further education under the GI Bill of Rights or could earn more in other fields. Typists earned 97 cents per hour while nurses averaged 74 cents. Compared with other jobs, nursing involved long hours, shift work and drudgery. Former nursing school director Helen Shull recalled that nurses were involved in menial and non-technical work—constantly sanitizing bedpans and bathing patients—and were not permitted to listen to chests or take blood pressures.

The national nurse shortage was estimated at 40,000 in 1948. Memorial hit a new low that year as well. It was forced to close eleven beds due to the shortage, while 20 on the seventh floor had never been opened. Nationally, nursing students made up more than 20 per cent of all hospital personnel in 1946 but by 1952 the percentage had dropped to 12. Like its peers, Memorial had always relied on students for the bulk of its nursing service. In 1946 there were twice as many students (114) as graduate nurses but it was also the final year that Cadet Corps students were enrolled. Student recruitment became both critical and challenging. The enrollment goal for the 1947 class was 35 but the school recruited only 23, for a total enroll-ment of 95, down 19 from the previous year. Board members actively encouraged candidates and organized recruitment began in earnest in 1948 with contacts at local high schools and a 15-minute recruitment program on WTAX radio. In 1952 Pauline Telford was hired to recruit nursing stu-dents, probably the first use of a paid recruiter. Though the number of nursing students rose slightly nationwide, the increase did not keep pace with the growing number of patients. Out of necessity hospitals hired aux-iliary workers for tasks formerly reserved for nurses. The number of these workers in U.S. hospitals nearly doubled between 1946 and 1952. From 1930 to 1947 the number of practical nurse schools also doubled, then grew from 36 to 296 by 1954.

At mid-century hospital-based nursing schools remained vital to their parent organizations. Veteran nurse Betty Snedigar recalled that only three registered nurses worked on each shift—one as shift supervisor, one in obstetrics (delivery), and the third in surgery. She noted that senior nursing students acted as unit supervisors (over a junior student, three nursing assistants and one orderly) and served 40 patients. A small staff could care for a large number of patients because the typical hospital stay was a week or more. That is, convalescence was slow and nursing care was not intense.

Another particularly persistent shortage occurred in anesthesia. As early as 1943 a registered nurse anesthetist, Sybil Stitt, was hired for $150 per month "plus full maintenance." Nevertheless, there was frequent discussion among medical staff and hospital officials about this shortage. In 1944 the board approved a measure which allowed doctors to bring their own anesthetists as long as they supplied written evidence of their training and registration. Late in 1947 Memorial's medical staff recommended hiring an anesthesiologist. They successfully argued that nurse anesthetists could not do emergencies and certain types of cases, notably brain and chest surgery. The anesthesia committee (Drs. James E. Graham, Robert J. Patton, and Walter Shriner) was finally able to recruit one, a woman, but she resigned after only two months. Eighteen months later Dr. O. G. Glesne was hired but he, too, stayed less than a year. With the severe nurse shortage, the hospital also had to do without nurse anesthetists, a serious situation which led to "several sad experiences" that might have been avoided if an anesthesiologist had been available. In 1951 the medical staff executive committee announced that doctors would sometimes be called in to serve as anesthetists in an emergency. Fortunately, several nurse anesthetists were finally recruited later that year.

Despite continual student recruitment challenges and radically changed social forces, the hospital and nursing school clung tenaciously to old patterns and mores. Prospective students were "carefully screened for commitment." Since 1944 the hospital had paid for "psychometric tests" to screen out "girls who were not fit for nursing." Even during severe wartime personnel shortages hospital officials exercised a long held moral authority which exacerbated their staffing problems. Two incidents in the early 1940s illustrate this propensity. In one instance, the board fired its only radiologist, with medical staff consent, for engaging in an extramarital affair with a hospital employee, who was also fired. It took nearly one year to replace the physician. A few months later five nursing students were discharged because they were not "fit" for nursing.

Closely aligned with staffing concerns were other deficiencies which the medical staff enumerated. The board adopted a rule in 1944 which automatically dropped doctors from the active staff at age 68 and placed them in the honorary staff category. However, when the medical staff presented its "major problems" to the board that year, age was not among them. Instead they listed a blood bank, a hospital formulary, delinquent medical records, and the need for a pathologist.

In 1943 the board had authorized the purchase of equipment for a blood bank but implementation followed slowly. Over a year later the executive director met with the medical staff's blood bank committee in order to decide "what technical method should be used in our proposed blood bank." At that time the hospital's blood and plasma room consisted of a single refrigerator and two nurses who were sent to St. Louis for training. Memorial's blood bank finally opened in 1945 and 535 transfusions were done in its first year. Apparently, policy required that two pints of blood be given for every pint received. In the early 1950s patients received weekly statements indicating how much blood they used and how much they "owed."

A lingering sectarianism also persisted at least through the 1950s. Until November 1950 Concordia Seminary students received the same discount for services as hospital employees, 25 per cent. Seminary students held many orderly jobs at Memorial and two nursing school graduates recalled joint dances and marriages with seminary students. One nurse graduate noted that many nursing students were Lutheran in the late 1950s because their parents remembered Memorial as a Lutheran institution. Former nursing school director Helen Shull noted that capping ceremonies were always held at a church, usually Lutheran, and on one occasion Lutheran ministers objected to Frank Shank's role in the ceremony and his presence on the platform because he was not Lutheran. In another example one board member offered the idea to pre-register "all the Protestants possible." The board agreed that the idea had public relations possibilities. Although not acted upon, this 1952 suggestion does illustrate the remarkable resilience of the early religious affiliation.

In the years following the 1943 move the hospital also had to adjust to demands for higher wages and better working conditions. Both the ranks of employees and the number of departments increased. Nurse salaries were

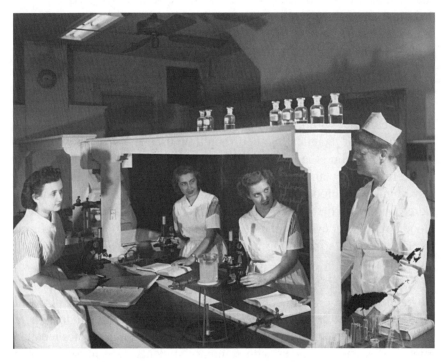

Nursing students learned the fundamentals of microscopy under the watchful eyes of an instructor and technician.

raised twice in 1946 but records occasionally note losses to the "neighboring" hospital, which offered higher pay. In January, February, and April 1948 nurses at Memorial requested shorter working hours and changes in the "conditions" of evening and night nurses. The board responded by surveying other community hospitals "to determine how far reaching this practice has become." Responses from St. John's and six other hospitals in Pekin, Peoria, and Champaign indicated that three of the seven, including St. John's, still maintained a 45-hour work week. The board concluded that the 40-hour week for nurses was "not prevalent in Illinois" and would "not produce more nurses." Citing the critical shortage, the board denied nurses' requests and continued its 45-hour and six-day policy at current salary scales. Nurses then submitted a counter request for a five-day work week on the evening shift. Apparently, no action was taken on this request though the issue continued to surface at subsequent meetings.

Indicative of the importance of nursing students, they comprised 28 per cent (114) of Memorial's 1946 payroll of 407 employees. In 1948 only 57 registered nurses were employed, five part-time. The nursing director's report to the board indicated that 75 nurses were needed to open all beds but 94 were needed if a five-day week was established. The board finally compromised with a 5 1/2-day week for evening and night employees in 1950. Day shift nurses were granted the same in 1952, when 72 nurses were employed. The five-day week eventually came for nurses late in 1953 with other personnel scheduled for gradual implementation.

Nurses routinely met to address staff and clinical issues. Wilma Fricke chaired the group when the pay issue surfaced and recalled that nurses contacted the Illinois Nurses Association (INA). Though not strictly a union, the INA was moving in that direction. Like most hospitals, Memorial was slow to modernize its labor practices but also worried about unionization, so administration and the board made occasional concessions. Personnel costs also edged upward when hospital employees became eligible for social security benefits in 1951.

Another postwar development, encouraged by physicians returning after the war, was a renewed interest in an internship program. Interns, also called "house staff," were physicians who were in the hospital on a 24-hour basis. Medical students sought internships as a way to acquire clinical experience following their M.D. degrees. Interns were already essential fixtures in large, urban hospitals as early as 1900. Urban hospitals were favored due to the large number of cases and the presence of prestigious and experienced physicians. Hospitals sought interns to ease the rotation burden on medical staff and also to acquire the aura of a teaching hospital, though most intern programs were not affiliated with medical schools. As early as 1917 the American Medical Association's Council on Medical Education published a list of acceptable internships. This action was one of several which led to the accreditation of hospitals. By 1960 virtually all large hospitals were of this "teaching type."

In February 1945 Memorial's medical staff designed a "mixed internship" program but the AMA denied approval because the hospital's eight per cent autopsy rate did not meet minimum requirements. The hospital later reapplied and received approval in December 1946 after it reported a 38 per cent autopsy rate. Among Memorial's notable early interns were Drs. Ann Martin Pearson, H. W. R. (Humphrey) Fluckiger, and David Chatara. With exceptions such as these, the intern program was beset with difficulties. The flood of postwar displaced persons included many M.D.s who sought internships as an entré to medical practice in their adopted country. Medical staff records revealed that most of the internship applicants in 1950 were foreign-born, and many spoke English poorly. The next year two alien interns were denied credit for their unsatisfactory performance. The medical staff resolved that "there will be no more foreign interns appointed and the appointments will be restricted entirely to American citizens." In 1952 the hospital was not able to recruit a single intern. In 1955 the AMA again rejected Memorial's proposal, citing an inadequate teaching program, poor medical records, a low autopsy rate, and insufficient experience with ambulatory patients. While the medical staff continued to express interest in an internship program, they concluded in 1957 that good interns were too scarce and the competition too keen.

Along with their efforts to add internships, the hospital board and medical staff worked for several years to establish a residency program. In July 1948 the first four resident physicians arrived. Among these was Dr. Glen Wichterman, who responded to a notice in the AMA's journal and was invited to visit Memorial, where he recalled being impressed with Victor Lindberg. Wichterman was on call at the hospital overnight every four nights and rotated through a variety of services, including surgery, medicine, obstetrics, and pediatrics. The residency was an arrangement made exclusively with Memorial, thereby limiting Wichterman's experience in pediatrics, a small unit at the hospital. Dr. Raymond Eveloff offered to take him on rounds at St. John's but the "Sister Superior said absolutely not." Wichterman recalled that "they wouldn't let us in at St. John's."

An Epidemic and a Cold War

More babies and fewer nurses were two demographic features of the postwar landscape which directly affected Memorial. Of lesser significance to the hospital were America's greatest postwar threats—poliomyelitis and communism. The Illinois polio epidemic peaked in the summer of 1949, when 249 cases were reported in one month, up from 81 the previous year. In Springfield three deaths in 10 days prompted a city-wide quarantine, declared on July 26. Summer camps were canceled and children under age 16 were barred from visiting Lake Springfield beaches, area swimming pools, and local hospitals. The city was sprayed with DDT three times by the third week of the quarantine, a "continuous" practice reported in the newspaper as late as December. The effort aimed to eliminate flies as "possible" germ carriers. Concern about adverse effects from DDT were overshadowed by the specter of polio. The epidemic, which preceded Rachel Carson's **Silent Spring** by a dozen years, riveted public attention as the 1949 Illinois toll was reported: 2,886 cases and 238 deaths. When the four-week quarantine was lifted, the **Journal** reported 58 Springfield victims.

The medical staff at Memorial adopted a policy in the summer of 1950 which recognized Memorial as a secondary polio facility. Acute polio cases were referred to the county contagious hospital operated by St. John's and built in 1926, in part with county and city funds. The Illinois Department of Public Health designated Memorial's use only when the number of acute cases exceeded 64. On August 4, 1949 St. John's admitted 90 patients, not all from Springfield. Memorial probably had patients that month as well. A veteran nurse recalled that Memorial had an iron lung but that it was not always in use because the hospital was not swamped with cases. Dr. Ann Pearson, however, remembered a "terrible polio epidemic," filling an entire floor at St. John's (a "contagion" ward) plus patients in hallways, many in iron lungs. She saw a few early, non-paralytic cases at Memorial as well. Dr. Humphrey Fluckiger recalled that many physicians purchased special polio insurance coverage due to the threat to their livelihood. He also recalled that polio patients were admitted to St. John's because that hospital had more space to isolate infectious diseases.

The epidemic exacerbated the nurse shortage. Too few nurses volunteered to care for polio patients and the local newspaper reported that each iron lung patient required assistance from three nurses. Both hos-

Summer Plague

The conquest of polio was the American success story of the 1950s and the "single most popular medical cause postwar." The epidemic reached its peak in the United States in 1952 with 57,628 cases. The country's first major epidemic had occurred in the New York state region in 1916, and in 1921 "the Crippler" struck Franklin D. Roosevelt, whose creation of a hydrotherapy center for polio victims heralded a crusade to defeat the disease. While polio was not the most prevalent disease nor among those with the highest mortality, it was the leading infectious killer of children, especially among the upper and middle classes. One victim described it as the disease which specialized in maiming people.

An early celebrity in the cause was an Australian, Sister Elizabeth Kenny. She developed her treatment methodologies by trial and error as a nurse in the Australian bush. She earned a reputation for achieving unlikely recoveries but her methods, which opposed the common medical practice of casting, were ridiculed by some (though not all) medical authorities. A mixture of healer and charlatan, Kenny was to therapy what Jonas Salk was to prevention.

Salk's research was funded by private donations through the immensely successful National Foundation for Infantile Paralysis, which raised more money than any other health campaign. The March of Dimes, as the Foundation was commonly known, was the "aggressively propagandist" forerunner of the modern tele-thon. The effort paid off with the 1954 Salk vaccine trial, the most extensive field trial in the history of medicine. One year later, when the vaccine was declared "safe, effective, and potent," there was delirious rejoicing. The 39-year-old Salk became an instant celebrity and reinforced the heroic image of doctors.

pitals reflected the American voluntary hospital commitment to care for the community in times of crisis by hosting training programs for nurses in the care of polio victims. Memorial sponsored a joint conference with St. John's to train staff. The local chapter of the Foundation for Infantile Paralysis donated equipment as well as funds to send Memorial staff for training in the Kenny method, a controversial therapy emphasizing hot packs and movement of individual muscles.

While polio patients were being encased in iron lungs, the iron curtain had descended in Europe. Memorial's medical staff met in 1950 to share advice and information regarding actions in the event of a nuclear bomb attack. The principal point was that "radiation is not as serious as the public feels it to be," and that "only 15 per cent" of people within an attack area were affected. The "rest of the casualties" were due to glass and flash heat. The advice was to avoid panic. In 1951 the Illinois Department of Public Health noted that Memorial had "surplus" beds at the nurses' home and officials were instructed to hold them for "stand-by service."

Reflecting the political landscape, the **Bulletin of the Sangamon County Medical Society** inaugurated a regular "civil defense" column in its February 1955 issue. Its purpose was to describe the medical community's plans in "war or other emergency." Early in 1962 Memorial was approached by local civil defense authorities to serve as a fallout shelter. The board denied the request because the hospital lacked the space necessary to shelter the required 200 citizens and provisions. The day before the Soviet Union announced it would dismantle missile bases in Cuba (November 1, 1962) hospital directors were sufficiently uneasy about the "world situation" that they discussed stockpiling drugs in case of an "extreme disaster."

Despite the menace of epidemic and attack, the exhilaration of victory in World War II carried over into a confident quest to conquer disease. President Roosevelt had described his intention to use federal funds for biomedical research as "the war of science against disease." The federal budget for medical research climbed from $3 million to $76 million between 1941 and 1951. Congress passed legislation funding research for specific diseases in what sociologist Paul Starr described as a "categorical approach" which was "very successful in opening the public's purse." The budget for the National Institutes of Health grew from $180,000 in 1945 to $46.3 million by 1950 and reached $400 million by 1960.

In little over a decade Memorial achieved the goals established by the Walsh report with stunning success, and entered the 1950s with a sense of accomplishment and no other goal but to maintain its hard won place in the community. Dedicated lay directors had spearheaded the institution's growth and improvement; a relentless demand for services and the infusion of federal funds ensured its success.

Memorial Milestones

1951	First African-American nurse and nursing students
1952	Charles H. Lanphier elected board president
	Frank R. Shank replaced by George Hendrix
1954	Nurse Education Unit
1955	Dr. Grant Johnson hired
	First personnel director, Gordon Miller
1958	A building
	First male nurse, Ed Quarry, RN
1961	ICU opened
	Hospital debt-free
	First cornea transplant
1966	Old hospital razed
	Medicare legislation in effect
1968	B building

Chapter Five

Expansionary Drift

In the third quarter of the twentieth century the United States assumed the role of international leader. In addition to its political power, America produced at least half the world's manufactured goods as well as a large share of its science, a new national asset. Fueled by federally funded construction and medical advances, as well as the growth in the insurance industry, hospitals enjoyed a "wave of expansion" between the Hill-Burton Act in 1946 and Medicare in 1965. From 1950 to 1970 expenditures for health care climbed from $13 to $72 billion and made it one of the nation's largest industries.

In manufacturing, wages increased more than 30 per cent in the decade following the war. That meant prosperity for industrial Springfield, whose major employers were Allis Chalmers, Pillsbury Mills, Sangamo Electric, Weaver Manufacturing, and International Shoe Company. Despite the 1947 passage of the Taft-Hartley Act, organized labor retained the right to bargain collectively for "conditions of employment." Several years later, the Supreme Court ruled that these included health benefits. By 1958, two of every three Americans had some kind of health insurance. Commercial insurers, which offered more variety than simply health coverage, split the market with Blue Cross. The widespread availability of insurance triggered an unprecedented demand for hospital services and allowed hospitals to increase staff, equipment, and facilities almost without regard to cost.

Total hospital expenditures and capital worth quadrupled from the late 1940s to the early 1960s, as spending and overuse of insurance benefits drove each other in an expansionary spiral.

Although it was already a large hospital by national standards—most had fewer than 100 beds in 1955—Memorial continued its twenty-five year postwar growth spurt. The hospital's roaring trade mirrored a national trend and, like its peers, it had evolved by the mid-1960s into a "complex, rapidly changing, technologic industry."

Industrial Model

A number of factors played a part in the evolution of the industrial model of health care. The burgeoning use of equipment and technical procedures assured that medicine was institutionalized in hospitals. The growth of hospitals into large physical plants staffed by many employees aped the industrial example and encouraged the participation of industrial leaders, who felt comfortable and competent to run their hometown hospitals.

In the quarter century after it constructed a modern and expansive facility, Memorial found it necessary to build five additions, bringing the reported bed count to 670. The construction was needed not only to accommodate patients but also to house nearly four times as many employees and a half dozen new, specialized services. This unparalled growth was not limited to Springfield. The ratio of personnel to patients in American hospitals grew from 1.5 in 1946 to 2.5 in 1965. Put another way, more than a million workers joined the health services industry between 1950 and 1960, a 54 per cent increase. As these numbers grew, the division of labor became sharply defined and specialized. One example of this trend was the large number of nurses' aides and practical nurses hired following the severe postwar nurse shortage. Memorial and St. John's jointly financed a school of practical nursing in 1958 in conjunction with the Springfield public school system. Although these aides assumed responsibility for the more menial tasks formerly performed by registered nurses, one Memorial nurse recalled that the school was controversial and that the registered nurses (RNs) feared they would lose their jobs.

As the hospital workforce grew so did the tasks and equipment required to maintain it. Indicative of the increased size and complexity of the staff, the board's executive committee approved personnel policies for the first time in 1956 and hired the first personnel director, Gordon Miller, two years later. Previously, each department had its own personnel rules and procedures. In an often repeated pattern, medical staff prodded the hospital in this progressive direction, though board records from the late 1950s-1960s revealed concerns about work-related injuries, health screening for new employees, and the need for a pension plan.

There was constant pressure to keep up with the rapid growth. In one instance, a board member urged the purchase of a check signer because of the "problem of signing 700 payroll checks twice a month." Veteran administrator William (Bill) Boyd recalled that three administrators personally signed these checks. Another sign of growth was a 1961 dinner meeting, held to provide members of the executive committee and department directors "the opportunity to get to know the work of the other." The board also discussed hiring a hostess to solve patients' problems by "cutting through all departmental lines and routine regulations." While the fate of this proposal is unknown, its mere mention demonstrated how times were changing.

Although Memorial was a more complex institution, one longtime employee remembered the 1950s administration as a fairly simple one. The executive director's title had changed in 1954 to administrator and by the late 1950s he had two assistants, Edna Huelskoetter and Bill Boyd. Despite the tremendous growth, day-to-day operations remained unsophisticated. Boyd recalled that it was commonplace, for economy's sake, to write letters rather than make long distance calls. In another example, hospital auditors Meyer and Van Meter persuaded board members to change Memorial's fiscal year from January 1 to October 1. The auditors preferred to do their work in the "off season." Accordingly, the board approved the change in August 1952.

As the size and diversity of the hospital workforce increased, a tripartite system of hospital control evolved, which included board members, administrators, and physicians. Conflict among these groups increased as the hospital evolved from a "doctors' workshop" into an institution with its own products. These tensions, still present in the hospital's centennial year, were exacerbated during the postwar years of rapid growth. One veteran nurse recalled being trained to respect the physician's stature and absolute authority. She rose when doctors approached, addressed them as "doctor" even when they were personal friends, and always responded with a "yes, sir" or "no, sir." While this particular style of professional relationship had a long history, the number of such hierarchical structures increased in the

1950s. Memorial and other hospitals were beset with constant jurisdictional disputes, tension with medical staff, and high turnover rates. Despite these differences, no one disputed the value of acquiring the latest equipment and services or the necessity of accommodating each other's needs. One historian described the primary characteristics of hospital operations in the 1950s as "conflict avoidance and expansionary drift." At Memorial, George Hendrix headed off the conflict and Chick Lanphier led the expansion.

Charles H. (Chick) Lanphier had served on the board of directors for eight years when he was elected president in December 1952. He joined shortly after the move to the new building, when technologically sophisticated hospitals throughout the nation attracted prestigious community leaders to their boards. Lanphier was president of Sangamo Electric, one of Springfield's leading employers, and a "very commanding figure in town." His tenure spanned nearly a third of Memorial's history, during which patient admissions tripled and several major building projects were completed.

The unremarkable Frank Shank was replaced by George K. Hendrix, who served as the hospital's principal administrator for nearly all of Lanphier's tenure. Hendrix had been employed by the Illinois Department of Public Health and tried to help the board locate a replacement when Shank left abruptly. The board eventually offered Hendrix the job. One veteran administrator recalled that Hendrix had been a consultant to the board and had supplied a candid analysis of "problems," presumably associated with Shank.

An engineer without formal hospital or business education, Hendrix was an enormously popular leader who visited frequently with staff. Fellow managers described him as "well-suited for his time," "down to earth" and "friendly and interested." Though the staff grew from 240 to 670 during his twenty-year term of service, Hendrix knew many of them by name.

Hendrix actually acted as executive director before he was formally hired. The board voted to employ him at its July 30, 1953 meeting, one month after he had signed an affidavit as executive director. The minutes of this meeting were signed by Hendrix, acting as secretary pro tempore. One month prior to the July 30 meeting, Hendrix was listed as a guest, though he participated as executive director in a resolution. These informal actions illustrated the fraternal atmosphere that permeated within the executive committee under Lanphier's leadership.

Charles H. Lanphier, III

Described as a "brilliant executive" and a man of "high energy and vision," Charles Henry Lanphier, III made an enormous contribution to Memorial and Springfield. Educated at Yale University, Chick Lanphier began his career as an electrical engineer at Sangamo Electric Company. A major Springfield employer for decades, the company was co-founded by Robert Carr Lanphier (his father) and Jacob Bunn, Jr. In its heyday, Sangamo employed about 5,000 workers, was listed on the New York Stock Exchange and had international affiliates. The plant initially manufactured electric meters then expanded to other electrical equipment and became the principal supplier of sonar submarine detection gear for the Navy.

Chick Lanphier followed his mother (Bertha O. Lanphier) on Memorial's board, serving for more than thirty years. He treated Memorial like a business facing unlimited growth prospects, and was considered a tough negotiator with new medical groups as well as the medical school. Although Lanphier did not trust doctors on the board, he earned their respect because he supported their requests for space and new equipment. His pipeline to physicians was Dr. Robert Patton, a cousin.

Lanphier obviously loved Memorial and felt a deep sense of responsibility for it. In its resolution at his death in 1978, the board saluted him as "uniquely responsible for the position of leadership which Memorial Medical Center holds among health care institutions throughout central and southern Illinois." In recognition of his "long and substantial interest" in the radiology department, the board re-named it the Charles H. Lanphier Department of Radiology.

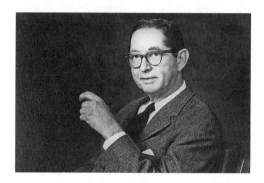

Charles Henry "Chick" Lanphier, III

According to one retired administrator, the real governance of the hospital was in the hands of the board's executive committee, which approved all major purchases, room rates, construction, and important personnel matters. In fact, for seventeen years the authority was exercised by Chick Lanphier and two of his key colleagues on the board, Bill Patton and Cecil Clark, the latter a fellow executive at Sangamo Electric. These three often met informally and kept no minutes. One board member compared Lanphier's executive committee to a "male fraternity" complete with off-color humor, profanity, and smoking. The president of the medical staff was permitted to attend only as a liaison. One board member recalled that these doctors "got bored" and did not attend frequently. Their boredom may have stemmed from the executive committee's habit of micro management, with long arguments over issues such as raising room rates 50 cents.

Dr. Grant Johnson, who directed Memorial's highly successful pathology department, recalled many chance meetings with Lanphier, who dropped by the hospital almost every weekday morning enroute to work. Johnson noted that Lanphier was "vitally interested" in the hospital and took a personal interest in upgrading the pathology department. Despite the evidence of mutual respect between the two, Lanphier clearly did not want doctors on the board. According to one observer, he suspected physicians would act out of self-interest and also betray board confidentiality. With an attitude typical of the period, Lanphier believed that the board was accountable to the community and must have a broader view than could be expected from the medical staff. When doctors expressed interest in attending each other's meetings, Lanphier visited theirs.

George Hendrix quickly established rapport with the physicians, though on at least one occasion his openness created tension. His habit of discussing matters with doctors prior to making decisions led to some confusion over the respective roles of medical staff and administration. The board minutes noted that the medical staff had gradually assumed that "these decisions were theirs to make." This was emphatically not the case with Lanphier's board, though he and Hendrix were supportive of physician initiatives, notably in radiology and pathology.

Bricks and Beds

The pathology department made a fateful turn when Dr. Grant Johnson was retained effective January 1, 1955. Under his leadership, the department developed from a "rock bottom" operation to the hospital's capstone. Johnson recalled that when he arrived quality had deteriorated, morale was in ruins, and St. John's pathology department was "far superior." He noted that Memorial's unit was so bad that doctors secretly pocketed tubes of blood from their Memorial patients and took them to St. John's for testing. While he found modern equipment, there were many defects in procedures. Johnson immediately instituted reform. New staff were hired and all procedures were refined and upgraded to ensure quality control. He also immediately planned an expansion.

Dr. Ann Pearson described the pathology department's rapid growth as "sort of like Topsy." The laboratory quickly evolved into a first rate department as it grew in both size and stature. Within his first year, Johnson's staff grew from nine to 33 technicians. In 1955 the laboratory performed 4,700 clinical tests; in 1970 (when the number of technicians had grown to 70) the total was 323,552. This phenomenal increase was also due in part to the rising use of the "pap" smear for the early detection of uterine cancer. Johnson also garnered a large volume of autopsies and coroner's cases, which were not only a major service to the region but also an excellent teaching resource and a public relations asset for the hospital. To accommodate the growing staff and equipment, Johnson managed to increase the laboratory's space five-fold by 1970. Much of this space had originally been assigned to the nursing school.

Two constant challenges of this period were physical expansion and physician demands. Indicative of the pace of growth, the 1943 structure was overcrowded in less than ten years, as were several subsequent addi-

Grant Johnson, M.D.

Dr. Grant Johnson was the enormously productive director of Memorial's superb pathology department for nearly forty years. He graduated from the Indiana University Medical School and, after residency, spent two years in the Army. Returning veterans glutted the pathology residencies so Johnson practiced medicine for two years while he awaited the opportunity to pursue his major interest.

He was finally able to get a pathology residency at the University of Chicago and St. Luke's Hospital, but this was interrupted with another two years in the Army, this time in Japan. Following the Korean War, Johnson joined the pathology faculty at the University of Illinois Medical School in Chicago. Two years later (1955) he moved to Memorial Hospital.

Always ambitious, Johnson continued his affiliation at the University of Illinois part-time. He taught there until he assumed a similar role at SIU School of Medicine. Johnson developed pathology museums for the purpose of teaching gross pathology at both the U of I and Memorial.

In pursuit of yet another of his many interests, Johnson was appointed coroner's physician in some thirty central Illinois counties. This service enabled him to perform numerous autopsies and testify in scores of trials. In the famous Hornstein-Worthington case, Johnson was able to identify the torso of a murder victim. He made many post-mortem determinations of cause and time of death and, in homicide cases, type of weapon. His medical-legal conferences, during which he shared slides and discussion of his forensic work, were packed with fascinated physicians. Johnson was also noted for his ghoulish sense of humor. He allegedly once sent Christmas cards which featured a severed and badly decayed hand, decorated with a sprig of holly.

continued ...

Students and staff feared him and many also loved him. Colleagues described Johnson in superlative terms, as a perfectionist who loved his work, an autocrat with his kingdom in the basement, an "irascible" man with professional standards "twice as high as anybody else's," and a "magnificent director of pathology." Dr. Richard Moy summed him up as "an absolute character." Dr. Grant Johnson died in February 1997.

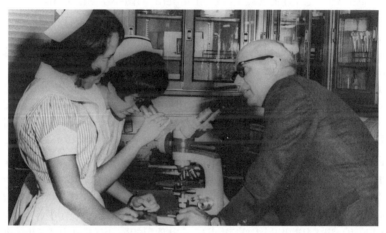

Legendary pathologist, Dr. Grant Johnson and student nurses

tions. Bill Boyd confirmed that the hospital outgrew its space every ten years during his career. As soon as the new hospital opened, the board had identified housing for nurses as its next construction priority. The old hospital had been converted to student living quarters, but required constant attention. The frame structure needed painting and was termite infested. At one point the fire marshal ordered the hospital to provide an exit from the basement because its classes qualified the structure as a public hall. As early as 1945 the board planned to construct a nurses' home at the new hospital site and expected it to attract students. The Women's Auxiliary sponsored several fund-raisers and, by 1950, $70,000 was available in a "nursing home building fund." As it turned out, the funds were not used for a nurses' home.

The November 29, 1953 **Illinois State Journal** announced the construction of a $250,000 building for the Memorial Hospital School of Nursing.

Funds were "an accumulation of contributions and bequests" over the years. The addition, known as the Memorial Hospital Nurse Education Unit, was located on the east side of the hospital, on First Street. The addition also expanded the laboratory by more than 50 per cent. A nurses' residence was still under consideration as part of a more ambitious construction plan. As a temporary measure, student housing at the old North Grand hospital was renovated at a cost of $11,140.

The Nurse Education Unit was completed in 1954, the same year that the board was awarded $525,000 in federal Hill-Burton funds for a two-wing extension at the rear of the 1943 building. The Memorial Hospital Citizens' Committee launched a $1.25 million campaign in March 1955 under the direction of board member Fred Schlitt. Echoing the hospital's earlier success, the goal was exceeded by 20 per cent. In a local press interview, Chick Lanphier noted that the additional funds would be used to accommodate more beds. In addition to the local campaign and federal funds, the hospital received $140,000 from the Ford Foundation. The $2.3 million building contract was awarded to Evans Construction Company.

The seven-story A addition, designed by Burnham and Hammond and completed in 1958, created 104 beds and housed more than 100 student nurses. The first floor accommodated apartments for two nursing school "housemothers" as well as "date rooms." Three floors were eventually devoted to an expanded psychiatric department, surgical patients, and a new rehabilitation center—the "only one of its kind" in Springfield. The latter service was designed for patients who required long convalescence and physical therapy, notably polio victims and paralytics.

While the A addition provided much needed space, it unfortunately brought some disappointment. The board initially refused to accept the building from the general contractor until the "generally poor workmanship" was corrected. Drs. Ann Pearson and Robert Patton both recalled that the design was a novel but bad idea. Narrow, inflexible patient rooms held two beds, foot to foot, with tiny bathrooms and no space for equipment.

Early in 1951 the board passed a number of successful measures to attract and retain nurses for the new wing. These measures were financed with room rate increases. In addition to a $50 per month raise, the board granted extra pay for evening, night, weekend, and holiday work. Other new professional staff were hired to work in the new or expanded programs in A wing, including physical and occupational therapists and an electroencephalography technician.

Mid-Century Nursing School

Though the 1943 move signaled a fresh start and prosperous new era for Memorial, the nursing school was never again considered on equal terms. A vitally important component of hospital business, the nursing school declined in the postwar years. A 1949 national ranking placed Memorial's school in the second quartile and, in two measurers of academic viability (instructor salaries and library services), the school's rank dipped to the third quartile. By mid-century the board noted the "very dangerous" enrollment level and took steps to improve both the school's ranking and enrollment. New members were appointed to the School of Nursing Advisory Committee and the board authorized a contract for "purchased teaching" of four science subjects with Springfield Junior College. Financial incentives were used to boost enrollment. Herbert B. Bartholf established a scholarship fund and the Women's Auxiliary initiated a loan fund.

While these actions brought improvement, the board credited the 1954 Nurse Education Unit with producing the highest enrollment (127) since wartime. A near tragedy probably encouraged board members to expedite construction of on-site housing. Students relied on a hospital shuttle bus for transportation among their North Grand living quarters, the hospital, and the junior college. Late one night, the bus stalled on railroad tracks at Third and Union Streets. The driver and all passengers escaped moments before a southbound train demolished the bus and dragged it several hundred feet.

Efforts to improve the school did not improve students' lifestyle. Veteran nurse Betty Snedigar described her student days as an eight-hour work shift and 5 hours of class daily, six days per week. In her final six months of school she received a stipend of less than $10 per week. Students had one hour of free time nightly but the adventuresome Snedigar recalled easily evading the curfew via a fire escape. Nursing and Concordia Seminary students congregated at Lee's Tavern, a neighborhood bar, or at Coutrokon's Ice Cream Soda Parlor.

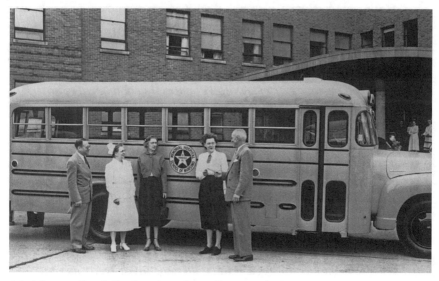

Administrator Frank Shank and members of Memorial's Nursing staff and Nursing School alumni with the bus that transported students to and from Memorial at First and Miller and the Nursing School, which remained at Fifth and North Grand for several years.

The addition also brought improved technology. A press report described new equipment that developed x-ray film in only six minutes instead of the usual 30. The A building was the first to have central air conditioning, though by this time the 1943 building had been outfitted with window units. Other innovations included piped in oxygen (rather than tanks) and some electrically operated beds. Most notable among these advances was a cobalt machine for the treatment of cancer patients. It was the third in the state and the only one outside the Chicago area.

Among Memorial's strongest departments at the time was radiology. Immediately after the board fired its only radiologist, a medical staff committee began searching for a replacement. It recommended Dr. J. Edward King, a Johns Hopkins graduate affiliated with Cook County Hospital. Effective May 1, 1943, Dr. King was hired for $600 per month and 35 per cent of the net profits of the department (not to exceed $10,000 annually). When King first arrived, he saw a dozen patients daily. By the time he retired in January 1970, the department had grown to include 5 radiologists and fifteen technicians who saw 180 patients daily.

In 1945 King replaced Dr. Harry Otten as director of the tumor clinic, the most active of three such clinics in Illinois. Dr. King's progressive service began treating patient with radioisotopes in July 1951. With radioisotope facilities in only 20 per cent of American hospitals by 1960, Dr. Grant Johnson accurately observed that King was "way ahead of his time."

With King's encouragement, the board won approval to train x-ray technicians in 1946. The same year, they granted Dr. King a one-year leave of absence for postgraduate study in "cancer and tumor diseases." Memorial hired an assistant for King (Dr. Ralph Theobald) in 1958 and 10 years later Dr. Charles Williams joined the department. King earned a reputation for hiring excellent staff, including Drs. David Lewis and William Sherrick. Colleagues described King as a "first rate radiologist" who was "always helpful." In 1969, after a long and distinguished career, he was "relieved" of his responsibilities as director of the department. Chick Lanphier arranged for him to be named Director Emeritus. Tragically, King collapsed and died at his testimonial dinner at the Leland Hotel. In a touching gesture, the hospital board's resolution was instead read at his funeral. The board then named the x-ray school the J. Edward King School of X-ray Technology. The school later moved to Lincoln Land Community College.

Integration and Additions

At mid-century the practice of racial segregation gained national attention when the Supreme Court, in *Brown v. Board of Education* (1954), held that segregated schools were unconstitutional. The nursing profession liberalized its views as early as 1950, when the American Nurses Association merged with the National Association of Colored Graduate Nurses. At that time only six per cent of nurses and nursing students were African Americans.

St. John's admitted "negro applicants" as early as 1948 and graduated its first nine in 1950. Memorial employed its first nurse (Marjorie Clem) and admitted three nursing students in 1951. These students were so successfully integrated that their peers supported them with a boycott similar to others in the United States. Former nursing director Helen Shull recalled that nursing students frequented a nearby drugstore until the druggist called the school to protest the black students' use of his business. The entire student body then refused to enter what used to be their favorite hangout.

Racial diversity was apparently not an issue for Memorial officials, because it merited only a single sentence in board records of the past century. The board suggested that "negroes be employed in the hospital up to the ratio that they are in population in the city of Springfield." No official policy enforced patient segregation but other sources confirmed that the practice existed. Jessie M. Finley (widow of Dr. Alonzo Kenniebrew) recalled that black patients were segregated at both hospitals and black visitors were barred from the cafeterias. Kenniebrew had opened his own hospital in Jacksonville after being refused membership on the medical staff at the local hospital. Kenniebrew, who was educated at Meharry Medical College and served as Booker T. Washington's personal physician, was also denied admitting privileges at both Springfield hospitals. Finley recalled that her husband's patients (most of whom were white) were admitted by other physicians, though Kenniebrew counseled their care. The situation had improved somewhat by 1944, a year after Kenniebrew's death, when Dr. Isaac B. English (an African American physician) performed Finley's surgery at Memorial.

Veteran nurse Wilma Fricke confirmed that patients were segregated at Memorial in the 1940s. Fricke was a head nurse when blacks were later integrated and had to handle objections from white patients and visitors. Geraldine Lee (widow of Dr. Edwin Lee) remembered that Memorial had a reputation for greater discrimination than St. John's, but that Memorial ended segregation earlier, "without any fanfare."

Acceptance of male nurses lagged further behind. Memorial hired its first male nurse, Ed Quarry, in 1958. Quarry had nurse training at St. Louis University, then at St. Francis in Peoria, and finally earned his master's degree at a California college. He met George Hendrix at a conference in St. Louis, where Hendrix informed him that Memorial had no male nurses: "why don't you give us a try?" Several months later Quarry applied and was hired. Within his first year he was appointed evening supervisor, then surgery supervisor. Quarry accepted his "pioneer" role and worked to open Memorial's school to males. The first three were admitted in 1963.

Memorial eventually overcame its objections to black and male nurses but clung to its bias against admitting married nursing students, a policy shared with most other nursing schools. The hospital formally admitted married students in 1961, two years before St. John's changed its policy. In 1957, St. John's allowed male students to marry upon admission but females could not marry until six months prior to completion. The prevalent bias against pregnant women was the likely source of this policy. Memorial graduate Helen Justison was allowed to marry four months before her graduation in 1961, soon after Memorial instituted the policy change. She recalled that students were not "allowed to be pregnant" and that the condition resulted in "automatic dismissal."

The professionalization of nursing occurred concurrently with the increased number and variety of health care workers. The 1948 Brown Report, prepared by Dr. Esther L. Brown and supported by the Russell Sage Foundation, had recommended changes in nursing education and had labeled hospitals "authoritarian." Graduates of Memorial's school agreed. One described her first day of nursing school as "a nightmare of sorts" that resembled army induction. The Brown Report was not well received by hospital administrators and physicians, but the postwar nurse shortage clearly revealed that the cheap labor pool had disappeared.

The remarkable increase in hospital admissions aggravated the nurse shortage so the government stepped in, once again, with the Health Amendments Act of 1956. It was the first federal aid to nurses since the war and fostered the professionalization effort by financing education in the fields of nursing administration and teaching. By 1964, appropriations for this program reached $7.3 million and fueled the movement toward baccalaureate nurse training.

Hospital-affiliated diploma schools admitted fewer than 80 per cent of professional nursing students for the first time in 1961 and about 14 per cent of that year's graduates came from baccalaureate programs. At first, some diploma schools converted to three-year junior college programs. Memorial followed this example by affiliating with the Catholic-sponsored Springfield Junior College, a move that would certainly have raised the ire of Memorial's Lutheran founders.

Along with financial aid to students, the Nurse Training Act authorized $90 million for the construction of nursing facilities in the same year that the National League for Nursing reported that the operation of nursing schools cost U.S. hospitals $250 million annually. Memorial's board was certainly aware of these issues. As early as 1955, in his annual report to the board, Chick Lanphier noted the "uncertainty of nursing education insofar as a three-year school is concerned." According to Lanphier, the board had decided to house students in the A building so that if the hospital "must close" its program, the space could be converted to patient use. Virtually the same language was repeated in records from 1962 and 1963. Then in

The Great Whale Hunt

Beginning with the world's smallest mammal (the pygmy shrew), Dr. Grant Johnson amassed a collection of mammalian hearts for his pathology museum at the University of Illinois Medical School in Chicago. His most challenging acquisition was a whale heart. He initially assumed that he could "go out there with a five gallon bucket and bring it back." Always adventuresome, Johnson spent three weeks aboard a whaler. The first few whales had butchered hearts due to the harpooners' practice of aiming for the thoracic cavity. Finally, a harpooner missed the heart and Johnson literally stepped in to remove it. "I got down inside this whale with a machete and I had blood up to my chin." Meanwhile, laborers removed the blubber with flensing tools. Johnson recalled that he had to be careful because these scythe-like blades "were flipping around over my head all the time and they kept up with their work while I was trying to cut this heart loose." A forklift removed the 600-pound heart to a refrigerated railroad car, which Johnson met in Chicago. When the heart eventually deteriorated, Johnson cut it up. Compared with his whale heart adventure, Johnson's efforts to move bricks and mortar for hospital laboratory space must have seemed tame.

1964, the same year as the new federal act, the board acknowledged that the total direct costs of the nursing education department and nurses' home were less than the total value of the services rendered by the students in patient care. At this meeting the board noted that an increase in the number of nursing students would "not increase costs appreciably" and would bring the expense of students and their value more "closely into balance." The meeting concluded with a vote to construct a separate building for the school, a decision which seemed to end several years of ambivalence. Bill Boyd recalled that the decision to move the students was prompted by a shortage of patient rooms.

The board continued to face pressure for additional space from all fronts. Dr. Johnson expanded the laboratory with breathtaking speed, patients filled the corridors, and more than 100 students lived at the hospital. Memorial spent more than $12 million on construction from 1943 to 1968 as the demand for beds and services continued unabated. Annual admissions tripled between 1944 and 1964, faster than the national rate, which doubled between 1935 and 1960. Private health insurance had created, then firmly entrenched, excessive utilization. Dr. Humphrey Fluckiger recalled that his patients "went in for a sniffle." Patients were admitted with minor injuries and ailments, which Fluckiger described as "nonsense stuff." He remembered that the hallways were filled with beds and that "getting a hospital bed in those days was like pulling teeth." With the exception of pediatric and obstetric patients, Memorial maintained a continual waiting list for patients to be admitted.

The occupancy rate was a key measure of the hospital's financial stability. Shortly after the A building was completed, the rate drifted lower—to 97 per cent—and generated considerable concern on the board. In August 1961, for no obvious reason, the rate reversed and by September, only three years after the completion of the A addition, beds were once again in the corridors. When the average occupancy rate rose to 101.7 per cent, (slightly higher than the 1941 rate) the board directed the medical staff to begin removing non-acute patients from the hospital in order to make room for acute cases. Several months later a medical staff utilization committee was established. The committee's actions had limited impact, as overcrowding continued for the next six years. On one occasion the hospital's capacity was exceeded by 42 patients, who were admitted to corridor beds on an emergency basis and were to remain for only one night. Memorial graduate Helen Justison spent "a good while" in labor with her first child

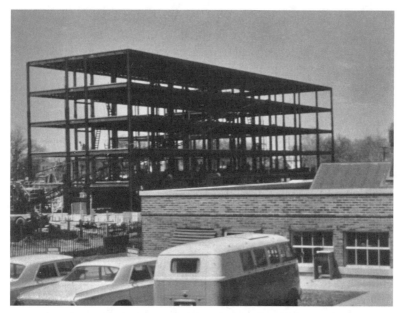

The Nurse Education Building (later renamed Medical Arts) under construction, 1953.

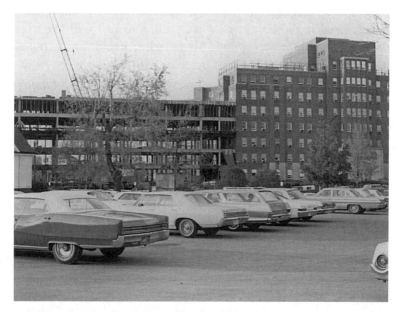

B Building under construction, 1966.

in a hallway bed. Such conditions were a strain on patients, visitors, and staff and forced the board to reject new services, including open heart surgery. The endless demand for beds and services led hospital officials to seek expert advice in planning.

The Chicago firm of Dr. Herman Smith was hired to develop a master plan, which was delivered late in 1963. Smith found "strong evidence" that Memorial's service area was expanding rapidly, the first clear indication of the hospital's movement to a regional market. He recommended increasing the number of beds by remodeling the A annex. This action was accomplished in 1964 and added 34 beds. The displaced nursing students were encouraged, for the first time, to live at home. When that action did not free enough space, rooms built for two students were converted to four-student use by welding twin beds into bunk beds.

The $750,000 five-story structure (later called the Medical Arts Building) was built north of the hospital and connected to it by a tunnel. When the school moved in 1965, the A addition was converted to add 102 beds to the hospital's complement. The old hospital had served as student housing until 1958. The original hospital site was sold to real estate developers in 1959 for $64,500. The new owners could neither sell nor maintain the old hospital. The city filed suit to force them to either demolish or repair it. The last vestige of the hospital's bleakest era disappeared when the building was razed in February 1967.

While the hospital simultaneously built the new nursing school and renovated both A and the Nursing Education Unit—the latter to again double laboratory space—it also planned another large addition. The **Illinois State Journal** detailed plans for a $7 million, eight-story B addition. The 200-bed facility was located to the southwest of the 1943 structure and was completed in June 1968. State law required windows in patient rooms so the B addition had a "double corridor" design with patient rooms around the entire periphery, racetrack style. Bill Boyd recalled that it was a fashionable layout in the 1960s and was the first and only Memorial building so designed. Despite problems with the A addition, the Burnham and Hammond firm was selected to design the B building.

The original chapel was moved to B, which also included the library, medical records department, and other administrative space. The remaining floors were devoted to patient rooms and services, notably rehabilitation and seven operating rooms. Space devoted to surgery and recovery nearly doubled. When the A wing had been converted, dietitian Eunice Scott warned that her space could not handle any more patients. She recalled that the hospital's postwar growth had virtually ignored dietary department limitations. The entire basement of the new B addition was devoted to food service and designed by a professional kitchen planner.

Although board members considered the concept "new and risky," they authorized a bond sale to finance the B addition. The hospital was able to afford the risk due to a run of remarkably good fortune. Memorial had suffered severe cash flow problems in the late 1950s. Officials occasionally used desperate tactics to sidestep these. In 1958 purchasing payments were withheld in order to meet the payroll, and the board borrowed more than $20,000 to pay its radiologist.

With an eye toward cost reduction, the board retained A. T. Kearney & Company to study the hospital's "non-professional" departments. These included the business office, accounting functions, dietary, housekeeping, laundry, and engineering. Kearney recommended a gradual staff reduction via normal attrition. Some recommendations seemed inevitable (such as using automated elevators instead of elevator operators) but others, notably in dietary, were protested in detail. Kearney suggested a reduction of 35-40 employees, for an annual savings of $76,000. The board apparently embraced few of the recommendations.

Then on a memorable May 31, 1963, Lanphier announced that the hospital again was "free of debt." The turnabout was due to the receipt of a number of substantial bequests. Among these was $275,000 from the Cora McGinnis estate. This good fortune continued for a decade with a $150,000 bequest from the Dr. George Palmer trust and $770,000 from the Stephen L. Littler estate. Hospital finances became so complicated that the accountant, Dwight McCormack, was invited to attend executive committee meetings. Despite its good fortune, the board reluctantly raised room rates to finance expenses associated with the latest addition because "no better method was offered." More staff were inevitably required because the B addition had incorporated Smith's recommendations for expansion of the laboratory, emergency suite, and the intensive care unit from six to ten beds. He had noted that "nothing will bring more public approbation and enthusiasm to the hospital than the Intensive Care Unit."

Technological Drift

In the United States, hospitals with the most technology enjoyed the highest status. Little thought was devoted to prevention or education because hospitals existed to treat the curable and were associated with the "critical life activities" of birth and death. By 1960 virtually all births and half of deaths occurred in hospitals. Faith in the miracles of medicine had evolved into an attitude that patients had a "right to a cure." The public and private funds that poured into health care did pay off in the 1955 polio vaccine, the rise of cancer research centers, and the emphasis on coronary care.

The polio vaccine led to the naive belief that other diseases, such as cancer, would soon be eradicated. The rise of cancer research centers was fueled with money from such foundations as Pew, Rockefeller, Sloan-Kettering, and Lasker. The shift from infectious to chronic diseases as the chief source of mortality created an increased public concern about cancer and heart disease. Between 1950 and 1965 hospitals responded by establishing specialty departments, such as radiotherapy and coronary care units, but the intensive care unit (ICU) was the most conspicuous sign of hospital technology in the 1950s. Sangamon County's first television station, WICS, went on the air in 1953, when Springfield residents shared the national fascination with "high tech" medicine, including the ICU. Coupled with the allure of television, this interest culminated in the early 1960s in programs such as *Dr. Kildare* and *Ben Casey* on each major network. In step with the national trend, Memorial's ICU was opened in 1961 and, at consultant Smith's suggestion, was expanded just three years later. Dr. John Denby recalled that the hospital was also pressured to expand its ICU and recovery areas by young surgeons who performed more complex surgical procedures and wanted special postoperative care for their patients. Memorial was far ahead of its peers in another program. The hospital received an American Cancer Society grant to develop an isotope program in 1955. Five years later, only 20 per cent of American hospitals had such a facility.

There was considerable public attention on prevention and early detection of cancer. A 1964 report by the Surgeon General led to an anti-smoking campaign and featured well-known victims, such as Nat King Cole, Babe Ruth, and Walt Disney. Anti-cancer campaigns also promoted pap tests and advertised the cancer warning signs. At the same time, President Lyndon B. Johnson established the Commission on Heart Disease, Cancer and Stroke, headed by Texas heart surgeon Michael E. DeBakey. The

William Boyd

At least once in its history, Memorial actually benefited from its financial constraints. Consultants had recommended hiring an assistant administrator but the board felt money was too tight and instead sought an intern. For $250 a month, Memorial hired William (Bill) Boyd in 1958 as an administrative resident. A navy veteran, he had earned his master's degree in health care administration from the University of Chicago and thus pioneered Memorial's modern tradition of administrative professionalism.

After only six months, he was retained as an assistant administrator with responsibility for professional departments. These included medical records, radiology, laboratory, and pharmacy. Boyd's title changed to associate administrator, then vice president. Twice, he briefly served as acting administrator. Colleagues described him as a "stabilizing" influence and "an outstanding administrator" who was "always fair, supportive, and respected." During the 1980s he guided Memorial's extensive land acquisition and construction projects.

Though he wore many hats during his tenure, Boyd's role as Memorial's "unofficial ombudsman" never changed. He was so well known for his kindly ear that staff and patients were voicing their complaints to him long after he was no longer responsible for patient relations. Boyd retired in 1992, after 34 years of dedicated service.

commission supported the notion of progress through technology and promulgated the idea of university-based regional medical centers to combat these diseases. Unaffiliated hospitals, however, continued to be places for short-term cures and for treating malfunctions and injuries. Most patients entered hospitals for surgical and obstetrical conditions. While public concern and cash poured into cancer and heart disease research, hospitals in the 1950s and early 1960s admitted more patients "for hemorrhoids than heart disease and more for hernia repair than cancer."

One historian described surgery during this time as a matter of "excellence through routine." Despite the growing volume, Memorial was slow to upgrade its surgical facilities, particularly in the 1943 structure, or G building, as it came to be known. The original operating rooms (ORs) were quite small because there was little use of auxiliary equipment. The seventh floor rooms had windows which could be opened for fresh air (and occasional moths, as Dr. Denby recalled). Dr. Humphrey Fluckiger recalled seeing not only insects but also pigeons strutting on the windowsills, which were covered with droppings. In 1957, George Hendrix successfully appealed to the board to replace the obsolete operating room tables for $17,000. One year later records indicate that the roof had leaked since new surgical lights were installed. An emergency roof repair was performed in order to prevent "contamination of the patient in surgery."

Denby described Memorial's surgery work in the late 1950s as "borderline adequate." There was little vascular surgery performed, no open heart work, and no postoperative recovery or ICU. When Memorial's ICU was created, the recovery area, which had been hastily converted from a four-bed ward in 1953, was enlarged to accommodate 12 patients. At that time there also were no residents, so general practitioners (family physicians) served as surgical assistants. Drs. Glen Wichterman and Humphrey Fluckiger did much of this work. The absence of residents also meant that surgeons made rounds at least once, often twice, daily. Despite these difficulties, the number of surgical patients increased more than 28 per cent in the four years following completion of the A building. Though surgery was largely routine, the increasing number of physician specialists assured that new techniques were occasionally used. In 1964 Springfield's first cornea transplant was performed at Memorial.

Surgical facility problems were aggravated by the continued difficulties in anesthesia. Unable to employ their own anesthesiologist, directors decided to recruit someone to carry on a private practice and reimburse the hospital for supplies and space. An anesthesiologist arrived in Springfield in March 1959 but stayed less than one month because he had "received such an unwanted welcome." Several surgeons had apparently told him that the anesthesia service was "good enough" and a physician was not needed. Anesthesiologists were generally available by 1960 but disputes continued over jurisdiction and fees.

Hospital officials clearly knew very little about what needed to be done to update or add clinical facilities. They relied almost exclusively on medical staff for this guidance and were vulnerable to their whims as well as their wisdom. When Dr. Denby wanted to establish a vascular surgery practice, he found officials were "very good at trying to modernize." He identified necessary equipment to nurses, who were able to procure it. Physicians also exploited the half century rivalry with St. John's to acquire desired services and equipment.

External Forces

Despite the guidelines for the distribution of services established under Hill-Burton, cooperative planning was difficult as hospitals became entrenched in their communities. Evidence of the success of the American community hospital model was obvious in the number of physicians, volunteers, and patients who developed a "fealty" to their hospitals. In Springfield, the rivalry between its two hospitals grew in proportion to their respective statures. Discussion of the need for cooperation between Memorial and St. John's sprinkled much of the record of the past century, but most of the attempts were superficial and short-lived. The rivalry often resembled benign competition of the high school athletics type. At times, fueled by rumors and suspicious personalities, it swelled to outright hostility.

One Memorial board member recalled that in the late 1950s the hospitals "weren't speaking" and secretly monitored each other's fees and rates. Hendrix wanted more dialogue but was unable to achieve it. Another administrator noted that Memorial was commonly viewed as "second best" and that a rumor persisted that St. John's would not permit the mention of its rival. Doctors reportedly encouraged the rivalry, and there is evidence in the written record to support this view. In 1957 two physicians promised to "prefer" Memorial if the hospital purchased certain equipment. The board agreed.

There is also some evidence of limited cooperation, particularly among nurses. Two retired nurses recalled joint continuing education programs, faculty cooperation, and combined student picnics. Nonetheless, a number of Memorial managers described the rivalry as "intense" from the 1940s through the 1960s. Records indicate that Memorial watched St. John's carefully and approached it sporadically—sometimes successfully—with issues of mutual interest. In a 1960 example the hospitals agreed to jointly determine whether to institute finance charges on unpaid bills.

For the most part, Memorial and St. John's, like many other American hospitals, duplicated services and spent their resources on construction and technology rather than on planning and coordination. Federal hospital policy of the era encouraged organizational growth, local control, and decentralization. It also ensured escalating costs.

Nationally, room rates tripled from 1948 to 1960 due in part to increased use of expensive new drugs, equipment, and techniques. As noted earlier, the most significant factor was the huge increase in payrolls, up 521 per cent during this period. Hospitals also passed on the costs of services, such as laboratory and x-ray, as additional charges and these increased 228 per cent. Memorial's room rates nearly doubled from 1947 to 1954, then nearly doubled again in only four years, in preparation for staffing the new A addition. Since rate increases generally accompanied nurse salary increases, hospitals were compelled to monitor rivals out of a legitimate fear of losing this scarce resource. The hospital closely monitored not only St. John's rates but also those of hospitals in Peoria and Decatur. According to one nurse, it was common gossip at Memorial that a nun spotted in the hallway meant that both hospitals would soon announce a rate increase. Chick Lanphier clearly believed that the board should "not be too concerned whether our rates are the same as those at St. John's," but the habit continued. A decade later, the board agreed to raise room rates to cover nurse raises "because St. John's is in the process of raising these."

The ideal of the voluntary, community hospital began to erode in the midst of the trend toward an industrial model. Americans had conflicting expectations for health care which included affordable care, access by the whole population, and unlimited technology. Until the early 1960s the prevailing notion was that community hospitals could be huge, technological complexes, but these expectations did not "match reality." The poor and elderly were not able to pay the increased costs of medical care.

It was obvious by 1960 that the expansion of hospital services had not cured "deficiencies in distribution." The Medicare legislation, effective in 1966, "attempted to improve distribution without reorganizing the system." When President Lyndon B. Johnson signed Medicare, Memorial officials surmised that they would have more older patients and would need additional personnel to handle the paperwork. One year later the hospital was several weeks behind in submitting Medicare bills due to their volume, and both personnel and space for this function were inadequate. Already, the hospital noted lengthy delays in receiving Medicare payments. One retired physician described the advent of Medicare as a "nightmare" that created "big, big, big, big, big problems" for physicians who attempted to collect claims. Veteran administrator Paul Smith observed that Medicare paid about half the cost of a nurse's salary, so the hospital, like its peers, had an incentive to hire at will.

As noted earlier, Chick Lanphier was the first board member to suggest a utilization review committee for the purpose of reducing the length of patient stays and freeing up beds. By 1966 such committees, designed to review appropriate use of services, were required by the federal government and the Joint Commission on Accreditation of Hospitals (JCAH). The autonomy of both doctors and hospitals had begun to erode.

Two developments, accreditation and the law, diluted hospitals' sense of accountability to the community. Instead, attention focused on meeting the requirements of external agencies. For years hospitals had participated in the American College of Surgeons (ACS) hospital standardization program not only to improve their services but also to pre-empt more intrusive government inspection. Memorial had been accredited by ACS since 1933. The Joint Commission on Accreditation of Hospitals originated in 1952 as a collaborative effort of the American Medical Association, the American Hospital Association, the American College of Surgeons, and the American College of Physicians. In 1954 JCAH became a private, not-for-profit organization and the only accreditor of hospitals. Though JCAH standards demanded intense planning and effort, accreditation became vitally important after the passage of Medicare, when it guaranteed participation in that federal program. In the 1950s, however, the Joint Commission's primary goal was to improve the organization of hospital medical staffs. It eventually succeeded at Memorial.

Accreditation was generally granted for three years but Memorial received only a one-year approval in 1957 (and again in 1968), due to the failure of the medical staff to meet requirements. In a meeting with the board's executive committee, medical staff representatives agreed with the JCAH assessment and were willing to take action "in order that the hospital might again be fully accredited." Apparently, medical staff credentials files were dated and committee minutes were inadequate. Chick Lanphier addressed a letter to medical staff in which he assured physicians of the board's determination to win a longer accreditation and suggested closer ties between the board and medical staff. Though he sought a "better liaison" with physicians, he did not invite them to join the board as members.

While Memorial's medical staff struggled with JCAH requirements, two court cases placed legal and financial responsibility for the quality of care on hospitals. One of these, *Darling v. Charleston Community Hospital,* originated in Illinois and made hospitals responsible for care given by medical staff. With this responsibility, hospitals began to pay closer attention to physician activities. This further threat to doctors' autonomy created more conflict and further eroded the familial sense of community dedication.

Despite the changes and tensions, Memorial remained very much a community hospital—albeit an ambitious one. In the same year that Congress passed Medicare, the Illinois legislature established a commission to survey the status of education in the health fields and identify the location for another medical school. The Campbell Commission, headed by Dr. James Campbell of Chicago's Presbyterian-St. Luke's Hospital, supported a model which trained medical students in a community hospital so that they would be "better able to identify with and serve community needs." It was an opportunity tailor-made for an aggressive, and somewhat rambunctious, institution.

Memorial Milestones

1966	First cardiac unit
1967	Reisch Brewery purchased
1968	Springfield selected for new medical school
	First physicians hired to staff emergency room
	Artificial kidney center opened
1970	First kidney transplant
	Marine Bank retained for data processing services
	Burn Unit opened
	Richard Moy, M.D. named Dean, SIU School of Medicine
1971	Reisch Brewery site sold to SIU School of Medicine
	St. John's designated trauma center
1972	George Phillips, Administrator
	Rosenfeld Associates hired for long-range plan
1973	*Roe v. Wade* decision
	George Hendrix resignation
	Nursing school 75th anniversary, closure announced
	Medical students arrived in Springfield
1974	Memorial Medical Center
	Final nursing school class graduation
1977	Regional Burn Center

Chapter Six

Turmoil and Transformation

Domestic and foreign conflicts were distinct features of the decade preceding the nation's 1976 bicentennial. The issue of "rights" permeated the period as a dissatisfied citizenry struggled with social inequities and questioned the status quo. Abortion was legalized in 1973 when the Supreme Court upheld *Roe v. Wade,* and protests accompanied the escalated war in Vietnam, as well as the civil rights and women's movements. President Lyndon B. Johnson's Great Society programs aimed to improve Americans' quality of life through measures such as Medicare, the war on poverty, and federal aid to housing and education.

In contrast to riot-torn cities, Springfield was involved in building and restoration. It celebrated the 1968 Illinois sesquicentennial with a number of events, including the dedication of the restored Old State Capitol building. This effort, as well as the restoration of the Executive Mansion, had the support of Governor Otto Kerner, who was notable both for his uncharacteristic participation in Springfield life and for his leadership of President Lyndon B. Johnson's National Advisory Commission on Civil Disorders (Kerner Commission), which attributed racial unrest to white racism. Between 1950 and 1970, construction boomed, with the number of Springfield building permits increasing 300 per cent. Personal income grew by 130 per cent, and Springfield won the All American City award for "incredible improvements in the quality of its civic and political life." The city's perimeter had expanded to three times its World War II size, while its workforce had transformed from largely blue to white collars. The Weaver Manufacturing and International Shoe companies had closed. These were replaced with thriving institutions in medicine, education, insurance, and government. By 1976 health care was the area's growth industry, with 600 jobs created that year alone in Sangamon and Menard counties.

Social changes affected health care as well. After decades of rising costs from investments in hospitals, technology, and research, Americans discovered that Europeans had higher life expectancies. Sociologist Paul Starr described American medicine of the 1970s as "overly specialized, over built and over-bedded." The technologies that enticed record numbers of Americans into hospital beds after the second world war were viewed with increasing skepticism. American attitudes began to shift from the omnipotent hero doctor image to one that considered the doctor as a partner and consultant. Public scrutiny illuminated disturbing instances of excessive therapy, that is, the system's tendency toward "therapeutic relentlessness" or what ethicist Daniel Callahan later described as "technological brinkmanship."

In the 1970s health care was the nation's third largest industry. The overwhelming cost increases drew attention to a faulty health care system and resulted in a backlash against the system's unquestioned autonomy. The health rights movement aimed to de-institutionalize medicine, particularly as it involved the primary life events of death and childbirth, a complete reversal of the postwar attitude. The movement embraced the concept of informed consent, the right to view one's medical record, and the right to participate in therapeutic decisions. Perhaps the most controversial outcome of the movement was the right to refuse treatment, included in the American Hospital Association's 1972 Patient's Bill of Rights. Several years later, Memorial created its first Patient Rights and Responsibilities policy.

Along with Medicare, Congress passed regional medical program legislation in 1965. Essentially a grant program, the act encouraged voluntary planning and cooperation among hospitals and medical schools and paved the way for the development of large medical complexes. Medical centers were clusters of institutions and services and usually included a hospital, clinic, medical school, pharmacy, nursing school, and specialty services such as heart or cancer. The concept assumed a regional rather than community market and was popular among large, progressive hospitals.

When Memorial officials expressed some bewilderment in 1965 about the future impact of Medicare, they could not have imagined what was on the horizon. Just three years later, Memorial was catapulted into a fast-paced, intricate, and politically charged era. Its struggles occurred against the backdrop of a medical system which had suffered a "stunning loss of confidence." The hospital was confronted with conflicting external pressures, namely a shift in government policy from expansion to containment at a time when its future depended on its ability to expand rapidly. Great Society programs were also in conflict with each other, particularly the tension between expanding services and controlling costs. Like the political and grass roots efforts to create a great society, Memorial found itself in turmoil and transformation.

A Crucial Affiliation

Memorial's physical growth paralleled Springfield's. With the completion of the B addition in 1968, the hospital had tripled its wartime size. While hospitals expanded rapidly after World War II, medical school enrollments did not. In 1957 American hospitals sought 12,000 interns but American medical schools graduated only 7,000 physicians. As noted previously, Memorial gave up its twelve-year struggle to recruit interns that year. Another Great Society effort, the 1963 federal Health Professions Educational Assistance Act, succeeded in augmenting the supply of physicians. Between 1965 and 1980 the number of medical schools grew from 88 to 126, while the number of graduates more than doubled.

While Congress signed Medicare into law, the Illinois legislature established the Campbell Commission in response to the 1964 Illinois Master Plan for Higher Education, which had recommended a survey of needs for facilities and educational programs in the health sciences. The subsequent "Campbell Report" made recommendations not only for medical education but also in nursing, allied health, public health, pharmacy, and related fields. Nearly a third of the commission's recommendations concerned medical education, specifically the "production" of physicians, innovations in curricula, and retention of physicians in Illinois. This emphasis on medical education was due to the commission's added responsibility to identify a downstate site for a new medical school by February 1968.

In a classic near miss of history, Springfield failed to send representatives to the Campbell Commission's hearings on proposed sites. More than a dozen cities expressed interest at the hearing held in Springfield, while that city's officials claimed ignorance. Not only had Springfield missed the hearing, but it also was not prepared to submit an application. Memorial board president Robert Oxtoby initiated dialogue with Sr. Jane Like at St. John's regarding the possibility of a medical school. Though they agreed on its value and continued to meet, the real push for a local medical school did not occur until physicians organized and prodded hospital and city officials. Following the missed hearing, the Sangamon County Medical Society quickly and unanimously voted to open discussion. It established a Committee for Medical Education chaired by Dr. Homer Kimmich, who was already a member of the Campbell Commission's State Advisory Board, as was Dr. Edwin A. Lee. Springfield Mayor Nelson Howarth sent a telegram to the Illinois Board of Higher Education (IBHE) to make application and request permission to present its case. A meeting among representatives of the city's two hospitals and the medical society was hastily scheduled. The Springfield presentation was slated for May 1967—only four months after the missed hearing.

Three months before the deadline, Memorial, St. John's, and the medical society jointly hired the Real Estate Research Corporation of Chicago to conduct a demographic analysis and evaluate Springfield as a suitable site for a medical school. Memorial's one-third share of the cost was $13,500. Two months later the "group working for the medical school" met at St. John's with Robert S. DeVoy of Real Estate Research to discuss the report. This working group included about a dozen physicians, the hospitals' administrators and board officials, and city council members.

Kimmich never allowed officials to become complacent about the Springfield application. At one Memorial board meeting he pointed out that Peoria already had 30 residents (physicians undergoing advanced training), and persuaded the board to establish several residency programs and to recruit a director of medical education. The inevitable room rate increase accompanied these decisions. Kimmich also urged the board to establish and pay full-time chiefs of service in surgery, medicine, pediatrics, and obstetrics. He was convinced that reorganization of the medical staff would sway the IBHE's decision. The medical staff revised its bylaws and constitution to incorporate provisions for the medical school in 1968 at the recommendation of the Real Estate Research Corporation. Kimmich told the executive committee, then under Oxtoby's leadership, that Champaign was the "hardest competition" and that a new medical school there or in Peoria would have a "disastrous effect on medical excellence" in Springfield.

Drs. Robert Patton and Chauncey Maher both credited Drs. Homer and Haydee Kimmich with successfully advocating Springfield as the site for the new medical school. Maher recalled that "Homer was a politician," a close friend of Governor Otto Kerner, and Mrs. Kerner's physician. Kimmich organized a large group of supporters, lobbied elected officials, and arranged delegations to address IBHE meetings in Chicago. A medical education symposium was held to promote Springfield as the best location. The Greater Springfield Chamber of Commerce enthusiastically supported the medical school and numerous local organizations and businesses wrote letters of support to accompany the city's application. Other notable promoters were Drs. Richard Herndon, John Standard, and Edwin A. Lee. According to Maher, Kimmich credited Dr. Hugh Howard with delivering the decisive speech at the final Chicago meeting. The frantic preparation ended when the Campbell Commission directed Southern Illinois University (SIU) to develop a medical school using the clinical facilities in Springfield.

Memorial officials worked diligently to be selected as a teaching hospital for the new medical school. Once this was accomplished the hospital was thrust almost overnight from its status as a progressive community hospital to an awkward and somewhat defensive one, confronted with its inadequacies and challenged by its inexperience as a teaching hospital. Its facilities and services had grown steadily since the close of the second world war and its officials were justifiably proud of their large and progressive hospital. New medical school officials, however, brought a new yardstick. The hospital that had measured up to community standards was, in some areas, found wanting by the new outsiders. The scramble to win the new medical school was quickly replaced by a more urgent struggle to maintain autonomy yet secure the largest stake hold in the school. Fear of losing its future to Peoria or Champaign gave way to fear of losing its future to St. John's Hospital.

The effort to prepare for medical students was a challenge that stretched Memorial's talent and resources. Dr. Robert Patton recalled that both hospitals were slow to fully accept the medical school and realize its potential value. Records of the period show that Memorial's board clearly knew the value of the school and was determined to win the bulk of medical school programs. However, Memorial was slow to accept the change in its culture from one of nearly complete control over its destiny to one in which decisions were shared or imposed. As in the health rights movement, the traditional distribution of power was challenged. To appreciate the magnitude of the challenge it is necessary to understand that the hospital's administrative staff had reached the limit of its expertise, its financial obligations increased along with an alarming increase in accounts receivable, and its clinical programs were uneven in quality and success.

Memorial did have some excellent services with which to attract SIU, notably radiology and pathology. Initially, pathology instruction was divided between the rival hospitals. Dr. Grant Johnson described it as a "clumsy sort of setup" until Dean Moy insisted that Johnson be the sole pathology chairman. Radiologists devised a different and more cooperative approach. Merging the two existing groups (one serving each hospital) was impractical, so they jointly formed a third entity, University Radiologists, to contract with SIU as the school's Radiology Department, chaired initially by Dr. William Sherrick. Memorial willingly upgraded substandard services and introduced new ones. A negative consequence of the medical school was increased cost; the benefits were an expanded range of services and improved quality of care.

Dr. Chauncey Maher recalled that Homer Kimmich also spearheaded the selection of a medical school dean. In late 1968, three members each from Memorial, St. John's and SIU formed a search committee for someone to "head the medical education program." From Memorial the representatives were Dr. Richard Herndon, board secretary Lewis Herndon, and George Hendrix. The board voted to approve the appointment of Dr. Richard Moy in September 1969, with each hospital paying 25 per cent of his salary. Moy recalled that the search committee evolved into a dean's advisory committee, which met with him monthly during his first year. The primary agenda was an affiliation agreement between the hospitals and the medical school. In 1968 SIU's vice president of academic affairs, Robert MacVicar, called for the appointment of two members from each hospital and one from SIU to a Joint Trustee Committee. The committee's charges were to draft a memorandum of agreement between SIU and the two hospitals and to act in an advisory capacity when disputes between any two parties occurred. Board president Robert Prather and Chick Lanphier represented Memorial.

The creation of the medical school affiliation agreement proved to be the first in a series of complex and politically delicate tasks. The role and effect of the medical school within the community created considerable insecurity among Springfield physicians, particularly "in-house" physicians, whose livelihoods depended on a hospital salary or a percentage of department income. Memorial's seventeen in-house physicians wanted a voice in the affiliation agreement. In a special 1969 meeting with the board they claimed that Dean Moy had the power to appoint whomever he pleased and therefore demanded their own contracts with Memorial. The board agreed.

Despite Lanphier's assurances to the contrary, the doctors were convinced that Moy planned to appoint SIU department chairs who would automatically head Memorial's departments. They repeatedly complained that they had no participation and that there was no policy on how these appointments were made. Moy published a description of his method in the **Bulletin of the Sangamon County Medical Society** but this article did little to assure in-house physicians, who continued to debate how and by whom they should be paid for the next three years. Records provide a lengthy account of a 1970 medical staff discussion of "the problems" that Memorial's in-house physicians had "with the medical school and specifically with Dr. Moy." Physicians were torn between anger with Moy and fear that his sudden departure would probably kill the medical school dream. Medical staff were concerned that SIU would dictate hospital policies and wanted Moy to provide written support of Memorial's renal program and St. John's cardiovascular program. In 1972, Memorial's board finally voted to employ the in-house physicians, in order to "obtain control," though the option was more expensive than others that were suggested.

A Chicago management consulting firm (Booz, Allen, and Hamilton) was hired to draft an affiliation agreement. Moy recalled that Lanphier's response to the draft was prompt and incisive, and that Memorial was prepared to sign by June 1970. St. John's was not ready until November. George R. Bunn reassured Moy, "that's the way the Sisters are," and agreements with both hospitals were signed in December 1970. Moy recalled that Chick Lanphier's goal was to make Memorial the "definitive tertiary hospital between Chicago and St. Louis," and that Lanphier often nudged him to make a bilateral deal, with Memorial as the teaching hospital.

As part of its agreement, Memorial pledged to construct an 80,000 square foot building for medical school faculty offices and clinics. Other

A Difficult Decision

Less than two months following the January 1973 Roe v. Wade decision, a special meeting of Memorial's Board of Directors was called to discuss "the policy of the hospital in regard to permitting abortion." Chick Lanphier felt it was simply another service that Memorial should provide, but George Hendrix expressed concern about public opinion. George Phillips read an Obstetrics and Gynecology Department opinion that only board certified obstetricians be permitted to perform abortions. After lengthy discussion, which included the issue of parental signatures on permits, the board directed administrators to poll the obstetrical staff for their preferences. Dr. John Standard had already spearheaded a movement to prohibit elective abortions at Memorial. Standard not only resisted abortion on religious grounds, but convinced Memorial that it risked becoming "an abortion mill." He successfully lobbied his fellow obstetrics and gynecology specialists as well as family physicians for support.

Memorial's Lutheran roots reappeared when a Concordia Seminary student requested permission to post a petition in George Phillips's office for employees who wished to oppose Memorial's involvement in abortion. The student's request was denied because the hospital had not yet made its decision.

Ultimately, Springfield's large Catholic population and the presence of a successful Catholic hospital made it politically too dangerous to perform abortions on demand. Former President Jack Cook confirmed that Memorial had a long-standing, unwritten position against elective abortion. Due to its competition for parity with St. John's, Memorial could not endanger its reputation. Physicians also chose not to risk their standing, supporting instead the referral of patients to abortion facilities within a two-hour drive of Springfield. Dr. Richard Moy recalled that the same sensitivity prevented SIU from offering elective abortions.

key points of the agreement called for Memorial to appoint hospital division chiefs with the advice and consent of the dean and to appoint future hospital-based physicians (those employed in hospital departments) only with the dean's concurrence. Veteran board member Walter (Bud) Lohman recalled that Dean Moy was very aggressive and successful at playing the two hospitals against each other in competition for SIU programs. Board minutes quote Moy's assertion that he was required to insist upon equal apportionment during development of the affiliation agreement, but after it was signed he was free to "vary somewhat from equal distribution." Two years later, Moy again expressed his preference to locate medical school programs at Memorial but wanted this idea to come from the Sangamon County Medical Society so that the medical school "would not be placed in the position of originating the idea." The same year, however, consultants for Memorial reported that the medical school "anticipates having its educational and patient care programs more closely identified with St. John's." Following a casual meeting with Moy, William Schnirring advised his fellow board members that St. John's had no desire to build an ambulatory services center and Memorial would get more SIU programs if it did so. The volley continued for years.

Inadvertently, the board had literally positioned SIU to locate its programs at Memorial. Realtor Frank Mason had approached board member Robert Oxtoby in 1964 to advise him that the Reisch brothers wished to sell their seven acre brewery property to Memorial. While it was located across Rutledge Street from the hospital, the board had no projected need for so much land. At that time, its purchases were limited to adjacent residential properties as these were needed for parking. Chick Lanphier and board treasurer Robert Saner favored the brewery purchase but several others on the board were skeptical. Oxtoby polled the members at a meeting and the final speaker, Louis Gillespie, offered a four word reply, "always buy contiguous property." By July 1966 Memorial had purchased the brewery for $330,000 and agreed to pay for demolition after the Lowenstein Company removed salvageable equipment. Former administrator Bill Boyd recalled that there was "no hint of SIU yet," but thanks to the land purchase, Memorial was well positioned to work with the medical school. Oxtoby agreed that the purchase gave Memorial enormous leverage in siting SIU.

Moy had money for an administrative building and library, but land between the two hospitals was close to railroad tracks, a poor location for sensitive laboratory equipment. The commercial real estate near St. John's was expensive but Memorial had seven acres, ready for construction. Lanphier cut a fast deal on the Reisch property. Moy recalled asking, "How much are you asking for it?" Lanphier countered, "Well, how much do you have for land?" When Moy replied, "a half million dollars," Lanphier concluded, "done." St. John's officials agreed it was a good deal. Memorial's board resolution was merely a formality that SIU required. Lanphier had already spoken. The sale was officially completed in 1971 for exactly a half million dollars, slightly more than Memorial's original purchase price and razing costs.

From Beds to Services

The publication of the Campbell Report had occurred concurrently with the completion of the B addition, the last structure built for the nearly exclusive purpose of adding beds for students or patients. Thereafter, Memorial concentrated on adding services.

One likely explanation for Memorial's initially slow response to the opportunity for a new medical school was its considerable preoccupation with internal operating issues. As noted in the previous chapter, it earned only provisional JCAH accreditation in 1968, not an auspicious start for a would-be teaching hospital. Memorial also continued to respond to physicians' requests for new equipment and services into the late 1960s. In the three years preceding the Campbell Report, it opened a half dozen new services and improved or expanded others.

For too many years Memorial lagged behind its rival and peers in emergency and trauma care. As late as the 1960s the "hodge-podge" emergency department was crowded into four rooms and lacked the latest equipment. The inefficient organization of the emergency room (ER) was dramatized by the plight of veteran board leader Chick Lanphier, who experienced lengthy delays there as a patient. Dr. Chauncey Maher recalled being "horrified" by Lanphier's experience and pushed for a new, streamlined emergency room. The difficulties were no doubt due to the huge increase in ER visits over the prior twenty years, from 649 in 1944 to 14,137 in 1965. The board approved hiring several physicians to provide full-time ER coverage in 1966 but recruitment efforts were unsuccessful. The following year an amendment to the medical staff bylaws required all medical staff to serve on the emergency room call list. This idea was neither popular nor effective and in late 1968 four full-time physicians were finally recruited to staff the emergency room, with Dr. Arthur Lindsay employed as chief physician and chair of the Department of Emergency Medicine. Earlier he had worked at Springfield Clinic and served on Memorial Hospital's medical staff. His task was to expand and modernize the unit, which occupied him for the next 15 years.

A fateful lost opportunity occurred in 1971, when the state announced a program to upgrade emergency care through designation of nine Illinois trauma centers, supported with public funds and a plan for rapid transportation of victims by ambulance or helicopter. Springfield was slated to have one such center, and both hospitals were encouraged to apply. To qualify, hospitals would have to upgrade their staffing and services, construct a heliport, and meet other exacting standards. Lindsay and several administrators argued in favor of an application, but Executive Director George Hendrix dismissed the program as costly window dressing.

SIU Dean Moy and others were "flabbergasted" by the decision, correctly judging it to be a serious strategic mistake. Progressive hospitals needed modern trauma care, and the public was enthralled (through television programs) by the glamour of heroic lifesaving exploits by emergency specialists. St. John's Hospital duly won recognition as the area's Regional Trauma Center, with an eye-catching heliport, newspaper attention, and highway direction signs.

Lindsay and other concerned officials found a more receptive audience with the new director, George Phillips, and his now energized board. A sharp decline in emergency admissions foretold the lingering consequences of a bad decision. Board members and hospital officials vainly sought action by the state to add Memorial to the state trauma network. Meanwhile, there were continued steps to improve the facility and its services.

Dr. Lindsay persevered through difficult times. By 1974 (when ER visits had increased 91 per cent since 1970) Lindsay had difficulty recruiting physicians due to a national shortage. In 1973, there were 20,000 vacant emergency medicine positions. By 1979, Memorial's emergency room employed six full-time physicians and 20 nurses.

With Dr. Lindsay's retirement in 1983, the need for strong leadership became even more acute. Hospital officials wisely chose Steve Kirk as Director of Emergency Medical Services. Although not a physician, he was "a very bright man" who had excellent experience as operator of a local ambulance service. Kirk wasted no time reorganizing the department and earning it certification to train paramedics. He also struggled to reverse a longstanding habit among city safety personnel to direct ambulances to St. John's, arguing that assignments should be split evenly between the two hospitals.

The improvements were substantial, and in 1988 Memorial applied to state public health officials for Level I standing, the highest possible rating for a trauma center. Protracted efforts produced a disappointing II rating, but at least this placed the hospital on a par with its crosstown rival. One measure of the center's enhanced standing was Kirk's final success in persuading city officials to specify Memorial as the destination for an equal share of all calls. It was a difficult and costly effort, but the Trauma Center finally reached parity.

While the hospital struggled to staff its ER in the 1960s, it also created a pulmonary care unit, opened in 1967 when the ICU was expanded. The ten-bed pulmonary unit consolidated care of these patients and immediately operated "at near capacity." Board records described it as the "second such unit outside Chicago." The service was the natural outgrowth of the hospital's Inhalation Therapy School, approved by the AMA in 1966.

The first cardiac unit was also launched in 1966. Medical staff appointed Dr. Gersham K. Greening chair of a committee to develop a cardiac unit at Memorial, and George Hendrix ordered cardiac monitoring equipment for an 8-bed unit. Two nurses were sent to both St. John's and the Miami Heart Institute for training that year. Initially, cardiology services grew, then came to a virtual standstill in 1971, the result of a physician boycott. Only four cardiac catheterizations were performed in nearly a year following the purchase of expensive equipment. The board had emulated its success with laboratory, radiology, and renal services by hiring two physicians, Drs. Paul Miller and William Lynch, to direct cardiology services. At issue was the control that radiologists exercised over scheduling the use of equipment. Close cooperation in these early years was vital between cardiologists and radiologists like Dr. William Sherrick, who worked on Memorial's first 50 coronary angiographies. The board acknowledged the unrest but blamed Dr. Miller's "personality," and did not renew his contract. His position was filled nearly a year later by Dr. Paul Smalley. Thereafter, close cooperation among the specialists and the acquisition of more equipment resolved the problem, and cardiac volume increased.

On July 24, 1968 (one month after the Campbell Report) the **Illinois State Journal** announced the establishment of an "artificial kidney center" at Memorial. Dialysis services began in 1963 when Dr. Herbert Henkel, Jr. donated an artificial kidney machine on behalf of his father, Dr. Herbert Henkel, Sr. Memorial was the selected recipient, though the equipment (for use with acute dialysis patients) was transported between the two rival hospitals. Eventually, Dr. Alton Morris, an internist, successfully proposed a dialysis and kidney transplant program. The board invested $250,000 in the program and recruited Dr. Antonio Versaci, from Chicago's Mount Sinai Hospital, to direct the program. The timing was fortunate. The Illinois General Assembly had already passed legislation to create two chronic dialysis centers, one in Chicago and the other "down state." Memorial was well positioned to qualify, and won the designation as an evaluation and treatment center. Memorial almost immediately had "problems" with Dr. Versaci, who was eventually replaced by Drs. Richard T. Bilinsky and Alton Morris.

Within five years, Memorial had opened eight renal "satellite" units, the first at Springfield Clinic then others as distant as Alton and Quincy. Dr. Chauncey Maher, who was president of the medical staff at the time, credits Dr. Morris with the satellite idea. Whenever a community had half a dozen chronic dialysis patients, Memorial encouraged the local hospital or clinic to house a satellite. Memorial paid for personnel, equipment and space while patients paid Memorial for the service. In addition to providing much needed care, the satellites supplied additional revenue and expanded the hospital's service region.

Dr. Morris envisioned transplant work when he first pushed for the dialysis program at Memorial. The first kidney transplant in Springfield occurred at Memorial on October 21, 1970, two months before the hospital signed an affiliation agreement with the SIU School of Medicine. Dr. Maher described the transplant program as a "major boost" for Memorial because the only other programs in the United States at that time were associated with major metropolitan teaching hospitals. A surgeon from Detroit traveled to Springfield to act as consultant on the first kidney transplants, which were performed by Springfield Drs. John Allen and John Denby. Nurse Wilma Fricke served on one of two transplant teams along with Drs. Morris and Bilinsky. The first kidney transplant was a successful five-hour surgery which allegedly made medical history because the patient had very recently undergone cardiac surgery, receiving an artificial heart valve nine months earlier at St. John's Hospital. The press coverage of this medical "first" stoked the rivalry with St. John's, which expressed "anger" when the article implied that the heart surgery had also occurred at Memorial.

A Standard of Excellence

Dr. John V. Standard, a leading area obstetrician and gynecologist, spent 30 years on Memorial's medical staff. A native Illinoisan, he earned his medical degree at Northwestern University and served two stints in the military before moving to Springfield.

Standard was a dedicated, demanding practitioner. In addition to sharpening his own skills, he pushed relentlessly to expand and upgrade the Ob-Gyn service at Memorial. On top of a busy practice he also found time to regularly lobby hospital officials for larger, better facilities and the latest equipment. Through voluminous correspondence, detailed reports and personal appearances before the board of directors, he sought to elevate the department's quality and stature above the mediocrity that had prevailed for many years.

Dr. Standard was no less determined in his expectations for fellow physicians. A disciple of rigorous peer review, he did not hesitate to discipline colleagues for substandard work. This commitment led naturally to his appointment in 1969 as the hospital's first division chairman in Ob-Gyn, a position he continued to hold for many years. He also was elected president of Memorial's medical staff in 1977, for a two year term.

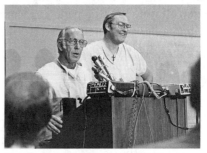

Dr. Standard (left) addresses the press after the birth of Governor James Thompson's (right) daughter, Samantha.

Standard lived long enough to observe great progress in obstetrical care at the hospital. In 1974 he was able to report that Memorial's maternal and infant mortality rates had declined, and were well below state and national figures. Sadly, his sudden death in 1986 at age 60 deprived him of the opportunity to see the culmination of his life's work, the construction of an advanced maternity suite that by the 1990s won Memorial high praise and the region's largest obstetrical volume.

The transplant program was an example of how SIU positively influenced the range and quality of medical services at Memorial. New medical school doctors were critical of local physicians' abilities to do kidney transplants. Tension developed among Dr. Robert Conn, SIU's new chairman of medicine, and Drs. Bilinsky and Morris. The latter two eventually left the renal program. Dr. Roland Folse, chairman of SIU's surgery department, recruited Dr. Alan Birtch from Boston as the assistant department chief. Birtch had transplant experience and was a valuable senior leader. It was money and not personalities that temporarily halted the kidney transplant program. Memorial stopped the transplants because they were expensive and not covered by Medicare. Executive Director George Hendrix calculated that Memorial lost $10,859 in one year on the dialysis program alone. Records note that $450,000 in renal dialysis service had been provided without payment. Hendrix told Dr. Birtch there would be no more transplants "unless the patients have sufficient financial backing." Fortunately, Congress obliged in 1972 when it extended Medicare coverage to kidney failure patients, including those under age 65.

As Dr. Morris prepared to open the renal unit, several surgeons approached George Hendrix to suggest that a burn center be established. The board noted that with "so many other things going on" it was not a good time to consider the service. The board recognized the regional need, however, and within a year William Schnirring recommended establishment of a burn unit. Dr. Jack Baldwin had conceived the idea and enlisted Schnirring to promote it to the board. Board records also noted that the unit would "improve the image of the hospital." This was one of several occasions when doctors promoted a new initiative by inviting an out-of-town expert to dinner at the Sangamo Club with the board. In January 1970 the board agreed to the burn unit but hedged its commitment with a six-month trial. A panel of surgeons had spent two years planning the five-bed unit, which was retained after the trial period.

From the outset, burn unit staffing was a chronic problem blamed on the "depressive nature of the nurses' work there." Despite this difficulty and though the unit was not profitable, the board continued to support it because it not only filled a critical gap in the region's medical services but also resulted in a deserved source of good public relations. John Denby noted that doctors were pleased to have a facility designed for cases that had troubled them for years. The unit, which immediately drew patients from as far north as Peoria and south to Alton, also boosted Memorial's regional reputation. Three years after the unit opened, the patient load had tripled but the service still lost money.

Dr. Baldwin served as the program's part-time director for six years. One nurse recalled that he "did a great job" because the burn unit was "his baby." Together with Drs. Edward J. Budil and Philip J. Haggerty, Baldwin personally trained the original burn nursing team. Betty Snedigar, formerly a head nurse on the unit, recalled that the staff continually sought ways to improve patient care. Among these was the use of a helicopter. She and others flew to accident sites to initiate the earliest possible treatment and transport of burn victims. Nurse Betty Ermann provided educational support to the unit.

Baldwin stepped down to associate director when a full-time leader, Dr. Edward Law, was recruited from the University of Cincinnati. Law joined the SIU faculty and Memorial contracted for 30 per cent of his time. Thereafter the burn service was largely taken over by the SIU Plastic Surgery Department. The change initially created hard feelings but was ultimately good for the program.

With a $40,000 Kellogg Foundation grant, the unit was renovated in 1977 and renamed the Regional Burn Center. A press account described the 17-member burn team as a "special breed" and noted that 600 patients were treated in the center's first seven years. When Dr. Law resigned in 1979, nurse recruitment remained a problem but the ever reliable Dr. Baldwin once again became the center's director.

In addition to these new, high profile programs, other less noticeable services also emerged in the early 1970s. These included the social services, speech therapy, communications, printing and graphics, and security departments, the latter "badly needed" due to theft and vandalism. Dr. Homer Kimmich, an ear, nose, and throat specialist, persuaded the board to invest $20,000 in an audiology program.

Two-Headed Monster

In recognition of his increased responsibilities brought by the medical school, George Hendrix was named Executive Vice President and Administrator in 1970. The size of the executive committee was expanded from 12 to 13 to accommodate the position. Around that time, he developed health problems and Dr. Chauncey Maher, his physician, encouraged him to retire. Board executives Lanphier and Oxtoby also unsuccessfully

Practice On A Pig

When Dr. Herbert Henkel donated a kidney dialysis machine for use with acute patients, Dr. Chauncey Maher and a group of internists got together to learn how to use it. The first generation dialysis machine was a "very primitive kind of open tub ... with a hundred gallon tank that you filled with electrolyte solutions." The physicians dialyzed some pigs, whose physiology was similar to humans.

Dr. Maher recalled the learning experience. "We formed a team, a dialysis team where each physician spent two hours in rotation ... A nurse, Betty Hankins ... would mix up the solution with a canoe paddle ... One patient (pig) we dialyzed for 60 hours, I remember, and learned how to use that dialysis machine." Board minutes of June 1963 noted that two teams were competent to run the "artificial kidney." The new service was announced to all "medical societies and hospitals" within a 150-mile radius of Springfield.

pressed Hendrix to retire. Dr. Moy recalled that Hendrix was a "nice guy" who did not fully understand the complexities of the medical school, an observation which others also made. Hendrix typically took direction from the board and apparently had made no effort to fully embrace the opportunity presented by the Campbell Commission. Less than two years later, in an effort to cope with his many duties, Hendrix successfully proposed dividing his position. He was to retain the title of executive vice president and handle external affairs, a "Mr. Outside." He suggested that a new administrator be hired as "Mr. Inside."

To that end, George Phillips was recruited from Boston's Massachusetts General Hospital early in 1972. He had earned his master's degree in health care administration from Duke University, where his mentor, Ray Brown, was a prominent hospital administration expert. Brown eventually moved to Northwestern University Medical School and knew George Hendrix. When Hendrix spoke of his need for someone to handle Memorial's "internal operations," Brown recommended Phillips. Board records foreshadowed trouble with the twin positions. Phillips was to "run the hospital on a day to day basis," but Hendrix noted that "it would not be easy to define Mr. Phillips's duties" as opposed to his own, and that the "separation will likely evolve over a period of time." Though Phillips was to function as "Mr. Inside," he was selected because of his medical school experience, a contradiction destined to create conflict. The board's action reflected its need for teaching hospital expertise but also a desire to ease Hendrix's eventual retirement. According to Bill Boyd, the action created a "two-headed monster." Dr. Richard Moy agreed that the dual leadership was a "disaster."

The ensuing year was charged with tension. When George Phillips arrived early in 1972 he was told that Memorial was pretty much a "carriage trade" institution, the hospital of choice for the area's non-Catholic, wealthy, and established families. He immediately observed that Memorial was a bit worn after much growth and particularly noted drafty windows, a congested entrance, and haphazard signage. When Phillips ordered a complete signage overhaul, at considerable expense, Hendrix complained to the board that this was a waste of money. Phillips moved quickly to modernize the hospital and made changes in financial systems, administration, the physical plant, personnel, and planning. The transition was a difficult one for Hendrix, who was not able to make a graceful exit. Phillips recalled that Hendrix envisioned retirement and intended to groom a successor.

Instead, he stayed on, took an office down the hall, and dogged Phillips. They shared a secretary but very little else. Phillips found deficiencies everywhere and Hendrix took umbrage at the tacit criticism.

The tension between Hendrix and Phillips was both personal and circumstantial. Phillips recalled that Dr. Moy had a "very, very ambitious" agenda which put pressure on Memorial to change rapidly. Recollections of board members, administrators, and physicians confirmed that Hendrix was totally unsuited to run a teaching hospital. There was also no clear line between the internal and external realms and staff tended to confer with Hendrix out of both habit and personal choice. Hendrix chafed at Phillips's decisions and even encouraged medical staff and others to bypass him. Veteran board member Robert Oxtoby noted that before long, Hendrix and Phillips were scarcely speaking, an impossible situation of Hendrix's making.

The pressure culminated in a testy meeting with doctors, the SIU department chairs, who were both critical and impatient. Hendrix apparently offered his resignation but Lanphier dissuaded him. The board held an informal, rump meeting and Lanphier solicited advice on resolving the tension. Though he liked Hendrix personally, Boyd advised Lanphier that Phillips was vital in dealing with SIU. Some board leaders were fed up with Hendrix and persuaded their colleagues to accept the resignation, giving Phillips full executive authority. Hendrix was allowed to "retire," apparently at his full pay of $45,000. Records indicate that Hendrix took a leave of absence from April to June 1973, when the board formally accepted his resignation "with regret."

The organization chart changed very little from 1952 to 1965 and, with few exceptions, the same people held key positions on the board and in administration. These leaders worked tirelessly to meet the demands for space and services but had no clear vision for the future. The previously mentioned 1963 Smith report was the first formal planning effort since the 1932 Walsh report. While Dr. Smith had advised the hospital to create a day care program for adults (as an alternative to nursing home care), his plan did little else but encourage facilities development. Fiscal incentives actually continued to discourage planning and cooperation despite the 1966 Federal Comprehensive Health Planning Act, which created a new state agency and divided Illinois into planning regions. Memorial was too preoccupied with the demand for its product to systematically address questions about its future. Late in 1964 George Hendrix had presented the board with proposed hospital "objectives" and a "philosophy." The board approved this statement but did not bother to include copies in the minutes. Their contents remain unknown but it is clear that the board's *modus operandi* was to respond to opportunities and problems as they arose.

Like Moy, Phillips observed that Memorial had some clinical strengths but that the entrepreneurial growth, such as the burn unit, had been haphazard. He found no budgeting process, no mission, and no plan. When he arrived, the board was ready to approve a $15 million building program, to which he responded, "for what?" Phillips correctly concluded that the hospital's growth prior to the advent of the medical school had resulted from patient demand, entrepreneurial physicians (such as Grant Johnson and Alton Morris), and competition with St. John's. Phillips's agenda included physical renovations, coordination with the medical school, and systematic planning based on functional priorities. He stressed the need for long range planning and persuaded the board to hire his mentor, Ray Brown, to "advise the hospital on its intermediate and long range plans." With Brown's assistance Phillips then convinced the board to engage a consultant to conduct a study of Memorial's needs. In a characteristically systematic fashion, Phillips prepared a detailed request for proposals and sent it to leading firms suggested by Brown, then a vice president at Northwestern University. In July 1972 the board signed a contract with New York based E. D. Rosenfeld Associates. Rosenfeld was a physician and the company's president; the project director was Thomas P. Weil, Ph.D. The study's objective was to create a 1973-1980 plan for Memorial to meet the needs "generated by its affiliation as a teaching hospital" of the SIU School of Medicine.

Blueprint for the Future

The overall challenge for Rosenfeld was to produce a document to guide Memorial through a major transition from a midsized community hospital to a comprehensive, regional teaching hospital. The consultants arrived at the climax of the Hendrix-Phillips crisis and in the midst of a furor between many community physicians and the medical school, specifically, Dr. Moy. The company also found that a key player, St. John's, was not interested in joint planning. A March 1973 interim report to the board stated that a valid plan needed to include St. John's because "to do otherwise would let the medical school play one hospital against the other." George Phillips described his relationship with St. John's as "kind of schizophrenic" because the hospitals continued to compete while cooperative programs were discussed. He had "made progress" in a discussion with Sr. Jane Like and successfully requested additional funds for Rosenfeld to develop a format for joint planning between the two hospitals. But by the fall of 1973, Dr. Weil recommended that Memorial cease efforts for joint planning because St. John's already had "considerable excess space" to establish medical school programs immediately and had no intention of joint planning with Memorial.

Phillips acted as point man in the intense interaction between Rosenfeld consultants and the board, medical staff, SIU, and others. The first phase of the effort resulted in more than 500 pages of detailed observations and recommendations. The first volume, a 200-page review of trends and data, was completed in six months. The board then directed Rosenfeld to develop a detailed master plan incorporating four initiatives suggested in volume one. These included bed reduction, a teaching affiliation with SIU, affiliations or mergers with other hospitals, and closure of the nursing school. The recommendations were foresighted, novel, controversial, and far reaching. With a few exceptions and some variations in timing, the Rosenfeld recommendations were carried out with remarkable precision. The study became the blueprint from which Memorial built its future.

In 1968, when it had become apparent that Springfield might be selected as the medical school site, Memorial had retained Dr. Robert L. Evans, a medical education director from Pennsylvania, to make recommendations on the transition to a teaching facility. Evans observed that Memorial's patient care was "good in the main, excellent in rare cases, and extremely poor in several others." Unfortunately, the Rosenfeld consultants found most of the same problems that Evans had identified five years earlier. When Moy assessed the quality of Springfield's medical care, he noted several outstanding physicians, including Robert Patton, Richard Herndon, and John Standard. He also recalled that many were competent "but unexceptional" and too many were "has-beens, never-weres, and fairly competent people." He observed that recruiting department chairs from outside Springfield stirred resistance but eventually raised medical standards.

Though Real Estate Research had recommended Springfield's clinical facilities for the new medical school, its study also concluded that these were "high in quantity and low in quality." The company attributed this to the large number of "nonconforming" beds (patient rooms which failed to meet state standards) and no intern or residency programs. Rosenfeld and medical school doctors were particularly critical of Memorial's pharmacy, nursing, and psychiatric services. Memorial was advised to convert the pharmacy from a "corner drug store." The pharmacy had no formulary, did not review its intravenous medication program, and did not use generic drugs. Criticism of nursing was not so specific, though records indicate that medical staff wrote to the board to complain about its poor organization. Rosenfeld recommended a "major reorganization."

The most serious deficiency came to light when new medical school psychiatrists indicated they would not be able to train medical students at Memorial. According to Dr. Moy, the hospital's psychiatric care was 20 years out of date. Electroconvulsive (shock) therapy was overused, nurses were inadequately trained, facilities were cheerless, and security was lax. The latter issue surfaced after a patient set fire to her bed. One former administrator recalled that many problems were due to the narrow space in the A building. The executive committee of the medical staff was given 60 days to prepare a report on the quality of the program and make recommendations for improvement. A sharp conflict arose between new SIU faculty and community psychiatrists, who were determined to maintain the medical model of psychiatry. Staffing and procedural matters were apparently resolved by early 1975. Hospital officials embraced the Rosenfeld recommendation to coordinate the "three major community mental health care giving systems," SIU's psychiatry department, Memorial's, and the Springfield Mental Health Association. The eventual turnaround in psychiatric services exemplified Memorial's determination to work with the medical school to transform its programs into stellar services.

The Rosenfeld recommendations were voluminous but only a relatively few key ones were far reaching. Among these was a gradual reduction in beds, from 617 to 500, by 1980. In fact, consultants noted that the hospital's service area already had excess beds and advised substantial bed reductions by both hospitals. Initially the board resisted this prophetic idea because members were proud of the large bed capacity and viewed reduction as a step backward. Nevertheless, Memorial's directors were shrewd civic leaders who successfully ran the hospital with one eye toward community service and another toward good business. The board's eventual acceptance of a reduced bed count illustrated its businesslike willingness to embrace innovation in the face of challenge.

A related concept proposed by the consultants was the development of ambulatory care services, a Springfield deficiency that the Real Estate Research Corporation had also noted. A corollary suggestion was to construct a physician's office building in the "immediate neighborhood." There had been some physician support for this notion several years earlier, when doctors hired an architect to draw plans for a building on hospital property. The board tactfully reminded the doctors that this was illegal.

Directors readily agreed to another significant recommendation, the corporate model of governance. A trend in this direction was already underway among progressive American hospitals. At Memorial, accustomed to the moderately industrial milieu introduced by Chick Lanphier's board, the corporate model was enthusiastically embraced. Throughout its history, Memorial had relied upon a small administrative staff which, with the exception of Bill Boyd, were untrained in hospital administration. As hospitals became more complex, the number of university programs in hospital administration increased, from nine in the 1940s to 33 in the 1960s. During this quarter century, Memorial remained largely a community hospital, led by a dedicated and autocratic industrialist. Two years before Rosenfeld was hired, Chick Lanphier had created seven board sub-committees to handle the increased quantity of work. Principal among these were a steering committee and two committees which divided clinical areas (Medical Services 'A' and 'B'). Again, doctors were allowed to serve only in an advisory capacity. Other committees, which met infrequently, were finance, business affairs, paramedical services, and service departments. This arrangement more closely resembled an administrative structure than a governing board structure. Memorial had outgrown the organizational framework that had changed very little over the past quarter century. Rosenfeld simply legitimized the need for change.

The proposed organizational restructuring closely paralleled commercial companies and thus suited board members, who were businessmen of high stature and represented Springfield's major economic entities, including each of the three downtown banks. Veteran board member Bud Lohman exemplified Memorial's long history of bank representation and succession on its board. Lohman was an Ashland, Illinois banker who moved to Springfield's First National Bank and eventually became president. His boss was William Patton, a long time Memorial board member. The bank had a health program for its employees through Memorial and managed the Littler trust. Patton wanted to preserve the bank's close ties with Memorial and had Lohman named to the board.

Memorial had managed in this mode for decades due to an active, involved board. Phillips, however, found the board's focus on detail "surprising." For example, he recalled that financial reports were in cents, not rounded numbers and that there were long discussions over room rates. He was also uncomfortable with the board's governance by anecdote rather than analysis, and recalled that board members often cited a "problem" that was overheard socially or in the lobby.

Hospital administration had become much more complex, as demonstrated by the number of consultants Memorial hired in the early 1970s. Their expertise was useful on insurance, taxes, planning, financial systems, interior decorating, and graphic design. The more businesslike the hospital became, the more it relied on experts, a motif repeated in other American hospitals as well. Phillips considered the hospital's five-member administrative staff very lean. They managed the hospital with considerable board input. Consultants, board members, administrators, and medical staff agreed that reorganization was necessary. Rosenfeld recommended the 27-member board, which met annually, be replaced by a larger executive committee. The board rejected the suggestion as well as one that would have restricted board service to ten consecutive annual terms. Since 1931 board membership had been tantamount to lifetime appointment, a circumstance that 30-year veteran Chick Lanphier enjoyed. Directors did approve board membership for the hospital's president, a new title that replaced "administrator." The position of executive vice president was eliminated.

The board also changed associate and assistant administrators to vice presidents in order to "greatly enhance the hospital's ability to recruit." This action symbolized acceptance of the corporate model and also signaled a key shift in the qualifications, experience, and perspective of Memorial's top management. The new cadre of administrators came with credentials and specialized knowledge. Chauncey Maher credited Phillips with the introduction of modern hospital management practices to Memorial. He built a large, hierarchical administrative staff, a process he initiated even before Rosenfeld suggested changes. The restructured administration created vice presidencies for professional services, administrative services, medical programs, and affiliation agreements. Vice presidents of finance (chief financial officer) and nursing as well as assistant vice presidents (health services) were added over the next few years. Directorships of

Chauncey Maher, M.D.

Among physicians who had long-standing, close ties to Memorial was Dr. Chauncey Maher. After graduating from Chicago's Pritzker School of Medicine in 1945, he accepted an internship at Presbyterian Hospital and then served two years in the U.S. Navy. He returned to the University of Chicago for his residency then moved to Ogden, Utah to join a classmate in medical practice. Maher's father (a "big-time cardiologist") and a "professional manager" later persuaded him that the move was a mistake. Maher acknowledged the error but credited his senior Utah colleague, Dr. Frank Bartlett, with teaching him the importance of "getting close to your patient," a skill not emphasized at the University of Chicago, where "science was the name of the game." Maher recalled that the professional manager persuaded him to contact Dr. Richard Allen of Springfield, Illinois, who was seeking an associate. The two established a highly successful practice and became "top admitters to Memorial."

As part of Memorial's administrative overhaul, Maher was hired as part-time Director of Medical Programs in 1972 and served as Vice President for more than a decade. He recalled, "I couldn't have gotten elected dog catcher... by the (medical) staff during those years" because he was "part of administration." He was relieved when Jack Cook fired him, with characteristic finesse. Maher recalled Cook's explanation that it was time to retire his jersey.

Maher was not only a top supplier of patients but also personal physician to George Hendrix, Chick Lanphier, Robert Oxtoby, and Bill Boyd. He joined the renal unit in 1973 and was among the cadre of entrepreneurial physicians who made it a success.

support services and ambulatory services also emerged during this reorganization. Phillips recruited "top" doctors as full-time employees in the department of medicine. These were Drs. Alton Morris, Richard Bilinsky, Paul Smalley, William Lynch and Chauncey Maher. The latter stayed for ten years as Vice President for Medical Programs. It had been Rosenfeld's idea to pay chiefs of staff and chiefs of service in order to cement the medical staff's ties to Memorial.

Modernization of financial systems was an essential corollary to the corporate model. George Phillips recalled that Memorial's financial systems were antiquated, an assessment shared by Paul Smith, who steadily rose through the financial ranks. Smith remembered that every patient charge was posted manually, a "horrendous task." In the late 1960s there were only five employees (including comptroller Dwight McCormack) who handled payroll, general ledger, and accounts payable. Payroll accounting was a "nightmare" that required long weekends every quarter to balance data on nearly 1,200 employees. Fortunately, the payroll function was in the hands of a "close knit group" guided by a veteran employee, Betty Carder.

Records of 1968 to 1970 include many grim references to the hospital's poor cash position, a repeat performance from the previous decade. The accounts receivable climbed steadily from $2.5 million in 1969 to nearly $6 million by 1972. At least $1 million was owed by the Medicare program. The hospital was again forced to hold checks due to lack of funds and had to cash in matured certificates of deposit. Memorial fortunately also continued to receive substantial gifts—$250,000 in 1969, which included a $50,000 bequest from Ella Clarkson. In fact, the board clearly counted on bequests, notably the Littler estate, to pay its debts. One of Memorial's largest gifts came in 1974 from the estate of prominent Springfield attorney, Henry A. Converse. Like Littler, he died a bachelor in 1951 and the funds were held in trust until the death of the last of his three siblings. Converse, who had consulted with early board members in its bleak Lutheran days, left Memorial two-thirds of the trust, $888,388.

Some of the financial difficulty was attributed to the method of preparing and presenting reports. In 1969 the board retained Arthur Anderson & Company to make recommendations regarding the use of computers for accounting, and in 1970 it engaged Marine Bank to generate patient bills. Marine Bank was selected because it had a large new computer center and was an important local vendor of data management services. The decision to contract out "batch processing" of accounts receivable rather than develop in-house capability saved the hospital large capital expenditures and expert staff.

Paul Smith credited George Phillips with instigating financial improvements. At Phillips's request, Smith developed the first budget, a simple effort that Smith described as a crude but crucial first step. For the first time, the hospital had a capital budget which anticipated equipment needs for an entire year. In addition to computer use, the board recruited Russell Beckwith as comptroller in 1972 and later promoted him to Vice President and Chief Financial Officer. Beckwith's background in hospital cost accounting met a key need. He and his staff prepared the institution's first annual report, in 1974.

The hospital also faced fiscal challenges brought about by reforms in personnel benefits and federal attempts to control runaway costs. Nurse salaries continued to rise in response to St. John's salary increases. In 1966 the board increased all employee salaries in anticipation of the 1967 Minimum Wage Act, which included hospital employees for the first time. Around that time St. John's announced a retirement plan for its personnel and prompted Memorial's board to follow suit. The pension plan went into effect in 1971 and shortly thereafter, Memorial was also required to contribute to unemployment compensation, costing about $135,000 in 1972. The passage of the Illinois income tax three years earlier had created "considerable unrest" among hospital employees. A delegation of the lowest paid employees pleaded their case to the administration, which agreed to raise all salaries. According to Paul Smith, the hospital was able to pass nearly half of these costs on to Medicare, a major cause of skyrocketing costs in the 1970s.

The changing of the guard in the financial arena was a key reason for Memorial's successful transition to a regional medical center. Russell Beckwith had a degree in accounting and finance as well as experience at the Ford Motor Company and a Detroit hospital. Beckwith, who recalled that Memorial's finances were in "shambles," made an enormous contribution. He took steps to reduce the huge level of accounts receivable. Payment delays shrank from 127 to 47 days and uncollectible debts dropped from 4 to 1.6 per cent. These two improvements netted Memorial over $20 million. Financial obligations to the medical school coincided with President Richard M. Nixon's wage and price controls. Beckwith found ways to legally increase both, producing a growing surplus in the 1970s. One way this was accomplished was by shifting costs to the state. Initially, Memorial paid a portion of SIU department chair salaries as well as residents' salaries. In July 1973 the state assumed all responsibility for faculty salaries. Beckwith also renegotiated leases with SIU, an action which netted nearly $500,000 annually.

Rosenfeld recommended a total makeover of Memorial's image as well as its corporate structure. Memorial agreed to create a new name, logo, letterhead, and signage. According to board member Norman Jones, the goal was to expand the hospital's name both functionally and geographically. The board quickly agreed to change the name from "hospital" to "medical center," to reflect its expanded functions as a teaching institution. Board member Robert Oxtoby explained it to the press as, "we're something more than a hospital now."

Discussion of a geographical qualifier ("of Springfield," for example) dragged on until Norman Jones suggested that it was unnecessary. In January 1974 the corporation name officially became Memorial Medical Center. The name symbolized the goal to become the definitive regional medical center. A new logo represented a multi-layered approach to medical care by means of a "cross with shadows of the cross receding into the background." The three crosses represented Memorial's three endeavors: patient care, teaching, and research. The crosses were open on one side to symbolize an attitude open to new ideas and change.

The Price of Progress

The Rosenfeld study encouraged Memorial to build its regional market, which the burn and renal units had initiated. The study defined St. John's and Memorial's primary service areas as Sangamon and its surrounding counties and noted that nine per cent of Memorial's patients came from outside this area. Rosenfeld predicted that the number of Memorial patients from outside this service area would increase to 15 per cent by 1980 if Memorial became the primary referral hospital, via affiliation agreements, with Carlinville, Hillsboro, Mason District, and Pana hospitals. Officials took no immediate action on this recommendation.

The least popular and most controversial Rosenfeld recommendation was to close the nursing school because it was neither cost effective nor necessary. They noted a shortage of other health professionals so the board agreed to convert the nursing building to an allied health school facility, hence the building's name change to the Medical Arts Building. Consultants predicted an "excess of registered nurses (RNs) in the Springfield area by 1980," and identified a "reservoir" of inactive nurses in Springfield. Rosenfeld had surveyed area physicians, who perceived a shortage of allied health and nursing staff, but instead relied upon data collected by the National Center for Health Statistics and the U.S. Consultant Group on Nursing. A 1968 Illinois Study Commission on Nursing had demonstrated a "great need" for additional nurses, the same year that Memorial instituted several innovative nurse recruitment efforts. Rosenfeld consultants attributed the conflicting viewpoints to Memorial's poorly organized nursing administration. Also, Lincoln Land Community College (LLCC) opened in 1967 and Sangamon State University (SSU) arrived, with the medical school, in 1970. These programs, along with St. John's nursing school, were expected to supply more than enough nurses.

Nationally, the number of active registered nurses grew more rapidly in the 1970s than at any other time in the century. At the same time, the number of hospital diploma schools declined at a rate of 30-40 programs per year, from 908 in 1960 to 288 in 1982. Consultants firmly advised Memorial to phase out its school as soon as the "Lincoln Land program is expanded and the Sangamon State University program becomes operational." Neither of these steps was accomplished in 1973. Dr. Maher recalled that the nursing school closure was a bad decision because Lincoln Land graduated only 25 students per year, while Memorial often graduated twice as many.

Rosenfeld's second reason to close the school was to save the $250,000 annual cost to maintain it. As mentioned previously, the board had calculated that the cost of the school was nearly equal to the value of the students' work for the hospital. One board member recalled that the school was a money loser, though not by much, but was also an administrative nuisance, with students, teachers, dormitories, rules, and space needs. Rosenfeld further advised Memorial to take advantage of an additional $200,000 per year in rental of the nursing school space to the medical school.

Another reason for the closure was Memorial's difficulty in recruiting qualified instructors. The Illinois Department of Registration and Education notified Memorial in 1969 that it could not accept students because it lacked qualified faculty and a director. An Indiana hospital where Memorial students fulfilled their psychiatric nursing rotation threatened to terminate the affiliation for the same reason. Board records of April 1969 note this problem but there was much more discussion about hiring physicians for non-existent medical school departments. Two months later, Hazel Kellams was hired to direct the nursing school for $22,000 while the board pledged $25,000 to renovate the burn center, which was clearly losing money. Despite Kellams' presence, the state refused to allow admission of students for the fall semester and rejected two faculty, one of whom Memorial had already hired. State approval did not come until September so the school admitted only 24 freshmen.

Memorial's board had tacitly accepted the closure of the nursing school at least two years before the Rosenfeld consultants were hired. In a September 1970 meeting directors reviewed an architect's timetable for SIU construction and noted that it required the "class of student nurses just admitted to be the last class." Members then agreed that a five-year timetable was more realistic, particularly because the new community college accepted only 25 students. Several months later, Hendrix warned the board that providing a floor of the nursing building to SIU would "signal the close of the diploma school." Despite their loyalty to the school, long term board members recognized that there were other means of acquiring nurses and that their future lay in accommodating the medical school. It was apparent that Memorial could not handle both programs, physically or financially, so the issue became merely a matter of timing.

In 1970 the board had already approved a plan to lease the top floor of the nursing education building to the medical school by early 1971 and, if the nursing school was "still in operation," to sell the building to SIU in 1974. Board records note that the Reisch property sale and the lease of the nursing school space would assure that the medical school was "firmly located thereafter" at Memorial rather that at St. John's. George Hendrix was the lone board supporter of the nursing school and reminded colleagues that LLCC was not ready to train the needed supply of nurses. Dr. Maher lamented the loss of the nursing school but was also convinced that it enabled Memorial to cement closer ties to SIU.

Despite the early agreement to close the school, no formal board action occurred until May 3, 1973. Lanphier suggested that no students be accepted for the fall class in 1973 but Boyd reminded him that half the students had already been accepted. Following a motion by Lanphier, the board agreed that no students would be accepted in the fall of 1974. Clearly, nursing school officials had no idea how tenuous was their program nor how imminent its demise. Just two days before the fateful board

George Hendrix

George Hendrix held the senior administrative position at Memorial for 20 years, longer than any other chief executive. His lengthy service is not notable for leadership or strategic accomplishments. Veteran board member Walter Lohman recalled that Hendrix actually followed the board's leadership. Nevertheless, Hendrix created and sustained a cohesive and community-oriented workforce. One nurse described him as a "wonderful administrator" who was "just one of the family."

As noted elsewhere, Hendrix had difficulty giving up his role, particularly to his antithesis, George Phillips. There is ample evidence that Memorial found the separation equally painful. Chick Lanphier prolonged Memorial's administrative agony by initially rejecting Hendrix's resignation. The board granted him a three-month leave of absence prior to accepting his resignation, undoubtedly to assure him exactly 20 years of service.

Six months after Hendrix left, Memorial nurses sponsored a dinner honoring him at the Illinois State Fairgrounds, and board member Robert Oxtoby commissioned a portrait of Hendrix which was presented to the board a year later. Even former President Jack Cook asked Bill Boyd to arrange for him to meet Hendrix in order to tap his knowledge of Memorial. Cook and Hendrix became good friends. Four years after Hendrix retired, Cook made him a special guest at the annual employee recognition dinner. Hendrix died in 1981.

meeting, school director Hazel Kellams proposed a tuition increase to George Phillips. The board's steering committee denied the request and indicated that closing the school was in the "best interest of the institution ... and fully recognized the emotional sentiments for retaining" the school. Phillips, a relative newcomer and outsider, was the only official who seemed to be unaware of the emotional attachment to the school.

Memorial Hospital School of Nursing celebrated its 75th anniversary on April Fool's Day, 1973. On May 16, George Phillips announced that it would close. The announcement triggered an angry response that caught Phillips by surprise. He received numerous calls and letters, especially from students and parents. He recalled it as "one of the most emotional (public) responses" that he had ever seen.

Once the decision was made, Memorial officials exerted pressure to close the school as quickly as possible. With approval from its accrediting agency, the National League for Nursing, the school adopted a quarter system and continued classes through the summer in order to accelerate the program. Normally a three-year program, it was compressed to two for the last class. The 78th and final class graduated at ceremonies held October 19, 1975 at the First Christian Church. Since its establishment in 1897, the school had graduated 1,551 nurses.

While all of the publicly expressed reasons for closing the school had some validity, they became the justification for terminating a program that was no longer a board priority. Officials viewed the nursing school as a burden which drained vitally important resources, including funds, space, and administrative attention. The nursing school closed because there was literally no room for it. George Phillips recalled that the nursing school was not cost effective for a teaching hospital and that space was at a premium. Rosenfeld predicted that the medical school would lead Memorial to the position of a regional health care center for central and southern Illinois.

Officials had discussed the closure for so long that they may have assumed that everyone else was aware that the school had to go. One nurse, however, believed that the information was deliberately kept secret. Veteran nurse manager Ed Quarry recalled that he and his fellow nurses learned of the closure from the newspaper and reacted with shock and distress. Dr. Fluckiger remembered that neither administrators nor board members consulted with doctors about the closure, which came as a surprise. Doctors were distressed because they had disagreed with Rosenfeld's assertion that the supply of nurses was adequate. Former nursing school director Helen Shull recalled that the closure also caught the alumnae by surprise. Her reaction was shared by many others. "I felt that was a tragedy."

In their determined attempts to accommodate SIU, Memorial officials announced the closure carelessly and abruptly. It came before Rosenfeld produced its final report and without consultation with key constituencies. In a pattern repeated at key intervals throughout its history, Memorial distanced itself from a past identity. These actions usually had positive results. For example, the hospital was revitalized by changes in its sponsorship and name. The nursing school was also sacrificed to a worthy cause, but this time the sacrifice was costly.

Memorial Milestones

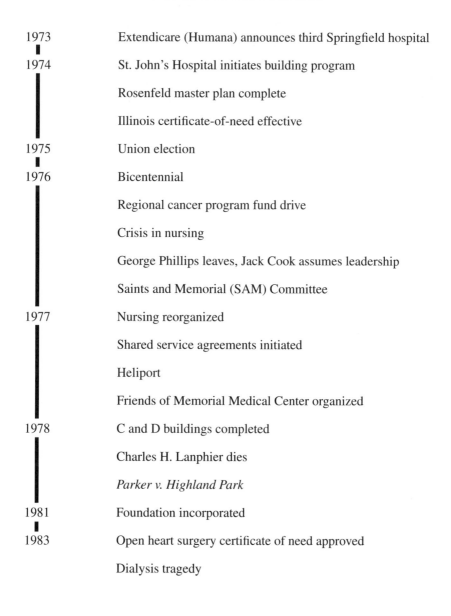

1973	Extendicare (Humana) announces third Springfield hospital
1974	St. John's Hospital initiates building program
	Rosenfeld master plan complete
	Illinois certificate-of-need effective
1975	Union election
1976	Bicentennial
	Regional cancer program fund drive
	Crisis in nursing
	George Phillips leaves, Jack Cook assumes leadership
	Saints and Memorial (SAM) Committee
1977	Nursing reorganized
	Shared service agreements initiated
	Heliport
	Friends of Memorial Medical Center organized
1978	C and D buildings completed
	Charles H. Lanphier dies
	Parker v. Highland Park
1981	Foundation incorporated
1983	Open heart surgery certificate of need approved
	Dialysis tragedy

Chapter Seven

Seeking Parity

Throughout the 1970s, Memorial faced a barrage of challenges. At a time when the medical center needed to expand rapidly in order to meet its ambitious goals, it faced significant cost increases, a relentless tide of regulation, unforeseen competition, and labor difficulties. Memorial's determination to become SIU's primary teaching hospital contained an implicit goal to best St. John's Hospital. Yet the medical center encountered a host of unprecedented challenges (some simultaneously) which delayed achievement of its primary goals by a decade.

Rosenfeld's extensive research convinced officials that Springfield already had a bed surplus and raised the specter of empty corridors. The board, confident that Memorial's success depended upon partnering with the medical school, struggled to catch up with one perceived St. John's advantage, space. A forthcoming joint meeting of both hospitals and SIU would identify separate institutional strengths in a funding request to the Illinois Board of Higher Education (IBHE). St. John's laid special claim to its family practice, pediatrics, trauma, neonatal, and cardiovascular medical and surgical programs. Memorial was to be the primary hospital for burn care, transplant care, renal dialysis, adult psychiatry, physical medicine and rehabilitation, and comprehensive mental health services. All other services were to be shared equally, though Memorial acknowledged St. John's "slight edge" in obstetrics and gynecology.

Memorial's board gave exaggerated attention to the apportionment of SIU programs. Officials were frustrated because they believed Memorial could win 85 per cent of SIU's programs if it had "physical facilities" equal to those at St. John's. Memorial board members instructed George Phillips to "get as much as possible" at the joint meeting, hoping that most SIU programs could be obtained once Rosenfeld's construction plan was completed. Indicative of this determination, it passed a resolution that "the proposed expansion program is consistent with the desire of Memorial Medical Center to eventually become a major university affiliated hospital for the SIU School of Medicine." This was a radical departure from the discussion which preceded the 1970 SIU affiliation agreement. Then it was "thoroughly understood" that there would be no attempt to turn the community hospitals into "university teaching hospitals."

The rivalry with St. John's in the late 1960s and early 1970s was particularly intense. Doctors joked that if they wanted some expensive new equipment at Memorial, all they had to do was to claim that St. John's already had it or soon would. Records note that a 1971 joint planning meeting between the two hospital laboratories was a "very poor one." St. John's not only had space already available for the medical school but also launched an ambitious building program a year ahead of Memorial. In October 1974 St. John's laid the cornerstone for a $30 million building program and started a $2.5 million fundraising campaign.

St. John's was not the only threat to Memorial's future. The economic incentives created by the Medicare program led to the rise of investor-owned (for-profit) hospital chains. By 1970 there were 29 chains nationally and their number grew more rapidly than the computer industry throughout the decade. In 1973 the Rosenfeld consultants had embarked on the second phase of their work, a detailed space plan, when the for-profit Extendicare Corporation (later called Humana) announced its intention to build a third hospital in Springfield. Extendicare based its decision on complaints from local doctors, who described "acute problems" getting on the hospitals' surgery schedules. Rosenfeld advised Memorial to adjust its plans from 500 to 400 beds if the proposed for-profit hospital was built, and urged officials to "take every action, including legal" to prevent the Extendicare Corporation's construction.

Both Memorial and St. John's firmly opposed the third hospital, but Governor Dan Walker favored it, an attitude typical of the 1970s market-oriented public policy. George Phillips brought both legal counsel and

Dr. Kenneth H. Schnepp, Librarian

Reliance on the medical literature accompanied improvements in medical education and scientific breakthroughs in medicine. Dr. Kenneth H. Schnepp deserved honorary recognition as Springfield's first medical librarian. What he lacked in formal library education, he made up for with a lifelong enthusiasm. As early as 1931 the Sangamon County Medical Society had established a small collection of medical periodicals and housed these at Lincoln Library. Schnepp, dissatisfied with this collection, convinced a small group of physicians to found the Springfield Medical Library Association in 1939. The Association, which still existed in Memorial's centennial year, collected dues from local physicians in order to improve their access to the medical literature.

Records note that Memorial's board held its meetings in the "medical library" after the 1943 move. Then, in response to a 1949 medical staff request, the board provided "library shelves and reading counters" in the doctors' lounge to house a third of the Medical Society's collection. The other two-thirds were sent to St. John's. The collection was reunited when the School of Medicine opened and it became the nucleus of that library's collection.

Never satisfied with the results of his efforts, Dr. Schnepp continued to seek funds for library development. In 1969 the medical staff rules and regulations were amended to fine doctors $5.00 per day per delinquent medical record. The proceeds were intended for the medical library. As late as 1972 the Sangamon County Medical Society contributed $1,000 to Memorial's medical library, very likely at the urging of former president Schnepp. Dr. Schnepp retired from practice in 1977 and a year later Dr. John Standard, on behalf of the medical staff executive committee, successfully requested that the board name Memorial's library after Dr. Schnepp. He continued to support local medical libraries, via donations and his membership on advisory committees, until his death in 1985.

Rosenfeld's extensive data to Humana's hearings, but to no avail. The **Illinois State Journal** described the controversy as the "culmination of a lengthy struggle in which the proposed hospital was declared by the Central Illinois Health Planning Council and the state Comprehensive Health Planning Agency to be unneeded here." But the state agency withdrew its objection after Governor Walker directed it to no longer "make findings on need." The Humana Corporation announced that it would break ground in April 1974 on the 200-bed, $9 million Springfield Community Hospital.

Rosenfeld's space plan was completed a month after construction started on the third hospital. When consultants began the plan in 1973 they did so with the understanding that Memorial would reduce its bed count to 500 by 1980 and would share medical school programs equally with St. John's. But in January 1974 the board directed consultants to change direction and assume that Memorial would become the "primary affiliated teaching hospital" with 575 beds. The change delayed the plan's completion by about six months and signaled officials' renewed determination to win all the SIU programs. Dr. Moy apparently did not share this ambition but he dangled the carrot for years. Just three months prior to completion of Rosenfeld's space plan, Phillips reported to the board that Dr. Moy had indicated two-thirds of the medical school programs would be located at Memorial. It was very likely just another of the many enticing speculations shared with the board over the prior six years. The board's ultimate refusal to significantly reduce beds was influenced by both the arrival of a third hospital and by St. John's refusal to give up any of its nearly 800 beds. In a pattern repeated in cities throughout the nation, Springfield's hospitals abandoned their modest cooperative efforts and intensified their rivalry.

Newspaper reporters and hospital board members seemed to be the only Springfield citizens concerned with an "overbedded" city. There was enthusiasm for beds of any kind in the bustling and progressive capital city. Ground breaking ceremonies for Springfield Community Hospital (later renamed Humana, then Doctors' Hospital) occurred the same year that the tallest building in Sangamon County, the Forum XXX Hotel, opened. The hotel (later the Springfield Hilton) was criticized not for the number of beds but for being taller than the capitol.

The board selected a Chicago firm, Perkins and Will, to develop the architectural component of the Rosenfeld master plan. The building plan, which included two floors for physician offices, was approved in mid-

1974. By then, the medical school and both other hospitals were already under construction. The pressure on Memorial to initiate its own construction was further increased by imminent regulatory legislation.

In the late 1970s, American hospitals drifted further from their identities as community organizations. Hospitals relied less on local gifts and formed alliances with other hospitals outside their local areas. Spiraling health care costs created a backlash against Great Society programs in the form of market competition, which not only created the "overbedded" city, but also invited regulation. New York was the first state to pass certificate-of-need (CON) legislation, in 1964. A form of "controlled competition" supported by the American Hospital Association, the legislation required hospitals to apply for state permission for construction and other capital investments. Nearly half the states adopted such legislation by 1972, and Illinois joined their ranks two years later. In Illinois the CON arbiter was called the Illinois Health Facilities Planning Board. Ironically, its first members were appointed by Governor Walker (who ignored their advice), and included the vice chairman of SIU School of Medicine in Carbondale, Dr. John Rendelman. Health planning agencies had little effect on either planning or costs. A study in the late 1970s showed that the CON laws reduced the number of beds but that hospitals spent more per existing bed. As one historian described the program, it involved "game playing at every level." Memorial had four months from its approval of the architectural plans to get construction underway. If it failed to do so, the most ambitious building program in its history could be further delayed or denied. Less than two months before the law's effective date, official records noted that the board was rushing to complete its plans before the regulations became effective. Other obstacles appeared only weeks from the planned groundbreaking.

Breaking New Ground

A $25.4 million building program was announced at the annual corporation meeting in January 1975. The **State Journal-Register** reported that the bulk of funding would come from the sale of $30 million in tax-exempt bonds through the City of Springfield. A zoning dispute disrupted these plans. In the summer of 1975, Memorial purchased most of the property on the north side of Klein Street for parking. A "politically influential" realtor owned property adjacent to the proposed parking area and protested the zoning change. Memorial made several unsuccessful attempts to reach agreement. The owner threatened legal action against the city, claiming the bond sale was not constitutional under home rule authority. Memorial was anxious to avert legal action, which would have prevented the bond sale. Officials faced a deadline on the expiration of construction bids and were under new CON regulations. A substantial federal grant as well as the prospect of higher winter construction costs compounded the difficulties. In a strategic and businesslike move, the board agreed to pursue a private bond sale. The financing was arranged quickly and quietly over one week-end to prevent court action. Memorial won good terms on the sale, which was arranged by the Illinois Health Facilities Authority, a state office created for such purposes. The underwriter, Chicago-based John Nuveen and Company, completed the sale in less than two weeks.

The board planned to augment its bond sale with state and federal grants for the medical school portion of the construction. In 1974 there was a major federal reorganization of health planning programs and, when Hill-Burton was folded into the National Health Planning and Resources Development Act, federal funds for hospital construction ceased. However, Memorial received $4 million from the federal Comprehensive Health Manpower and Training Act, a 1971 law which once again aimed to augment the supply of health care professionals and supported construction of medical school facilities. Together with St. John's and Doctors' Hospital in Carbondale, Memorial also applied for funds to the Illinois Board of Higher Education. Memorial's request for $13.5 million was twice as much as St. John's request. Dr. Moy told George Phillips that he would endorse only $8.4 million because the IBHE thought Memorial was using the medical school to fund its patient services. Though George Phillips denied the allegation, Chick Lanphier went on record one month later that his "patient consumer" viewpoint agreed that Memorial was asking the state to pay for the expansion of its services. If there was any disagreement with Lanphier, it was not recorded in the minutes.

While plans were underway for the groundbreaking, Memorial completed renovation of the Nurse Education Building. The medical school occupied about 90 per cent of the building, which was renamed the Medical Arts Building (MAB). The new construction program included two buildings, C and D, but these were actually designed, built, and operated as a single unit. Another portion, called AW or A West, was a two-story addition to the north side of the 1958 A wing and adjacent to both the C and

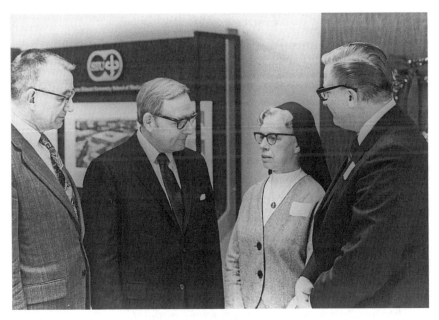

The presence of a new medical school spurred some cooperative dialogue. Executives George Hendrix (left), Sister Jane Like of St. John's Hospital and SIU Dean Richard Moy confer with Governor Richard Ogilvie (second from left), circa 1970.

George Phillips

George Phillips' four-year tenure as the senior administrator was a whirlwind of change, accomplishment, and controversy. Phillips' action-oriented and ambitious agenda, coupled with his remote demeanor, clashed with the status quo.

When the overall score was tallied, however, Phillips successfully transformed Memorial into a teaching hospital in record time. Memorial went from zero to 45 residencies in two years, overhauled financial systems, and recruited a cadre of able physicians and administrators. Under his leadership, the Rosenfeld consultants developed a master plan which led Memorial to regional prominence.

Phillips recalled that the staff and board treated him fairly and he felt no bitterness toward his experience. He was justifiably proud to have "laid the foundation" for Memorial to become "a very sophisticated teaching hospital."

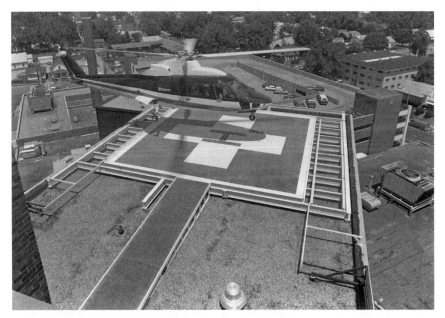

The intense effort to upgrade Memorial's emergency care services included construction of a heliport in 1983, helping earn the hospital a Level II Trauma Center rating.

D buildings. Together, the three new additions had a pinwheel shape. Both architects and administrators intended to leave empty an open space created by the new buildings. Dr. Chauncey Maher instead lobbied successfully to create an outdoor courtyard adjacent to a small, new cafe. He was inspired by his frequent trips to Europe, where he enjoyed dining at outdoor tables. The popular courtyard cost about $60,000 and included umbrella tables, plants, and a fountain. Administration contacted various service providers (including McDonald's and Steak 'n Shake) to operate the small cafe. When they declined, Memorial contracted with a popular local restaurant, the Dairy Rose.

Memorial's multi-level structure added no beds but greatly expanded clinical facilities. The emergency, intensive care, radiology, and nuclear medicine areas were expanded. Plans featured reflective glass, a 193-car parking ramp, and a pneumatic tube transmission system. The new addition faced Rutledge Street and the visitor entrance was moved there from its original 1943 location on Miller Street. The 220,000 square foot addition was one-third larger than the 1943 G building.

In 1970 the board had rejected George Hendrix's suggestion to construct a heliport, but by 1977 competition led the board to select the roof of the G building for one. It opened in November and linked Memorial to the statewide emergency medical services heliport network. A new cancer facility was occupied in May and other services moved into the new buildings during the summer of 1978. Existing space and services (including the Regional Burn Center) were also refurbished. As in 1943, a special supplement to the **State Journal-Register** featured detailed stories, photographs, and congratulatory advertisements in recognition of the September 24 open house.

While the new buildings were a boost to Memorial's progress and stature, some criticism was almost immediate. The new lobby, located on the lower level of C, was obscured by the new parking ramp and officials immediately regretted the poor entrance and image. Once visitors found the entrance, they were often lost in a maze. Staff were also confused. Dr. Donald Ross, who had arrived at Memorial as a surgery resident in 1975, recalled that he got lost one night when he was on call. When he was paged to emergency, he could not figure out how to get through the hospital. He went outside and walked around the block.

As part of the construction project, Memorial launched its regional cancer program, a strategically significant effort. Memorial's market had already

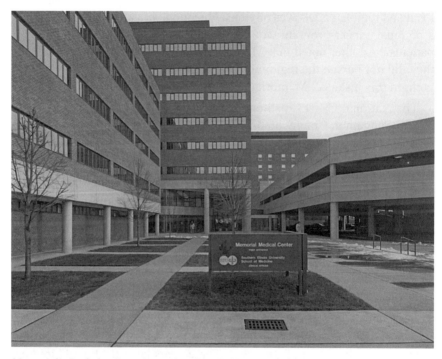

Memorial's Rutledge Street entrance in the 1980s. Its visual obstruction by a parking ramp proved to be a major disappointment.

expanded beyond Springfield when entrepreneurial physicians pushed its dialysis, kidney transplant, and pathology services. The regional cancer program, however, was the watershed between Memorial's local focus and its conscious determination to be the hospital of choice in an ever widening region. At one 1975 board meeting the tension between Memorial's local and regional goals was obvious. One member expressed concern that a regional cancer program would come at the expense of "care for local patients." Another noted that Memorial's inpatient census would suffer if they did not pursue the regional market. The market won to the benefit of both. In this instance, Memorial's timing was perfect.

The National Cancer Institute had just published a cancer atlas which named Sangamon County among the 200 United States counties with the highest cancer death rate. Nationally, the public focus on cancer began in the 1960s and reached its peak in the 1970s. In January 1971 President Richard M. Nixon announced an all-out campaign, with a sharp rise in National Cancer Institute funding. Popular culture both reflected and fed this heightened attention with enormously successful movies like **Love Story** and **Brian's Song.** Surgery for breast cancer came 'out of the closet' with the well publicized experiences of Shirley Temple and Betty Ford, while fad cures (laetrile) and occupational cancer hazards filled the news.

Late in 1969 Memorial radiologists and board members met at the St. Nicholas Hotel to discuss the possibility of establishing a radiation therapy service. George Hendrix had apparently met with St. John's executive vice president, Sr. Jane Like, and agreed that Memorial would proceed with construction of a radiation unit. Three years later, the board hired the firm of Will, Folsum, and Smith to conduct a fund drive feasibility study. Finally, Memorial launched a $1.6 million regional cancer program fund drive in 1976. Radiologist Dr. David Lewis, a pioneering area specialist in computerized tomography (CT), spearheaded the planning effort. In addition to funding space, the drive aimed to support the purchase of an EMI head scanner (for diagnosis) and a linear accelerator (for therapy). The board had already approved the purchase of the linear accelerator in 1975. The EMI scanner, the first such equipment in Illinois between St. Louis and Chicago, was purchased in 1976. Campaign funds were also used to initiate a regional tumor registry in 1977. The registry arrangement was with the University of Illinois. Initially, St. John's did not participate.

The board hired a fund raising firm, Ketchum, Inc., to run the campaign. Costs were expected to exceed $100,000, a considerable investment given

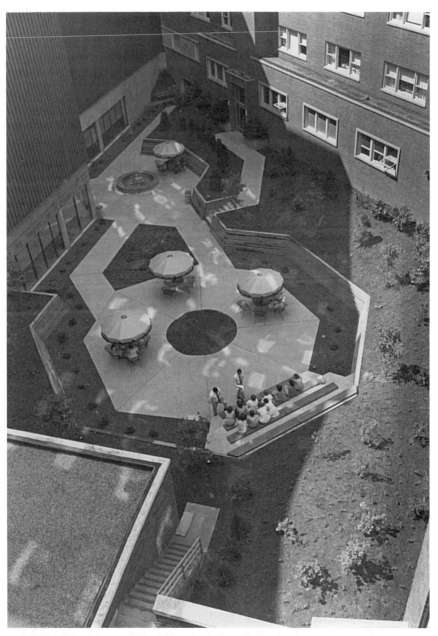

New building additions created vacant space that Dr. Chauncey Maher recommended developing into a courtyard adjacent to a small café. This inexpensive project was an instant success.

Memorial's tenuous financial situation. The drive was a resounding success. More than 400 fundraising volunteers were determined to decrease Sangamon County's cancer death rate. The campaign was chaired by Jack Watson with the assistance of Robert V. Prather, Jr., George E. Hatmaker, John Brubaker, Bruce Campbell, Jack Lisenbee, Lois Davis, and Judith Stephens. Though the campaign officially ended in December 1976, gifts and pledges continued for at least two more years. The Masons, an organization noted for its support of Protestant and secular hospitals, continued their tradition of generous support to Memorial with a $20,000 contribution. A victory celebration was scheduled at William Schnirring's rural property in July 1976, an appropriate commemoration of the nation's bicentennial. By late 1978 gifts exceeded $1,977,000.

Crisis in Nursing

In the half year between groundbreaking for a third Springfield hospital and Memorial's announcement of its own building program, it encountered another obstacle. Though the number of persons employed in the health care industry rose 55 per cent from 1970 to 1979, salaries across the country remained lower than the all-industry average. When hospitals moved to a market orientation, they caught the attention of organized labor. Due to their charitable role, hospitals had been exempted from the 1947 Taft-Hartley Act. Amendments made in August 1974 made hospitals subject to the law. In June, two months before the law became effective, the International Brotherhood of Laborers attempted to organize Memorial employees. The federal wage freeze had been lifted only a few months earlier, in April, and the board had immediately approved both wage and price increases, effective at the start of its next fiscal year in October. Memorial's circumstances were exacerbated by the recently granted wage increase at St. John's, which was effective earlier due to that hospital's July to June fiscal year. Phillips noted that Memorial lost personnel to both St. John's and Springfield Community Hospital.

Room rate increases were expected to generate an additional $1,800,000 per year and employees received an eight per cent wage increase. Late in 1974, room rates were again increased, this time in response to St. John's increase. The pending wage increase failed to derail unionization efforts. The campaign caught Memorial officials off guard as they grappled with fierce medical school, marketplace, financial, and regulatory pressures.

The National Labor Relations Board (NLRB) determined that all nonprofessional staff except clerical (856 employees) were eligible to vote in the election, which it conducted on January 31, 1975. The union lost by 102 votes.

The election did force Memorial to attend to labor issues that it had neglected due to other concerns. Board records listed a few areas in which the medical center may have been in violation of labor law. There were discrepancies in pay for similar work, notably aides versus orderlies and maids versus janitors. Some employees had been clocking in too early without being paid overtime, and the night shift was not allowed to take a lunch break away from the work area. The latter issue was attributed to too few employees, a situation that should have alerted officials to another smoldering issue. Departments with significant problems included dietary, housekeeping, nursing, and personnel. The unionization effort also resulted in improved salaries and employee benefits. Memorial reached a settlement with the federal Wage and Hour Division, which cost more than $110,000 in the first year. The effort did not completely satisfy the equal pay for equal work issue, which Memorial was required to accomplish by January 1, 1976. Employees had already been granted personal days in July 1975 and these measures strained the already shaky 1975 financial picture. As noted earlier, Phillips initiated a hiring freeze (except for graduates of the last nursing school class) in order to "reduce expenses."

Labor relations problems did not end with the union election. In another cost saving measure, Memorial entered into a contract with ServiceMaster, Inc. for housekeeping services in July 1976. The contract saved the medical center $109,000 in its first year, but created a reservoir of discontented employees. Records also note organizing activity that year in the engineering department.

Officials met the challenges created by the medical school and new federal laws and regulations with dogged determination. The pace and pressure of these demands caused the board to double the frequency of its meetings and probably contributed to its failure to notice the severe unrest that developed in nursing. The uproar surrounding the unpopular decision to close the nursing school was tame in comparison to the bitter and emotional controversy that erupted just seven months after the final graduation. There was already a nurse shortage when the school closure was announced. Nursing director Jean Nickels reported a shortage of more than 50 nurses to the medical staff executive committee in August 1971.

This problem was obscured by a unit staffing model that functioned poorly, and by the Rosenfeld consultants' reliance on national statistics that failed to reflect Memorial's dramatic growth. In the spring of 1976, there was tacit acknowledgment of difficulty in nursing when the board approved the employment of additional administrative staff to do "business and clerical functions" in order to relieve nurses of this burden. The shortage probably would not have grown to crisis proportions if the medical center had moved more cautiously and deliberately to phase out the school. Instead, officials bowed to the medical school's unrelenting pressure and initiated Rosenfeld's new concepts with insufficient consideration of the institution's history and culture. Memorial edged closer to a crisis that was at first invisible and then ignored.

About the time the school's closure was announced in 1973, New York passed the first nurse practice act, which recognized nursing as an autonomous profession. All states licensed professional nurses but the practice act went beyond licensure to provide statutory authority for the practice of nursing. Nurses enthusiastically embraced their professional autonomy and sought recognition for their vital contribution to health care. Nurse administrators assured the availability and quality of nursing care, an aspect of service which "could make or break a hospital's public image," a lesson Memorial learned the hard way. Dr. Humphrey Fluckiger witnessed the change in roles from the 1960s, when nurses were primarily care-givers, to an increased managerial role in the 1970s. He recalled that the best doctors paid close attention to what nurses said. As events unfolded at Memorial in 1976, this was also wise advice for administrators.

When Rosenfeld consultant Thomas Weil recommended a "major" reorganization of nursing, the board created a new position, assistant administrator of nursing (later changed to vice president). In keeping with both consultant recommendations as well as his own efforts to professionalize administration, George Phillips recruited Isabel (Peg) Letcher, who had experience in a teaching hospital and who held a master's degree in nursing. Creation of Letcher's position essentially caused Jean Nickels' demotion. Nickels, who had hired and worked with most of the nursing staff, was quite popular among them. The action spawned a sense of mistrust and insecurity among nurses.

Letcher introduced higher educational standards for head nurses. The idea was reasonable, as this was a national trend and a primary reason for her appointment. Phillips correctly observed that as Memorial grew, it needed more nurses with advanced skills and specialized experience. He believed that Springfield's traditional nurse providers (the two hospitals) could not supply these. According to Phillips, Rosenfeld's solution was to raise salaries and standards in order to recruit and retain this higher level nurse. Veteran nurses were threatened by the new specialists with higher pay, and they resisted the higher standards.

Unfortunately, Letcher (like Phillips) was a poor communicator and managed the transition poorly. One physician described her as "an ex-army type" who was "very authoritarian." Phillips verified that Letcher had a military background and discovered that she was, indeed, autocratic. According to veteran nurse Ed Quarry, Letcher implemented a "wheel approach" in nursing. With Letcher at the hub, key tasks were assigned to the spokes on the wheel. Tasks performed competently for years by non-degreed nurses were directed only to those with baccalaureate degrees. Letcher had correctly assumed that her role was to elevate nursing skills at Memorial and so required all supervisors to have baccalaureate degrees.

Instead of developing a cadre of nurses with specialized skills, Letcher's efforts had the opposite effect. As frustrated registered nurses resigned in unprecedented numbers and with no Memorial graduates to replace them, nursing heads were forced to adjust the skill mix to accommodate additional practical nurses and nursing assistants. As the medical school affiliation brought more complex procedures and equipment, the skill mix situation was disastrous. In addition to long hours, registered nurses were also forced to become "on-the-job teachers." They had already assumed this role with new medical students, described by one veteran nurse as "little whipper snappers." The shortage and dissension created a crisis which quickly spiraled out of control.

One administrator recalled that Letcher refused to make rounds or leave her office. It may have been fortunate that she rarely interacted with nurses. Quarry noted that she terrorized nurses, who avoided her because she constantly criticized and yelled at them, and swore in meetings. One physician recalled that Letcher and her senior managers stonewalled most requests for personnel and equipment and viewed those who made requests as "troublemakers."

When the shortage reached an acute point, the administration contacted doctors and urged them to dismiss patients early. Paul Smith, who was later appointed chief financial officer, resisted the decision and recommended that "we throw off our suit jackets and go empty bed pans." His advice went unheeded and the message to doctors sent alarm rumors racing around town and into the newspaper. In addition to the negative press, Phillips' young daughter received a death threat over the telephone. By chance, Phillips was out of town when the fight went public. While officials lamented the leak to the press, the scope and intensity of the controversy hardly lent itself to secrecy. Phillips recalled that he returned home to find "the whole place was in an uproar."

Press accounts cited a 30 per cent nursing shortage, with four to six beds in each of 22 nursing units closed due to lack of personnel. Nurses discussed a strike and Illinois Nurses Association representatives held several union organizational meetings with them. Quarry remembered that nurses complained to doctors because they did not dare complain to the administration. Nurse Wilma Fricke confirmed that doctors, particularly Chauncey Maher, supported nurses against Phillips and Letcher. Maher noted that board members had heard reports of trouble from many sources. He met with a dozen head nurses, all about to quit, approached Letcher several times to no avail, and finally warned Phillips of serious trouble. Phillips and other board members were already aware of the gravity of the situation. Several weeks prior to the press coverage, he reported receipt of two letters from the Laborers International Union, notifying Memorial of its intent to organize nurses.

Phillips maintained that the shortage issue was overblown, issues were taken out of context, and rumors exacerbated the problem. His credibility was destroyed, however, when he publicly denied that all nurse supervisors were required to hold degrees, only to discover that the policy was printed in Letcher's handbook. Phillips claimed that Letcher misrepresented hospital policy on credentials to him and trapped him in public embarrassment. While he did not create the policy, he acquiesced and thus was held responsible. A second protested policy required part-time nursing staff to "float" assignments and shifts.

At a June 18, 1976 meeting of the board's steering committee, Phillips recommended and members unanimously agreed to suspend the two nursing policies immediately. Chick Lanphier, Bill Schnirring, and Robert Prather, who were present at this meeting, also agreed to require resignations from Letcher and both the director and associate director of clinical nursing. The latter two, caught in political purgatory, were offered the opportunity to reapply for other nursing positions, an offer both refused.

Just two weeks earlier, the board planned to recognize one of these managers, the director of clinical nursing, for her outstanding job as co-organizer of the employee fund drive. The employee portion of the cancer fund drive had set a goal of $150,000 and exceeded it by $100,000.

Letcher's exit was cause for celebration by nurses, who continued for several years to bring cakes in honor of the event. Medical staff president John Allen approached Ed Quarry to suggest that he succeed Letcher, then accompanied him to discuss the appointment with Phillips. At Quarry's insistence Phillips met with nurses, a heated meeting with open hostility to Phillips. When he had met with board members, Phillips announced his intention to meet with both the medical staff executive committee and with nurses and, if he did not have their support, he would resign. With a characteristically standoffish approach, Phillips asked Boyd to test staff opinion. Boyd later reported, "George, they say you've got to go." Phillips offered his resignation at a medical staff meeting. Drs. John Allen and John Standard were particularly insistent that Phillips had to leave.

When Phillips formally submitted his resignation to the board at their next meeting, the board invited supporters to speak on his behalf. The support was insufficient. One board member thought Phillips probably hoped that his resignation would not be accepted and that if Phillips had sought board support he might have gotten it. Bill Schnirring, however, noted that Phillips "acted with great courage." Veteran board member Walter Lohman recalled that the board was so preoccupied with the crisis that they met informally at a social gathering to discuss it. Key medical staff were apparently also there. Dr. John Denby recalled that this secret, rump meeting occurred at Bill Schnirring's weekend property, which had been prepared for his daughter's wedding. There, under a bridal canopy, the group decided to accept Phillips' resignation. Schnirring, who also recalled meeting with medical staff at his home, noted that the board was at first divided over Phillips' resignation but finally concluded that he could not reverse the situation. He had failed to step in, then remained passive and detached as the crisis mounted. By temperament, he was ill-suited to placate or reassure people.

When asked to analyze the situation which developed in nursing, former medical center president Jack Cook noted that the crisis which occurred in 1976 stemmed directly from the nursing school closure and was immensely aggravated by Letcher's hard line and remoteness. The school's closure not only shut off the pipeline of new nurses but also deprived Memorial of the

Jack Cook

In his role as President of Memorial Medical Center, Jack Cook concentrated on building cordial relations. He was remarkably adept at it. He could afford to concentrate on public relations because, as he observed, "the place was being well run before I got to be CEO." At the time he was appointed president, he knew Bill Schnirring (from church) but no other board members. Cook recalled, "I got to be CEO at that hospital because I was popular with the doctors. It was that simple." In marked contrast to George Phillips, Cook enjoyed a broad base of support, from doctors, nurses, the community, the press, patients, and board members. He was also politically astute. Dr. Chauncey Maher described him as a "real nice guy" with "the manners of a southern gentleman and the instincts of a barracuda."

Even his staunchest allies noted weaknesses, including a hesitancy to push Memorial to new plateaus or pursue risky opportunities. The downside of his focus on public relations was a tendency to defer or avoid prickly issues. He happily let Russell Beckwith be the administration "heavy." Cook was the right man for his time but was not a dynamic leader for the nineties. For example, one former administrator observed that Memorial was not as well prepared for the prospective payment system as it might have been.

Nurse Ed Quarry noted that Cook had a "personal touch you would not believe." He toured the hospital daily, knew employees' first names, noted their birthdays, and asked about their families. He established a variety of goodwill programs, including an annual employee service dinner, public recognition of donors and board members, etc. Cook considered the shared service agreements his greatest achievements. Dr. Grant Johnson summed him up as an "entirely trustworthy" and "good and competent man."

students who had always served as nursing aides. Ed Quarry recalled that he and other nurses worked 16 and 20-hour days and that patients had to be shifted from understaffed wings. Another nurse manager, Wilma Fricke, confirmed that the school's closure made hiring a constant challenge and one of her "biggest headaches." She, too, recalled that nurses often worked overtime and double shifts.

Paul Smith described the crisis as "not a pretty situation." A president, vice president, and two other managers were terminated. Smith noted, "I was spending a good deal of time writing severance checks." With Memorial's capital campaign underway, it was a particularly awkward time for a public uproar. To Bill Schnirring, who had been board chairman for only four months, "it seemed like everything … was going wrong."

Let the Kid Do It

Former vice president Russell Beckwith felt that the crisis was not only overblown but also a pretext for disgruntled nurses, doctors, and board members to fire Phillips, "an excuse to get rid of him." Both Phillips and Letcher had built walls instead of bridges and Phillips was unpopular with many longtime doctors, who associated him with the threatening influx of new SIU doctors. After formally approving Phillips' resignation, the board immediately appointed Jack Cook, who had been at Memorial for only two years and had less experience and seniority than other administrators. This abrupt action was unusual, and a reflection of the crisis condition.

A factor which may have contributed to Phillips' demise was Jack Cook's popularity. As vice president for professional services, he had developed close ties with staff and physicians. Russell Beckwith recalled that Cook's presence made it easier to take the risk of ousting Phillips and observed "they liked Jack better than they liked George." Like Phillips, Cook held a graduate degree in hospital administration from Duke University.

While Dr. John Allen worked to recruit Ed Quarry as nursing head, medical staff president-elect John Standard also took matters into his own hands. Without the board's knowledge, he reached Cook, who was vacationing in South Carolina, to announce that Phillips would lose his job and asked if he would be interested. It was an awkward moment for Cook, who got along well with Phillips and did not wish to undermine him. Phillips had also called Cook to let him know "how bad it was." Cook made it clear to Standard that he would be interested only if Phillips was "out." Standard then reassured the board that Cook would do a good job and urged them to "let the kid do it." A few days later, Bill Schnirring called to offer the job to 31-year-old Cook, who immediately cut short his vacation and flew back to Springfield.

There was some concern among board members whether Cook had enough experience to be president, so they made the appointment temporary, with the title of executive vice president. Schnirring devised this plan and candidly explained to Cook that too much damage had already occurred. He promised that the board would protect him (assure him a position) but that they wanted to be able to appoint a different president if that became necessary.

Cook developed a strategy for reversing the crisis and was determined first to obtain board and top management support, then calm nurses and medical staff. Upon his return, he immediately met with department heads in a basement room of the Medical Arts Building, ironically the former Nurse Education Unit. The atmosphere was rife with speculation and rumors. It was a dramatic moment and turning point for Memorial as Cook announced the terminations and his interim appointment. He asked for their patience, calm and support.

Cook won the board's support so quickly that he was officially named president in only a few months. In order to gain credibility with top management, some of whom doubted that he had the necessary experience, he convened them and directly enlisted their support, only one of many examples of his forthright manner. Notably with John Standard's assistance, Cook relied upon his ties with medical staff to calm the turbulence. He delayed naming a new vice president for nursing because he thought it would create further anxiety. Instead, he appointed Lincoln (Link) Tumey to act in the role and promoted Ed Quarry to director of nursing. Jim Rigby was promoted to Cook's prior position. Rigby had earned his graduate degree in hospital administration from the University of Missouri, where his mentor was Thomas Weil, Rosenfeld's principal consultant at Memorial. Rigby had been hired during the 1973 reorganization as Director of Support Services under Bill Boyd.

According to Quarry, Cook met with him immediately to pledge his assistance, "anytime, day or night," and implored Quarry to take all possible steps to persuade nurses to return to Memorial. Quarry visited nurses

Memorial Meals

Though Memorial's services became more diverse and sophisticated with the medical school's arrival, its outreach efforts continued to focus on basic community needs. Veteran dietitian Eunice Scott recalled that Memorial's dietary staff prepared Springfield's first Meals on Wheels in March 1973. A local nursing home owner, Clarence Ramshaw, initiated the community effort and dietitian Marguerite Saxer represented Memorial on a planning committee. St. John's was in the midst of a building program so Memorial assumed sole responsibility for meal preparation. Scott recalled, "We served one meal the first week, two the second, three the third." Eventually, Memorial prepared thousands of meals. Conn's Catering and St. John's later assisted. Scott concluded, "we are indeed proud, as a department, to reach out with our services to the community."

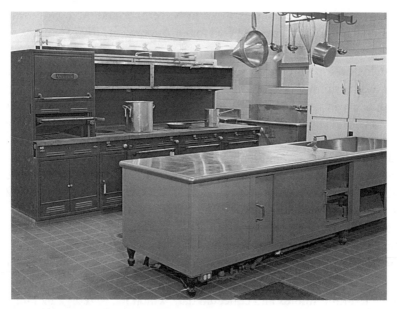

Dietary staff had ample space and the latest equipment when they moved to the new building in 1943.

in their homes and persuaded many to return with full restoration of benefits. He recalled that Cook desperately wanted to avert unionization, conferred with him daily, and frequently accompanied him on rounds. Cook worked around the clock, seven days a week, and Quarry described him as a "wonderful man" who "pulled us through" the crisis. Schnirring concurred that Cook did a "miraculous job."

Only one week after the three nurses were fired the board reported that morale had "greatly improved." Within the first month, Cook held a press conference and outlined his strategy for a complete makeover of the nursing department. He also met with the nursing school Alumni Association, at its request, to share the goals already in progress. These included a reorganization of the nursing department in a more simplified structure, revision of all nursing job descriptions, and the addition of more nursing staff. Within three weeks of Letcher's departure in June, 45 RNs and LPNs (licensed practical nurses) as well as 49 nursing assistants had been hired. Though this brought the number of nursing staff to its budgeted level, Cook considered the number inadequate for the higher patient acuity in a teaching hospital. At least 73 beds were closed at the peak of the crisis. A number of these remained closed in November and the board declared that nurse recruitment would be a "major priority" in 1977.

In order to meet his goals, Cook brought in a consulting firm, Ernst & Ernst, to develop a program to improve nurse staffing practices, and initiated vigorous recruitment efforts. Records note the presence of a nurse recruiter, Jeri Easley, in September. She and other Memorial representatives traveled to Canada and New York to recruit nurses. Quarry recalled hiring nine nurses in Toronto. Memorial paid their relocation expenses, helped them find housing, and assisted them with preparation for state board examinations. At the time of the crisis, Memorial's turnover rate was 27 per cent (still lower than the national average of 35 per cent), but it dropped to 22.5 per cent one year later. By 1980 the rate was a miraculous 19 per cent compared to the national rate of 31 per cent. Quarry attributed the reduced turnover rates to steadily improving nurse salaries and benefits.

Ernst & Ernst identified problems with low weekend staffing and an inability to adjust day to day staffing levels. Quarry and these consultants conducted time studies and collected data which led to reorganization and reallocation of nursing staff. An acuity system (a means to allocate staff based on the level of care required by patients) was installed as well as a new nursing care delivery model, modular nursing. Sometimes called "block nursing," modular nursing was a radical departure from Letcher's dictatorship. It gave nurses the opportunity to exercise judgment and autonomy and replaced the directive management style with mentoring. A nurse from Rush-Presbyterian-St. Luke's Hospital in Chicago worked with consultants to train Memorial nurses on the new concept. The new modality of care was instituted in May 1977 and created small groups of nurses to care for small groups of patients. Quarry described it as total nursing care, in which a single nurse performed all procedures rather than the team nursing approach in which some nurses specialized in medication, others in testing, etc.

Though Memorial's challenges remained, the crisis was over. Ironically, many enduring achievements originated immediately in the wake of the 1976 crisis. Several years of breakneck change and turmoil had preceded it. Difficult as it was, the crisis had a cathartic effect on Memorial. The medical center which emerged was a more mature and thoughtful institution, one that had made it through adolescence and embarked on a new post-Lanphier era.

In the mid-1970s Memorial's board was restive. Several members agreed that the pace set in the 1940s no longer worked. Both Phillips and Cook recalled Lanphier's casual, anecdotal, and rambling meetings. His domineering style was also outmoded and new board members resented it. Schnirring, who had joined the board in 1968 after Fred Schlitt's death, was tapped for the board due to his "strong involvement" with the Masons, a characteristic he shared with Schlitt. As noted earlier, the Masons contributed generously when Schlitt and, later, Schnirring served on the board.

Lanphier became ill in 1975 and asked Schnirring to chair the board in 1976, probably because Memorial was about to launch a capital fund drive and Schnirring had fundraising experience as head of Springfield's 1975 United Way campaign. Phillips was considered Lanphier's man because Lanphier had selected him. In what looked like a 'palace coup,' the Schnirring faction accepted Phillips' resignation and hired Cook while Lanphier was ill and in Michigan. Though Lanphier continued to serve on the board until his death in 1978, the action signaled the end of the Lanphier era. His illness removed him from an active role, and Schnirring rose to leadership. Despite their differences in style, Schnirring kept Lanphier informed about board business while he was in Michigan.

Jack Cook recalled at least two occasions when his style collided with Lanphier's. As already noted, Lanphier responded to complaints or problems that he heard at social gatherings. One Sunday morning, Cook received a call from Lanphier, who demanded immediate action on a problem he heard about at a cocktail party the previous evening. Cook knew that the problem was a chronic one and refused to jump at gossip. He recalled saying, "Mr. Lanphier, if you want to run this hospital on cocktail gossip, you'd better have me at the cocktail party."

During this time, Memorial expanded its market via the development of shared service agreements with outlying hospitals. The medical center shared a variety of services, both clinical and managerial, with 20 hospitals and 16 nursing homes in the region. Cook sought board approval for each new hospital agreement. He remembered that the Pittsfield hospital agreement was pending board approval when Lanphier stopped at his office to chat. Lanphier abruptly said, "You may think you know what you're doing here, but you're not prepared to run any hospital outside of Springfield, and we're not going to do that." Lanphier had drawn a line in the sand, only to watch it wash away in a tidal shift in the board's behavior. Lanphier's was the only "no" vote on the Pittsfield agreement. In the past, there would not even have been a vote if Lanphier expressed opposition. In 1977, Memorial signed a one-year management contract with Illini Community Hospital in Pittsfield. By 1979, Memorial had 90 service agreements.

Bill Schnirring came to the board with an agenda, and his record was impressive. He influenced the positive outcome of the nursing crisis with his support of Cook, and the capital campaign during his tenure was among the most successful in Memorial's history. More important, though, were the positive and enduring changes which still remained visible in Memorial's centennial year. As the nation celebrated the 200th anniversary of its revolution, Schnirring and Cook led Memorial through a crisis and into a new era.

Era of Good Feeling

Under Schnirring's leadership the board developed structure and routine. Cook sent monthly written reports and other materials to members before meetings, which began and ended punctually. There was a precise agenda which included only a few issues for discussion. A strong committee and reporting system was developed and the board focused on overall policy and drifted away from micro management. The most significant shift, however, was in the board's attitude toward physicians. Schnirring recalled that when he arrived on the board there was a deep-seated "paranoia" against doctors on the board, especially by Lanphier, who feared that doctors would divulge confidential matters to St. John's. Cook described it as a "mind set" sacred to Lanphier. Veteran board member Walter Lohman noted that the addition of physicians to the board was "long overdue." As early as 1973 Schnirring suggested that the medical staff president and president elect be invited to board meetings at least quarterly to discuss any topic of their choosing. During the 1976 fund drive, Schnirring met with the medical staff and was amazed by how "uninformed" they were. Both Cook and Schnirring frequently invited them to meetings, a practice that was formalized in 1981, when Drs. William Sherrick and John Denby attended regularly as official "guests." Further incremental change came in 1983, when Denby and John Allen were listed as "ex-officio" members. By 1986, when Allen and Barry Free served, the medical staff officers had full voting status. Fortunately, Memorial had a series of particularly capable and conscientious medical staff presidents during this period, including Drs. John Allen, John Standard, Charles Wabner, William Sherrick, and John Denby.

While Memorial changed, so did its milieu. Before the 1970s, voluntary community hospitals operated as quasi-public institutions and enjoyed a number of privileges and exemptions. When hospitals embraced the corporate model they forfeited some of these advantages. In a landmark 1978 Michigan case, *Parker v. Highland Park,* the court declared that all hospitals were businesses and were subject to tort liability.

At the same time, the successful 1976 capital campaign led to enduring achievements. Walter Lohman urged the creation of an arms-length endowment entity to protect Memorial from future government claims that it had its own assets. Schnirring was a key leader in the creation of the Memorial Medical Center Foundation, first approved by the board in 1976. Initially, the board formed the Community Relations and Fund Development committee chaired by Schnirring. There were sub-committees on annual giving, deferred giving (estates), recognition of donors, and others which regularly reported to the board. The foundation was incorporated in August 1981, when lawyers advised the board to reorganize Memorial's corporate structure and legally separate its various distinct activities. The restructuring protected the medical center's non-patient services from rate review regulations and enabled it to add new services readily by creating a parent organization (holding company) and a multi-institutional structure. It also sheltered the foundation's assets. Schnirring was the first foundation chair and received assistance from board member and lawyer Norman Jones.

Discussion of changes to the organizational structure occurred throughout the summer and were approved in September 1981. The old 14-member executive committee was eliminated and redesignated as the new board of directors of Memorial Medical Center, a change originally suggested by Rosenfeld. The medical center became a controlled affiliate of the parent corporation while the foundation gained its own board. The majority of the foundation's board members could not be from Memorial. The separate foundation also enabled Memorial to ensure that contributions were tax deductible. In 1982 the Internal Revenue Service accepted the foundation's tax exempt status. In its first four years the foundation raised more than $2 million.

Friends of Memorial Medical Center was also born in the capital campaign and was closely linked to development efforts. Cook and Bill Boyd worked with Judy (Mrs. Harvey B.) Stephens, Shirley (Mrs. Robert C. III) Lanphier, and Elaine (Mrs. Lawrence) Hoff to reorganize the auxiliary and volunteer programs in 1977. According to Schnirring, Memorial needed more external exposure and goodwill. He looked toward the creation of a more aggressive and creative citizen's group that would provide community services such as health education.

Friends replaced both the hospital auxiliary and hospital club. In less than a year, it had 400 dues paying members. In addition to fundraising, the organization sponsored many community events and medical center activities, including health seminars, hospital tours, scholarships for hospital employees' children, an "art" cart for patients, Tel-Med (automated, telephone health information), and numerous others. One extremely successful Friends program was "Medical Madness." The aim of the program was both fundraising and community goodwill, the latter to showcase hospital staff and doctors in a different light, as entertainers. Bonnie (Mrs. Charles) Wabner was a key organizer and the original chorus of entertainers included Cook, Beckwith, and Drs. Sherrick, Glen Pittman, and Alan Birtch. Friends quickly became a large and invaluable group of Memorial ambassadors.

Diplomatic relations with St. John's also improved. Schnirring was pivotal in opening dialog with St. John's after what he described as a period of "really bad" relations, fraught with gossip, name calling, contempt, and silence. Even the intense rivalry of the 1960s and early 1970s was peppered with notable attempts to bridge the gap. Veteran board member Bob Oxtoby recalled that his 1960s overture to Sr. Jane Like was greeted cordially. George Hendrix and Bill Boyd also had successful meetings with Sr. Jane. Late in 1967 Memorial's board had approved a Joint Conference Committee, intended for joint meetings with St. John's board on matters related to "which hospital provides which service." The most successful cooperative efforts were those conducted well below that administrative level, notably among nursing staff and with St. John's School of Dietetics.

These efforts, however, did not overcome the pressures of the marketplace, intensified by the third hospital, the medical school, and doctors. The rivalry resulted in excellent quality and availability of services but higher hospital costs. Services were duplicated and unprofitable ones were embraced for prestige and competitive advantage. Ironically, SIU spurred both competition and cooperation between its two teaching hospitals and the arrival of Humana created a common enemy as well as increased competition.

In 1976 there occurred a notable shift in the hospitals' relationship. Schnirring and Cook made the era of rapprochement possible. Following a 1976 meeting of the First National Bank board, Jack Clarke (St. John's lay advisory board) approached Schnirring with his concern about Memorial's capital drive for a regional cancer program and the duplication of services it created. Clarke said, "We should try to get the hospitals together." Schnirring and Walter Lohman readily agreed, though other Memorial board members would have resisted this effort. Schnirring met with Carl Forth, president of St. John's lay advisory board, to discuss opening a dialog. Hugh Graham (St. John's) hosted a luncheon at the Illini Country Club on April 28, 1976. Members of the two boards aired many issues and agreed to continue meeting and to rotate hosts. Meetings with St. John's improved further with Cook's arrival and Bob Oxtoby's assistance. Schnirring recalled that this informal group was later dubbed the SAM committee (Saints And Memorial) and that "a lot of good came from it."

Friends

Memorial's first organized group of volunteers, the Springfield Hospital Club, was organized in 1909 then changed its name in concert with the hospital's, first to Memorial Hospital Club, then the Medical Center Guild. Meanwhile, with a charter membership of 74 women, the Women's Auxiliary was founded in 1932, an outgrowth of the hospital non-sectarian reorganization. Unlike the Club, the Auxiliary reported to the Board of Directors and had a vital role in funding, furnishing, and staffing the 1943 hospital. Auxiliary membership appears to have peaked in the late 1950s with about 2800 members.

The Auxiliary met monthly at the Masonic Temple for many years to fold bandages, sew hospital bedding, and make patient tray favors. The 1945 president, Pauline (Mrs. Alan) Myers, cited additional accomplishments such as redecorating and furnishing the Nurses Home. Another important early Auxiliary leader was Katherine L. (Mrs. Harry W.) Watson, who served at least 5 terms as president. The organization raised thousands of dollars for construction, a nursing school bus, automatic washers and other appliances, and student loans. In addition to dues and ice cream socials, the Auxiliary's concerts were particularly successful fundraisers. Audiences were enthralled by Lily Pons, the Hour of Charm All Girl Orchestra, and Nelson Eddy, who was so impressed with the Auxiliary's enthusiasm that he donated $500 to his own concert fund-raiser. In 1960 the Springfield Junior League initiated a two-year trial program to recruit volunteers for Memorial and successfully generated 29,555 hours donated by 427 volunteers. At that time the Director of Housekeeping also directed volunteers and in 1963 the board voted to create a separate department and hired Elaine Hoff as first director.

continued ...

With the changing of the guard in 1976, Jack Cook, Bill Schnirring, and Bill Boyd hoped to also reorganize and reinvigorate volunteer programs. The JCAH had recommended by-laws changes to better organize the "two ancillary women's organizations," the Auxiliary and the Guild. The Guild disbanded in February 1977 due to its inability to recruit new officers. Later that year, a reorganization luncheon was held at the Sangamo Club. Judy Stephens was a key organizer. The newly merged organization, Friends of Memorial Medical Center, soon boasted 400 members. The women who organized Friends were leaders whose business acumen showed in the breadth and success of their endeavors. A newsletter and logo set the tone. The logo's three interlocking rings represented Memorial, the community, and health care and symbolized a broader commitment to education and community service. The Friends organization was the quintessential example of Memorial's community partnerships.

A Seat at the Table

Prior to the medical school's opening, Memorial had passed up the opportunity to pioneer cardiac surgery in Springfield. The board took no action in 1964 when Dr. James Graham approached them to suggest the establishment of cardiac diagnostic and surgical services. He also approached St. John's. Graham had recruited two physicians to Springfield Clinic who had "expertise in this field," Drs. Robert A. Harp and Paul Smalley. Dr. Graham estimated hospital costs at $125,000 as well as required changes in facilities.

According to both Bill Boyd and Dr. Chauncey Maher, Harp and Smalley first approached Memorial but officials balked at the heavy investment in space and equipment. Evidently the board felt that prospects for cardiac service were not promising in a small city like Springfield. Maher also noted that Springfield Clinic had traditionally been more closely tied with St. John's and that the doctors would probably have favored that hospital anyway.

By the late 1970s the climate had changed. Memorial's new and enlarged cadre of businessmen formed a phalanx determined to overcome a 75-year reputation as the hospital always a step behind St. John's. Former administrator Jim Rigby remembered Memorial as the "kid brother" always seeking parity. Heart surgery was glamorous, profitable, and prestigious. Under Jack Cook's youthful and ambitious leadership, Memorial made a concerted effort to shed its 'Avis complex.' As Cook recalled, "we deserved a seat at the table in cardiac surgery."

In 1973 Rosenfeld had recommended that cardiac surgery be performed "solely at St. John's Hospital" until the number of cases justified consideration at Memorial. By 1979 the time seemed ripe. St. John's surgery schedule reached capacity and created delays, a condition which apparently persisted for several years. Doctors who were dissatisfied with delays supported cardiac surgery at Memorial. Cook acknowledged that local cardiac physicians manipulated Memorial for both personal gain and leverage at St. John's. He accepted this with a characteristically positive outlook. "Memorial needed to come up a notch or two in its sophistication to really go into the world." In turn, Memorial officials used cardiologists and surgeons as their ratchet.

Memorial transferred its cardiac catheterization patients to St. John's for surgery and administrators concluded that 38 per cent of St. John's heart surgery patients had been catheterized at Memorial. The addition of cardiac surgery was considered an important, patient-focused service. Patients, however, were not as vocal as physicians. One veteran administrator recalled that the "non-Prairie" thoracic surgeons and cardiologists (those not associated with either Prairie Cardiovascular Consultants, Ltd. or Prairie Thoracic and Cardiovascular Surgeons) chafed at playing "second fiddle" and prodded Memorial to start a program.

Dr. Robert McGann approached Jack Cook on several occasions in 1979 to express interest in open heart surgery at Memorial. Cook then requested letters of support from cardiac surgeons. Late that year Memorial hired Touche Ross, Inc. to conduct a feasibility study. Theodore Druhot, St. John's executive vice president, shared data with the firm, which reported that the demand was sufficient and the service could be established for only $183,000. The board voted to proceed with a certificate of need in February 1980.

Two months later, board records noted that St. John's intended to oppose Memorial's effort. Willard Bunn, chairman of St. John's lay advisory board, wrote a letter published in the **State Journal-Register,** publicly opposing Memorial's plan. Despite opposition and unanswered questions, Memorial's board was already committed to open heart surgery in 1980. Bill Schnirring stated that it was only a question of "when." By July the board had amended its master plan to reflect this intent.

The first effort was apparently thwarted by disagreements with doctors, though these are not explained in records. Then Dr. Anthony Hawe renewed board interest with a presentation in late 1981. Cook made it clear at that board meeting that cardiac surgery, if done, would be done on Memorial's terms and "not on the terms of the cardiac surgeons" specified two years earlier. A special committee was created to study the proposed service. In the midst of the effort to complete its feasibility study, Memorial also won certificate of need approval for a second catheterization lab, to augment the approximately 200 procedures performed annually and to improve the existing lab, which was overcrowded and had eight-year-old equipment.

In January 1982, Chicago architects Perkins & Will were retained to design two additional floors to the D building. Echoing earlier conflicts, complaints from local architects led to an invitation for them to also make presentations. Bill Boyd recalled that Memorial's failure to use local architects was a "bit of a sore point." Local architects lacked experience in hospital design and construction, so Memorial tended to favor them only for small and unspecialized projects. The board estimated that the addition would cost $4 million. On May 12, 1982 it deferred a final decision but authorized administration to proceed with architectural plans, a financial study, and preparation of a certificate of need application. Updates on the plans were presented at nearly every board meeting.

The board discussed the issue at length at its meeting on October 13, 1982. The estimated cost, which required an additional two floors on the D building, had risen to $6 million. New, dedicated operating rooms were required and existing catheterization labs had to be relocated. With an optimism and determination that imitated the 1942 board's building effort, members expected to fund 80 per cent of the cost ($4.8 million) from contributions, with remaining funds to be absorbed by the 1983 and 1984 capital budgets. Representatives from Price Waterhouse were present to affirm the financial feasibility. Several physicians, including Drs. Hawe, Sherrick, Allen and Denby, answered board questions. Cook recommended action and the board finally approved the submission of the certificate of need.

Though many administrators and nursing officials were involved in data collection for the CON application, Jim Rigby was pivotal in developing the documents. He speculated that Memorial's application may have been the state's first one for heart surgery because St. John's program started prior to the certificate of need rules. He noted that Memorial had the further advantage of an established cardiac catheterization program that illustrated both demand and competence. The application, a large document that Rigby described as a "book," addressed projected needs and financing. It first was presented for approval to the regional Health Planning Agency (HSA) and then to the state HSA.

Preparation of the CON application was only part of the process to win approval of the open heart surgery service. Memorial officials made careful plans to win the "political battle" as well. Key physician allies were Drs. Hawe, McGann, Roland Folse (SIU), and William Lynch. Blue Cross, however, actively and publicly opposed Memorial on the grounds of cost and duplication of services. Jack Clarke, **State Journal-Register** publisher and a member of St. John's lay advisory board, spoke against the plan at a Memorial board meeting, and also informed members that he had assigned a reporter to investigate the issue. Generally, St. John's opposition was quiet, perhaps because, as one administrator recalled, Memorial's service would not seriously dent St. John's workload. As late as one month prior to the first CON hearing, Memorial board members agreed that St. John's opposition was "limited." Cook assured board members that he had staff actively seeking community support and asked them to attend the regional HSA hearing, scheduled February 3, 1983 at the city council chamber in Jacksonville.

In a carefully orchestrated strategy, Memorial "packed the room" with supporters. Ted Druhot and others from St. John's were forced to stand outside. Rigby made the presentation because Cook could not. He happened to serve on the HSA, which voted 11 to 3 in favor of the application. A nearly identical strategy worked in Chicago at the state Planning Board hearing, where the application won approval on a 11 to 0 vote, with one abstention. Both Jim Rigby and Jack Cook recalled that the CON approval was a "big step" in converting Memorial to a tertiary care center, equal in stature to St. John's.

At the same meeting at which they approved open heart surgery, the board also heard a disturbing report on a freak accident in the renal dialysis unit. As part of a routine winterization process, maintenance workers added antifreeze to pipes in a rooftop water tower. The system was not meant to be connected to hospital plumbing but, by some mix-up, the antifreeze entered dialysis unit water lines. Jack Cook recalled that the plumbing plans had been approved by the State. Six dialysis patients accidentally received ethylene glycol solution (antifreeze). A physician quickly observed that something was terribly wrong and instituted immediate counter action. The source of the problem was discovered by a toxicology technician in Memorial's pathology department. Dr. Grant Johnson described it as a "sharp observation."

Following the tragic incident, Memorial immediately engaged an engineering consultant to inspect the facility and design a fail-safe system. Though one patient later died, an autopsy failed to attribute death to the accident. Hospital officials had immediately notified families and "were straightforward" about the incident. Jack Cook recalled that the tragedy, which was reported in the **Wall Street Journal,** was a huge embarrassment. Inevitably, lawsuits followed but were settled out of court.

Despite setbacks and challenges, Memorial Medical Center had made immense and impressive progress. Bill Schnirring attributed Memorial's success in achieving parity with St. John's to SIU's growth. He acknowledged that SIU did not favor Memorial but that the medical center's proximity and faster response than St. John's was a major boost. With its open heart surgery victory, Memorial crossed a symbolic border. No longer the hospital always a step behind, Memorial had become a resilient and tough competitor.

Memorial Milestones

1983	Robert Clarke succeeds Jack Cook as president
	New Medicare payment plan (DRGs)
1984	Humana Hospital antitrust suit
	First open heart surgery
	Membership in Voluntary Hospitals of America
	New long range plan
1986	Installation of first downstate lithotripter
	Abortive HMO: "Pro Health Illinois"
1990	E Building construction (1987-1991)
1992	Family Maternity Suites
	New name: Memorial Health System
	Joint venture: Baylis Medical Building
	"Independence Square"
1994	Healthcare Network Associates (HCNA)
	HMO: "Health Alliance"
	Lincoln and Taylorville hospital affiliations
	Affiliation: Mental Health Centers of Central Illinois
	Joint venture: Heritage Enterprises
1997	Centennial

Chapter Eight

Quiet Revolution

As Memorial Medical Center approached its tenth decade, profound changes and challenges lay ahead for the nation's health care industry. Dubbed by some experts as a "quiet revolution," these manifold trends were destined to wreak havoc on the habits and norms that had brought unprecedented growth and prosperity to American hospitals and physicians since World War II. Fierce marketplace competition, stringent new federal cost controls, shrinking occupancy levels and the spread of health maintenance organizations (HMOs) were just some of the startling developments that would test the wits and resources of hospital governing boards, executives, physicians and employees in the closing years of the 20th century.

Memorial confronted the successive waves of change with a new administrative team and a vigorous board that generally managed to overcome all perils and capitalize on all opportunities. Their numerous accomplishments positioned the institution for growth and success in uncertain times. They quickly adapted to the new financial realities imposed by Washington and third party payers. They modernized governance and administrative affairs and also cemented good working relations with SIU Medical School and their neighboring rival, St. John's Hospital.

They responded to the erosion of traditional inpatient demand by expanding outpatient services. Recognizing a need for diversification, they acquired auxiliary enterprises and pursued joint ventures much in the manner of an aggressive conglomerate. They emulated successful business organizations through focused attention to long range planning and comprehensive marketing. In an era of cost containment they still managed to upgrade and expand various medical and surgical services, creating "centers of excellence" that won Memorial stature as a regional tertiary care center.

Such an impressive record of success exacted its own price in the form of high administrative turnover and a few missteps and setbacks. But as the millennium approached, Memorial could face its own second century from an enviable position of financial strength, heightened stature and clear vision.

Challenge and Change

After eight years at the hospital and six as president, Jack Cook was ready for a career move. His adroit management of the 1976 crisis and his many steps to improve staff morale were known in health care circles and among executive search firms. Late in 1982 he informed board chairman Robert Saner and key colleagues that he was under consideration for a metropolitan hospital position. The next April he left Memorial for the presidency of Christ Hospital in Cincinnati, Ohio. The timing was propitious; Cook had largely accomplished his own agenda, and there were new challenges on the health care horizon that would require a different executive style and outlook. During the interregnum veteran administrator Bill Boyd was asked to serve as acting president. Never interested in the job on a permanent basis, Boyd was a natural choice because of his wide experience and high standing throughout the hospital and the community.

Saner headed a search committee that included other board members and several physicians. An executive search firm recruited external candidates and screened the pool, which included two internal applicants, Russell Beckwith and Jim Rigby. Beckwith was the more seasoned of the two, and he enjoyed support among several board members. The narrowed field of finalists included him and Robert T. Clarke, executive vice president and chief operating officer at Community Hospital in Indianapolis, Indiana. Clarke held a master's degree in Hospital Administration from the University of Michigan, and he had risen steadily through the ranks during his 15 years at Community Hospital.

The Clarke Imprint

By 2007 Robert T. Clarke had spent 24 eventful years as president and CEO of Memorial Health System. It was a volatile and risky age for hospital executives, and his lengthy tenure was atypical. Several board members attributed this to the comfortable fit between his strengths and Memorial's needs. Aggressive, competitive, demanding, mentally systematic and highly focused, Clarke had both a clear vision and a firm hand on the institution's future. No one in the sprawling enterprise could honestly speculate over who was in charge.

A hard edge in his professional dealings belied Clarke's cordial and engaging personality. Even those former subordinates whom he encouraged or forced to leave spoke respectfully of his leadership. Officials at St. John's Hospital and SIU School of Medicine regarded him as a tough but reasonable negotiator who kept his word.

As head of a large regional health system, Clarke readily sensed both the responsibility and the opportunity to be active in professional, civic and public affairs. Among many assignments and honors, he is a Fellow of the American College of Healthcare Executives, member of the AHA House of Delegates, board member of the National Council of Community Hospitals and charter board member of VHA Great Rivers, Inc. Previously he served as chairman of VHA Great Rivers, president of the Association of Community Cancer Centers, and chairman of the Illinois Hospital Association's board of trustees. His many civic assignments have included board memberships for Downtown Springfield, the Council of Teaching Hospitals of the Association of American Medical Colleges, the Greater Springfield Chamber of Commerce and the United Way of Central Illinois. Upon his retirement, Clarke became an Emeritus member of the MHS board of directors.

In a difficult choice between two highly regarded candidates, the board selected the outsider Clarke, who offered broader administrative experience than Beckwith, whose career had been limited to financial positions. Clarke began work in August, 1983. He proved, as one close observer noted, to be "the right person at the time" to lead Memorial Medical Center to a higher plateau of quality and stature. Labeled by another observer as "a great visionary" who fully understood the dynamics of the health care industry, he also was "a mover and a shaker," never evading tough decisions.

Temperamentally Clarke stood in contrast to the casual, even laid-back manner of his predecessor. More detached and businesslike than Cook, he set high standards for his staff, then gave them the authority and responsibility to deliver. Focusing on an ambitious agenda and strategic planning, he reduced the frequency and length of staff meetings, and was disinclined to spend time roaming the corridors for casual conversation with employees and patients. Preferring a more structured and efficient way to meet Memorial's many employees, he scheduled a series of meetings with departmental staffs, to directly acquaint them with his style and goals.

In contrast to the crisis conditions of 1976, the hospital in 1983 was functioning smoothly. Nevertheless, Clarke, his board and staff had plenty to think and worry about. First, there were numerous ongoing tasks and challenges, notably the recently approved initiative to offer open heart surgery and related cardiac services. Second, there were major regulatory and socioeconomic changes underway, most urgently a fundamental revision of federal Medicare reimbursement. Third, Clarke quickly developed his own agenda of organizational and programmatic goals, all designed to address weaknesses or build on strengths. Chief among these were the inauguration of strategic planning, improvements in the physical plant, a careful review of certain existing and proposed medical services, linkages with area medical facilities and emerging health networks, and reshaping both the governance and administrative structures.

Clarke lost no time apprising board members of his ambitious agenda and his activist approach. Early in August, at their first meeting together, directors heard him preview several pet ideas. One month later, he told them of rapid and fundamental changes in health care that would force Memorial to either adapt or risk perishing. With 300,000 empty beds in the nation's 7,000 hospitals, it was not possible to survive by relying exclusively on acute care. Instead, hospitals needed to diversify into other health services, welcome joint ventures with staff physicians, join a national network to realize economies in purchasing and capital formation, and gain a competitive edge through enhanced quality, convenience and pricing. The drumbeat of new ideas continued, when in October Clarke reported on several additional concerns and initiatives.

Board members were unaccustomed to such energy and gravity. A gentlemen's club air of informality had prevailed for many years, and it took some time for directors to adjust to the new regime and tempo. Clarke later recalled "a rocky first year" during which he had to tackle several difficult issues and also—as an outsider—earn the board's trust. Fortunately, everyone wanted him to succeed and they sensed the need for change. Bud Lohman of the First National Bank had followed Saner as chairman, and he was a patient and supportive counselor. Other particularly dedicated directors in that first year were Robert Lanphier, Robert Oxtoby, and bankers John Brubaker and Alvin Becker.

The year 1983 was notable for the return of women to board governance. Sylvie (Mrs. James) Barge broke a male monopoly that had persisted for 35 years, since the Mildred Bunn era. She served for three years, and was succeeded by Linda Culver, a banker at First of America, who served long and ably, rising ultimately to the chairman's position. While women remained a small minority, they altered not only the board's composition but also its conduct, in a constructive manner. In addition, Clarke asked his secretary, Kathy Bird, to attend all board meetings and prepare the minutes, and later named her assistant to the president.

As noted in the previous chapter, Jack Cook had instigated another break with tradition, having two physicians serve ex-officio on the board. Under Clarke this welcome trend continued; doctors received full voting rights and by 1994 their ranks grew to six. The presence of women and medical doctors broadened and enriched board deliberations, and broke the constraints that had prevailed during Chick Lanphier's long tenure.

Operating in the manner of a modern corporate board, directors willingly left personnel and administrative matters fully in the president's hands, and focused exclusively on broad policy issues. Clarke reinforced this habit by reshaping and formalizing the monthly agenda. One innovation was "Board Continuing Education," the first order of business, which featured presentations by Clarke, staff members or visitors on timely medical topics and issues. Regular staff and committee reports consumed the remainder of each meeting, except when a special issue required attention.

Judging by the minutes, board deliberations were intensive, with wide-spread participation by attending directors and top administrators.

It was a sign of the changing times that four topics dominated board discussion during these years: financial trends, strategic planning, marketing and litigation. No longer did directors devote hours to a proposed $5.00 increase in room rates, or anecdotal criticism of a nurse's behavior, or micro management of the kitchen; now the subjects were of a breadth and complexity to challenge even the most seasoned lay director.

President Clarke faced several early administrative challenges. One was his strained relationship with Russell Beckwith, deeply pained by his failure to be named president. Major financial changes in medical reimbursement were underway, and Memorial needed decisive team leadership to accommodate them. Beckwith was an able financial manager, and he had strong local ties, but colleagues viewed him as abrasive and divisive. The awkward situation ended early in 1984, when he resigned to launch a highly successful medical service company.

Much more threatening and fateful were state and federal efforts to contain escalating medical reimbursement costs. State officials and legislators began considering proposals for regulatory review of hospital rates, a disturbing sign. Even more ominous were developments in Washington. Nearly one half of Memorial's patients were eligible for either Medicare or Medicaid assistance, making Uncle Sam the dominant source of operating revenues. Hospitals had flourished for nearly 20 years under a generous and open-ended cost reimbursement system for Medicare and Medicaid patient care. Soaring federal deficits led Congress and health officials to make drastic revisions. The 1981 Budget Act, for example, set the reimbursement ceiling for all Medicaid inpatients and outpatients at only 65 per cent of Memorial's actual costs. Hospital officials calculated that the net impact would be a $1.4 million drop in income.

The major blow came in 1983, when Washington adopted a radically different Medicare reimbursement plan, the prospective payment system, using Diagnosis-Related Groups (DRGs). Rather than reimburse actual costs, the government annually set flat fees for 467 distinct medical and surgical conditions. Uncoupling a hospital's Medicare revenue from its demonstrated costs for equipment, supplies and personnel dramatically transformed old free spending habits into draconian steps at cost control. The impact, both immediate and enduring, was "awesome," as hospital officials overnight had a disincentive rather than an incentive to acquire new technology, hire new staff specialists, or encourage lengthy patient stays. Nothing less than an entirely new system of medical cost accounting was the only way hospitals could recover a reasonable portion of the expense to treat older patients.

The DRG scheme took effect in October of 1983, with a graduated payment calendar that gave hospitals three years to steadily tighten cost controls before payments declined to the national median cost of each diagnostic group. Fortunately for its new president's sake, Memorial Medical Center already had excellent financial systems and cost analysis resources in place, and therefore was able to adjust promptly and successfully, though with great effort. Russell Beckwith's financial deputy, assistant vice president Paul Smith, had primary responsibility for the conversion, spending fully half of his time on this one assignment. He developed the in-house systems and expertise to perform detailed cost analyses of every medical procedure and service. In fact, this task gave Smith the opportunity to devise analytical and forecasting programs that in later years would establish him and Memorial as leaders in health finance administration.

DRGs were a managerial headache, and in time they would drastically curtail hospital growth, but at Memorial in 1983-84 they provided a one-time revenue windfall of nearly $4 million. Because of the first year's relatively generous allocation formula, hospitals with good financial controls already in place could recover a high proportion of their actual costs. Memorial's Medicare revenue was 94 per cent of the billed charges, a very high reimbursement level. In later years the share dropped, especially after the payment formulas changed to favor metropolitan and small rural hospitals at the expense of middle-sized community institutions like Memorial. By 1994 shrinking DRG payment levels were enabling the hospital to recover only 78 per cent of its billed charges. Moreover, DRGs affected much more than the hospital's operating results; the entire calculus of decisionmaking was transformed by the iron law of cost-effectiveness. President Clarke and his top staff had to educate physicians and others as well as themselves on the new realities of marketplace medicine. Operationally, every unit and department was instructed to improve efficiency, streamline procedures, and reduce to a minimum each patient's length of stay. Before long, the DRG regime even presaged a complete reorganization of Memorial's administrative structure. The halcyon days of risk-free hospital finance and administration were over.

Systematic long-range planning was a forte and special concern of the new president. By placing this focus at the top of his agenda, Clarke ensured that the hospital would position itself strategically for the powerful changes already underway and yet to be discerned on the horizon of health care. One novel step he took to inculcate a planning mindset was to invite board members and selected physicians to accompany him to national conferences and seminars on medicine's future. In this manner he exposed key associates to the ferment of new ideas, and he also had the opportunity to develop personal ties and credibility with his peers, to whom he otherwise might have remained an unfamiliar successor to the popular Jack Cook.

Strategic planning began with senior administrators, so Clarke held a planning retreat for them late in 1983. From that brainstorming session he assigned various tasks to his vice presidents, and then began working with the board. Several years earlier it had conducted its own planning effort through a special board committee, "MMC 2000," headed by Robert Lanphier. This had led to a new mission statement in 1981 and the selection in 1982 of a Chicago architectural firm for long-range facilities planning. This was a useful backdrop, but Clarke wanted to reinvigorate the process and make it a continuing board priority.

He began by reassigning facilities planning to an Indianapolis firm that he knew and respected. Through monthly briefings he alerted directors to new trends on the health care landscape. It took several years, but by 1985 a new blueprint for Memorial was taking shape. The three-year plan identified four strategic goals. In an increasingly cost-conscious environment Memorial would maintain price competitiveness. Second, it would take steps to clearly differentiate itself from other area institutions through superior services and advanced programs. It also would aggressively diversify into new but related health care activities as a hedge against declining inpatient trends. Finally, it would join networking ventures and alternative delivery systems to reach consumers. These goals—price competitiveness, differentiation, diversification and networking—became bywords as Memorial entered its centennial decade. Two years later the plan was refined to designate medical "centers of excellence" that would emphatically mark the hospital's distinctive stature. There were to be six centers of excellence, building on existing strengths: cancer care, plastic surgery, the kidney program, women's health, cardiopulmonary medicine, and physical rehabilitation services. Relatively simple to identify, these hallmarks of Memorial health care would require a heavy investment of effort and funds to reach the desired level of regional prestige.

It was the special responsibility of top administrators to implement this ambitious plan. To clearly denote this task, Clarke won board approval in 1984 to create a new tier of three senior vice presidents, with executive responsibilities in three broad areas: operations, finance, and corporate development. To fill the three new positions Clarke promoted one incumbent officer and recruited the other two. The insider was Jim Rigby, previously vice president for professional services, who now also had a second title, chief operating officer. In that capacity he oversaw the personnel office, nursing, medical relations and programs, and the many support activities lumped under "administrative services." This was a handsome promotion for the young Rigby, and a measure of the trust he had earned with Clarke and others.

For chief financial officer Clarke in 1984 believed he needed someone with advanced academic credentials, so he went outside rather than promote the talented Paul Smith. His choice was Gary Zara, who unfortunately had to resign two years later, for health reasons. Later Smith would hold the top financial job. The CFO also directed Memorial's rapidly growing data systems operation.

Replacing an ill-defined division known as Community Services was a new entity, Corporate Services, which Clarke envisioned as the driving force behind his diversification and networking plans. For this senior vice presidency he hired Robert Porter, who had previous experience with a medical supply company. Corporate Services (later renamed Corporate Development) included planning, marketing, management agreements with neighboring small town hospitals, and regional or national affiliation opportunities.

During this mid-decade period there were several other vice presidential appointments, including a nursing director and Mitchell Johnson (from Pekin Memorial Hospital) to manage the marketing. Therefore, within his first year Robert Clarke lost no time reorganizing the hospital's administration and filling its top positions with his own people.

By the end of the decade a complete organizational overhaul was in order. Instead of the traditional functional arrangement (nursing, laboratory, etc.), why not organize the staff from a patient-centered perspective? Memorial would form administrative units around "products" (areas of medical care) such as cardiac, physical rehabilitation and cancer. Not only would this simplify DRG cost analyses, but it also would encourage better and more coordinated care through teams of physicians, nurses, technicians and support staff.

Such a radical scheme could not be implemented, let alone accepted, quickly, so Clarke and his senior colleagues installed it gradually over a period of several years. Employees had to shed old habits and reporting relationships for the product line approach to succeed. For example, the nursing division stayed in place, but was limited to such general concerns as recruitment, retention and quality assurance. Operational authority over nurses—their staffing assignments, scheduling and direct supervision—was allocated among the various product lines. Nurses in cardiac care worked under that unit's chief administrator, and so forth.

Memorial's table of organization therefore changed dramatically in the 1990s, with newly established operating units: cancer, cardiac, ambulatory, rehabilitation, nephrology, psychiatry, neurological, etc. Once fully implemented, this approach paid dividends through staff team-building, continuity of care, and favorable patient surveys. Interestingly, it soon became commonplace in the nation's progressive hospitals.

Many other administrative departures and appointments occurred during Clarke's first decade in office. Jim Rigby was highly regarded, but left to take a CEO's position in Ohio. Succeeding him for several years was Jo Adkins, who originally came to direct nursing but later was promoted to chief operating officer. After leaving abruptly in 1994, she was followed by Ed Curtis, who began at Memorial as a nurse, won successive promotions, and became one of Clarke's "shining stars." The affable Bill Boyd retired from his longtime service as vice president for administrative services and later, facilities management. Senior vice president Robert Porter left his Corporate Development position in 1990, and Mitchell Johnson succeeded him.

A common refrain at Memorial, especially among physicians, was to complain about a proliferation of administrators during the Clarke years. In part this trend was characteristic of complex organizations in contemporary America, and certainly of modern hospitals. Bureaucratization was a universal phenomenon of the "quiet revolution" in health care wrought by Medicare and HMOs. At Memorial, however, it had a special resonance resulting from the CEO's aggressive steps to reorganize the staff and seek new talent from outside.

Sensitive to these concerns, Clarke and the board commissioned a consultant's study that yielded some disturbing data. One general finding was that no fewer than eight administrative layers existed between the governing board at one end and the typical patient at the other. While not markedly different from peer hospitals, this figure conjured images of excessive bureaucracy. There were 253 employees in administrative positions, which (in a total payroll of 2,500) meant one manager for every 8.7 full-time staff members. Both the board and Clarke agreed that steps were necessary to curb administrative growth.

Exercising leadership over a modern comprehensive hospital in a time of change was a special aptitude of President Robert Clarke. Fully conversant with the latest concepts and practices in health care management, he acted decisively and often briskly to diversify and strengthen the board, manage the DRG shift, recruit hardworking administrators, hold them to exacting standards, invigorate long range planning, and set programmatic goals that would steer Memorial to new levels of achievement. With a new administrative infrastructure in hand, he could tackle the many challenges on his ambitious agenda.

Competition and Cooperation

For most of their histories, Springfield's two hospitals had competed fiercely and even engaged in mutual invective. As noted earlier, a rapprochement developed in the 1970s, when broad-minded board members and executives at both hospitals, spurred by the new SIU School of Medicine, initiated a dialogue that led to the joint affiliation agreement over medical education, and also the informal "SAM" committee for continuing board member dialogue. Still highly competitive and protective of their respective areas of superiority, Memorial and St. John's hospitals began a new era of consultation and cooperation, with SIU an active third partner.

This constructive development confronted an institutional and legal obstacle in 1984, when Humana Hospital officials filed a federal antitrust lawsuit against Memorial and SIU for conspiring to prevent the upstart newcomer from effectively competing in Springfield's patient market. For some reason St. John's was not named as a defendant, but clearly the new era of bilateral cooperation was at risk under the specter of antitrust litigation.

Humana claimed that its effort to secure a toehold had been resisted from the outset by Memorial and SIU, which, it insisted, had coerced staff physicians to neither join the Humana staff nor refer patients there. Consequently, it struggled at 30 per cent bed occupancy and suffered operating losses.

For Bob Clarke in his second year as CEO, this was an unanticipated and highly unwelcome development that endangered close ties with St. John's and SIU, and also threatened to paint Memorial as an unfair bully or Goliath in the public eye. The urgent concern was getting good legal representation. Memorial turned to the antitrust specialists at Chicago's prestigious (and expensive) firm of Jenner & Block.

Trial preliminaries and exploratory discussions with the plaintiff consumed three anxious years until late in 1987, when Humana agreed to drop its suit. While this saved Memorial the expense and possible embarrassment of a trial, and also the threat of damages, the affair still exacted a painful price. Legal fees approached a whopping $800,000, and the SAM committee was disbanded. One thing that did not change was a pervasive enmity among officials and loyal physicians at Memorial and St. John's against Humana and its successor facility, Doctors Hospital.

A sign of the litigious times, the antitrust suit heralded a conspicuous increase in legal actions and issues at Memorial and hospitals generally. By the late 1980s, a regular agenda item at board meetings was the report on threatened or pending litigation. At any given time there were active lawsuits against staff physicians, plus occasional disputes with vendors, patients, former employees and property owners. At one distressing high point (1988), Memorial was a party to 21 pending suits and 45 potential claims. Such figures were not unusual for a large modern hospital, but that offered scant comfort.

The bewildering variety of legal issues, some highly specialized, made it impractical to employ in-house counsel. For property, zoning, workmen's compensation and routine liability actions Memorial relied upon the local firm of Brown, Hay & Stephens, which had represented it for many years. Various Chicago firms handled specialties like bond issues and labor relations. McDermott, Will & Emery, also of that city, consulted on the legal and regulatory aspects of complex new ventures. A Pittsburgh, Pennsylvania specialist managed malpractice suits against the medical staff. The annual cost of this legal assistance hovered close to $1 million, which directors (including several lawyers) reluctantly accepted as a cost of doing business in modern times.

While cooperative dialogue with St. John's Hospital was stalled and somewhat curtailed as a result of the antitrust suit, it did continue in at least a cautious mode. Inter-staff discussions were permissible on safe topics like disciplinary standards for doctors with overdue patient records, certain workplace rules for nurses, and a coordinated ban on smoking. At the executive level, the degree of communication depended somewhat on changing personalities. Bob Clarke's interaction with top administrator Sr. Ann Pitzenberger (to 1990) was satisfactory but not cordial. With her successor, Al Laabs, he enjoyed "an outstanding collegial relationship." Their frequent informal meetings were an opportunity to share some data, exchange concerns and maintain a healthy dialogue. This spirit of cooperation was much in order by the 1990s, when mergers, HMOs and joint ventures became commonplace in the health care industry. In this more relaxed setting there was talk at the board level of restoring the SAM committee and perhaps developing other formal ties.

A hospital consultant in 1992 described as "peaceful coexistence" the relationship between Memorial and St. John's. What had begun nearly a century earlier as sectarian warfare now consisted of keen but friendly competition. For most of its history Memorial had struggled to match the size and civic reputation of its north side rival. Reaching parity or superiority with St. John's in the most prestigious medical specialties had been a prime goal of successive chief executives. After many years of effort, each hospital had its unchallenged winners: pediatrics and cardiac care at St. John's, renal and cancer care at Memorial. But the competition in these and other areas continued. Critics often complained about costly duplication of service, but both an expanding regional demand and the higher quality owing to competition justified the expense.

After many decades as the underdog, Memorial now enjoyed several structural advantages that helped close the gap. One was its proximity to, and "persistent, positive working relationship" with the medical school. A quarter century earlier, when SIU first approached the two hospitals, Memorial was quicker and more enthusiastic in its response, and it had a large land parcel to sell. From this tactical edge there flowed countless small decisions and commitments that worked to Memorial's competitive advantage. For example, by 1989 70 per cent of SIU's clinical facilities were housed at Memorial, double the quantity at St. John's. Moreover, Clarke was able to negotiate an ingenious agreement with Dean Moy to build badly needed clinical space on Memorial's land, then lease it to the medical school. Fittingly named the Richard H. Moy Building, this facility reinforced the bond between the two institutions and further enhanced Memorial's rising stature.

VIP Patients

At least three of Illinois' first families of modern times chose Memorial Medical Center for scheduled or emergency attention. Early in 1962 Shirley Stratton, wife of former Governor William G. Stratton, gave birth to the couple's daughter Nancy. Medical complications required a lengthy three-month convalescence for the former First Lady, so Governor Stratton arranged to stay in an adjoining room. Longstanding director Robert Oxtoby recalled often seeing Stratton conduct business from his temporary quarters during the spring of 1962.

Another blessed gubernatorial event occurred in August of 1978, when Jayne Thompson, wife of Governor James Thompson, gave birth to "First Baby" Samantha. The Cesarean delivery was performed by Dr. John Standard in the newly expanded and remodeled obstetrical wing. Hospital officials were "honored" that the Thompsons chose Memorial rather than a hospital in their home city of Chicago. While mother and daughter remained as patients for nearly a week, the governor resumed work and his reelection campaign.

Governor Jim Edgar was admitted twice midway through his first term for brief and unplanned medical procedures. Discovery of a blocked artery in October 1992 led to immediate hospitalization and a balloon angioplasty performed by cardiologist Dr. Randolph Martin. Intense press coverage and security efforts made Memorial a beehive of activity during Edgar's four-day hospital recovery. This was a presidential campaign season, and the governor received cheerful messages from President George Bush (by telephone) and Vice President Dan Quayle (in person).

The following summer Governor Edgar returned for surgery to remove his gallbladder. Dr. Keith Wichterman performed the relatively simple procedure, and Edgar was able to convalesce at home after only one night in the hospital. Again, however, there was great press interest, largely due to surprise over the sudden hospitalization of a young and otherwise healthy public figure.

A second structural advantage lay in the two hospitals' governing systems. Part of a large regional system, St. John's lacked the autonomy to move quickly to seize opportunities. Furthermore, its lay board was advisory in nature, denying it the clout or prestige that a board of directors can enjoy. Time and again Memorial's board of civic leaders proved able to respond decisively and flexibly to programmatic opportunities. Dean Moy had many occasions to observe the two institutions react to problems or invitations that he impartially presented; almost invariably Memorial's directors and officials beat their rival with a timelier and more creative response.

CEO Clarke's four-point long range plan and his focus on centers of medical excellence all pointed toward maintaining the intense competition with St. John's while still exploring all reasonable avenues of cooperation. At long last, after decades of vitriolic animosity and unequal rivalry, the two institutions competed as equals and communicated in myriad ways. Both the competition and the cooperation were healthy in their own right, and evidence of sensible leadership at the two institutions.

The principal spur to competition was the nation's dwindling supply of patients and the shrinking length of their hospital stays. This was a nationwide trend, caused primarily by stricter regulations and reimbursement levels for Medicare, Medicaid and insurance-covered patients. Nationally, inpatient hospital usage began dropping sharply after peaking in 1981. That year Memorial operated comfortably with an 85 per cent occupancy rate and an average hospital stay of just over eight days. The numbers thereafter began slipping. By 1983 occupancy was below 80 per cent, and patient days had declined by six per cent.

Much like their anxious forebears decades earlier at Springfield Hospital and Training School, Memorial administrators and directors began tracking admission and bed count figures constantly, comparing them to peer institutions, and exploring countermoves. Through most of the 1980s the hospital fared better than the average throughout Illinois, but that cushion shrank after a group of Springfield physicians purchased Humana Hospital (renamed Doctors Hospital) and began referring fewer of their patients to Memorial and St. John's.

Memorial administrators fashioned a dual strategy to address the alarming pattern. One recourse was to convert excess inpatient rooms to other, more productive uses. A silver lining in the usage trends was a countervailing rise in outpatient services. Between 1982 and 1987 the hospital experienced a sharp 34 per cent outpatient increase. Moreover, there were other claimants for hospital space, so the board approved plans to reduce Memorial's inpatient capacity by eight per cent, to 553 beds, thereby providing prime space for examination rooms, support services and classrooms. Further conversions lowered the capacity to 519 beds by 1992. That year occupancy stabilized temporarily at 75 per cent, with the average patient stay at 7.8 days and the total of outpatient visits up still further, to 140,000. Thereafter patient days steadily diminished, in accordance with national trends.

A second initiative was to adopt modern business theories and practices, in order to position the hospital to maximize its penetration of the regional health care market. If such language seemed more apt for a soap company than a hospital, it was because institutions like Memorial found themselves squarely in a highly competitive environment. Like their private sector counterparts, hospitals intent on surviving had to gauge their "customers," design products and services to suit them, and influence their shopping decisions through advertising.

In 1986, under Clarke's prodding, Memorial developed a comprehensive marketing program, and this became a regular agenda item at monthly board meetings. Mitchell Johnson was recruited to fill a new vice presidency overseeing the effort. A primary theme of the campaign was to persuade citizens that Memorial was much more than a hospital for sick people; it was a total system offering "a continuum of care." A panoply of wellness programs, diagnostic services, disease prevention offerings and auxiliary activities underscored the promotional theme for print and electronic ads: "Memorial Medical Center—So Much Care—So Many Ways of Showing It."

The marketing approach permeated hospital operations. A "Quality Assurance" program was inaugurated to monitor patient care, pursue complaints, and inculcate staff members with a "patient first" outlook. Every month directors heard reports on this campaign. Similarly, a new Guest Relations office produced user-friendly patient brochures and conducted client satisfaction surveys. Use of the word "guest" revealed how serious officials were about emulating the service credo of the hotel industry and creating patient goodwill. Another effort was the development and prominent display of Memorial's "Statement of Values," a pledge of superior service.

There were other components of this bold new approach. A rising advertising budget highlighted the designated centers of excellence, spreading

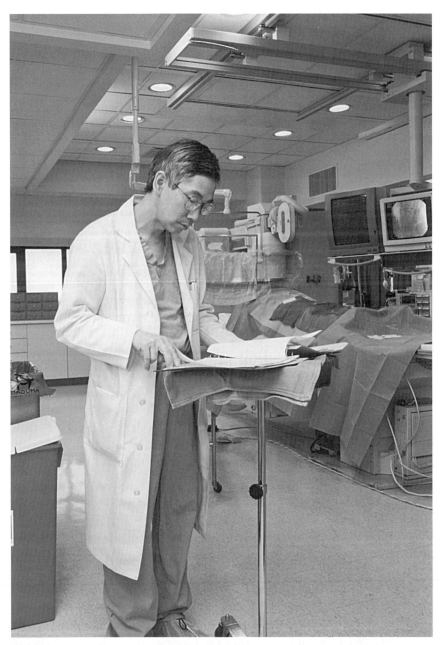

Cardiac services grew rapidly in Memorial's ninth and tenth decades. Here Dr. Wilfred Lam works in the catheterization laboratory.

the message that Memorial was a first-rate institution for the most complex and demanding procedures. Women's health became a special focus, with an annual Women's Fitness Fest drawing 700 people in 1987. Altogether 7,000 women attended special hospital programs and workshops that year. Older citizens were another market niche. Memorial's "Gold Club" had 9,000 enrollees, and its "Seniors' Health Fair" attracted hundreds of guests. Wellness was promoted through free cholesterol screening and blood pressure testing at shopping malls.

Demographic data and opinion sampling were collected through telephone surveys, patient questionnaires, and focus groups. MMC distributed an informational and subtly promotional health newsletter to doctors' offices. Just how far hospitals had progressed in adopting a business approach was revealed in board discussion of a proposed renovation of the Psychiatric Department. Phrases from the minutes included "strategic evaluation ... Revenues are good ... an opportunity to capture the market ... loss of market share." In short order the language of modern marketing had invaded the once-altruistic rhetoric of community hospitals. Intense competition was a powerful motivator, warning hospitals to adapt or wither.

Medical Milestones

No amount of promotion or public relations could help an institution unless it had resources and programs worthy of the attention. Bob Clarke, his governing directors and his top staff were determined to raise Memorial to new heights of quality and even distinction, so that it would be commonly regarded as a superior tertiary care medical center offering a comprehensive array of programs and services.

Open heart surgery and related cardiac services represented a crucial step in Memorial's competitive strategy. Cook and Rigby had spearheaded the successful campaign to enlist support and neutralize criticism of their application for a Certificate of Need. When Clarke arrived the extensive construction program was underway and plans were being made to train cardiac nurses and technicians. However, all was not well, as medical politics confronted the new president with a serious challenge.

Rumors flew late in 1983 about which of the rival cardiovascular doctor groups Clarke would favor with the lucrative work that would begin the next year. As a newcomer without allies or trusted advisors, he innocently was entering a political mine field that imperiled him as well as the

The Modern Medical Staff

By 2007 Memorial's medical staff numbered over 500, more than forty times larger than the small band of charter physicians who launched Springfield Hospital and Training School. Not only more numerous, today's staff is much more differentiated by specialty and immeasurably more proficient. Also, its members (especially those in high demand specialties) can exert considerable influence over hospital decisionmaking through their leverage and stature.

CEO Robert Clarke and his top executives have taken various steps to integrate staff physicians as active partners with a mutual stake in Memorial's success. One important accomplishment, initiated by Jack Cook, was to add medical staff officers as voting board members. Another was to introduce stipends for all elected chiefs of service, thereby cementing their institutional allegiance. Clarke also inaugurated a modern concept, the appointment of a paid medical director from staff ranks. This board appointee plays a key role in strengthening communication between hospital executives and physicians.

In further seeking to enlist the medical staff in strategic policymaking, Clarke regularly invited key physicians to accompany him to national medical conferences. He thereby exposed dozens of doctors to current trends and issues, and also developed cordial social ties with them. Consequently much of the traditional suspicion and animosity disappeared, as a growing cadre of staff leaders appreciated the linkage between their professional welfare and the hospital's. Physicians like John Allen, John Denby, Barry Free, William Sherrick and others became Memorial advocates, "our front line of defense." Clarke welcomed this profound change, which views the medical staff as a major asset rather than the necessary nuisance that his predecessors perceived.

embryonic program. At least one influential physician bluntly warned him that the wrong choice would quickly cost him his job. The crisis passed when he made a well-considered decision, bolstered it with assurances of evenhanded treatment, and won the support of his board.

Construction progressed through the summer of 1984, and the necessary preparations and training occurred on schedule. Late in September the new Cardiology Department opened on the seventh floor of D building, with surgery one floor below. When the board met in mid-October, officials proudly reported 12 cardiac surgeries in the unit's first two weeks. Surprising those skeptics who had doubted there was sufficient demand to sustain two open heart centers in Springfield, Memorial soon averaged one open heart operation daily, and an equal number of other cardiac procedures. These figures increased modestly but steadily in the following years, reaching over 400 open heart operations and more than 3,000 catheterizations in 1991. Demand was sufficient to enlarge the bed space by 20 per cent, construct a new catheterization laboratory, and add another surgical suite. In 1996 Memorial reached a milestone with 800 open heart operations, still below St. John's (the state's largest program), but enough for third rank in Illinois. With these achievements cardiac care earned stature as one of the hospital's centers of excellence.

Dating back at least 50 years to the weekly tumor clinics for staff doctors, cancer care had been a focus of special attention at Memorial. Mounting public concern over the dread disease and growing government support underscored its priority status in the 1980s. Most of the attention and federal funds had been channeled to the nationally recognized cancer centers in a few major metropolitan areas. The need for a parallel effort in smaller cities spurred formation of the Association of Community Cancer Centers (ACCC). Millions of cancer patients needed access to the latest treatments by experienced oncologists without the burden of extended stays in distant cities. A milestone in ACCC's campaign was persuading the National Cancer Institute (NCI) to siphon some of its research funds to community cancer centers, where most of the nation's cancer patients were treated.

By chance Bob Clarke, while at Community Hospital, had been an early appointee to ACCC's board, and thus knew the organization's mission and its leaders. Thus informed and inspired, he quickly initiated staff planning and board deliberation to promote the concept at Memorial. A feasibility study revealed that the hospital already captured 29 per cent of the cancer patients in the nine-county region. Stressing comprehensive care, planners envisioned combining all elements of cancer detection, treatment, rehabilitation, hospice care and research in one facility. To direct this ambitious effort Clarke recommended Dr. Gale Katterhagen, an acquaintance from his ACCC days. Katterhagen was a charter member and former president of ACCC, and enjoyed national standing. The board approved both the plan and the appointment in 1986, and Memorial's Regional Cancer Center was born.

An enthusiastic apostle of the regional approach, Katterhagen promptly turned to planning and staffing the new facility. Like the 51 other community oncology centers in 31 states, Memorial would serve as a downstate "hub" of diagnosis, treatment and public information. A major goal was to convince citizens that many cancers were curable, and that Memorial offered the cures.

In 1987 hospital directors approved plans for a large new facility, and NCI awarded Memorial a coveted three-year, $240,000 research grant. A central tenet of the support was the regional approach; Memorial would work closely with rural hospitals in a coordinated effort. The public would be educated through a cancer newsletter, a hotline, and a free hemoccult screening program. Periodic oncology conferences and a weekly Tumor Board (shades of the tumor clinic) would update physicians on current research and practices.

Construction of the new facility was part of the construction program for E building, and took three years, 1988-91. It was designed to provide easy ground floor access for patients, and "one stop service" to ensure comfort and privacy. Included in the plans were a surgical suite, a 30-bed unit of private rooms, a hospice lounge and beds, and space for radiation therapy, hyperthermia, bone marrow transplants and the new field of biotherapy. The center opened with fanfare in May of 1991. In the short space of six years Memorial had managed to vault to the front ranks of community cancer care, and to create another center of excellence. The visionary Dr. Katterhagen resigned in the early 1990s, but was succeeded by another nationally prominent oncology specialist, Dr. John Yarbro. Previously acquainted with Clarke, Yarbro had directed NCI's comprehensive cancer center program.

Another area of concerted effort was Rehabilitation Services, earlier known as Physical Therapy. For many years relegated to a ground level corner space in A building, its growing patient volume dictated a move in the 1970s to larger quarters on the third floor of G building. This made it possible to consolidate scattered programs in physical therapy, audiology, occupational therapy and speech therapy. Patient demand, coupled with more specialists with new techniques and equipment, led to further expansion and remodeling the next decade.

Singled out as one of Memorial's centers of excellence in the 1980s, Rehabilitation Services continued to grow. It gained referrals and status as downstate's only accredited spinal cord and head injury center. To enlarge the regional pool of trained specialists, Memorial joined five other Illinois hospitals in helping underwrite the cost of physical therapy training at Bradley University in Peoria. Further growth and several added services led in the 1990s to yet another new departmental rubric: Neuromuscular Sciences. The department, in addition to existing programs, featured both inpatient and outpatient facilities, sports care, psychology, and clinics for specific neurological conditions.

A notable achievement for the department was construction of "Independence Square," offering state-of-the-art concepts and furnishings to help patients regain skills for independent living. Designed to simulate routine daily experiences, this ingenious facility provided such challenges as using kitchen appliances, boarding a bus, walking on different ground surfaces, and shopping. Area businesses donated $300,000 to furnish and equip Independence Square. Interdisciplinary, multifaceted and "very sophisticated," Neuromuscular Sciences filled a vital need for thousands of downstate citizens.

As noted earlier, the Trauma Center had experienced dramatic growth and improvement in the 1980s. This progress continued during the Clarke years, to the point of surpassing St. John's Hospital in volume. In 1996, for example, Memorial captured 54 percent of the emergency admissions to the two hospitals. In the cost-conscious 1990s there was some irony in this success story. Operating a high-level trauma center required 24 hour medical staffing and other costly services. Even the rising emergency admission figures could not counterweigh a "terribly expensive" unit. Trauma work remained exciting and glamourous, and it enhanced the hospital's community image, but its financial return was poor in comparison with other medical services.

Another medical department that had traditionally lagged behind St. John's in size and standing was Obstetrics. Consistent with its concerted attention to women's health as a center of excellence, Memorial's board in 1991 approved a $5 million relocation and modernization, to accommodate over 1,400 births a year. Planning consultants persuaded Memorial officials to create a boldly different, state-of-the-art facility. Traditionally maternal care patients had to be transported through four separate locations for the labor, delivery, recovery and post-partum stages. In conformity with Memorial's new patient-centered and continuous-care approach, expectant mothers were placed in one of the department's new multipurpose Family Maternity Suites. In this comfortable and attractive one-stop setting they could receive medical and nursing attention through all four stages.

The new facility was an instant success, and Memorial's maternity admissions rose dramatically, by over 50 per cent. In 1996 it boasted 1,900 births, surpassing its crosstown rival and longtime obstetrical leader. The biggest challenge was in the selection and training of qualified nurses, who now needed skills and the aptitude to provide pediatric and general as well as obstetrical care. The maternal team approach took hold, however, and Memorial now boasted a premier obstetrical service.

There never was doubt about the outstanding reputation enjoyed by the Kidney Center. Renal dialysis and kidney transplantation were longstanding Memorial specialties, and a satellite dialysis network was welcomed by thousands of area residents. Determined to protect this asset, officials decided in 1984 to lead downstate Illinois by acquiring the latest equipment, a lithotripter. This machine used ultrasonic waves for the non-surgical removal of kidney stones. After regulatory delays, the board authorized spending $1.4 million to purchase an advanced version, which was manufactured in Germany. It was installed during the summer of 1986, and went into operation that September.

The lithotripter was an immediate success, performing 300 procedures a year by 1988. These results prompted Memorial to reach more patients by placing the equipment on a semi-trailer that could travel to distant downstate hospitals. The cost of a truck and installation was estimated at $650,000, but projected annual usage would rise to 550, nearly doubling the output. Mobile lithotripsy service began soon after, bringing advanced treatment to kidney stone patients in eight locations throughout Illinois, plus one in Indiana.

Capitalizing on its medical expertise and broad experience, the Kidney Center received approval in 1996 to perform a rare surgical procedure, combined pancreas-kidney transplants. That August doctors conducted the first such operation in Illinois outside Chicago. A large and profitable department, the center maintained its stature as one of Memorial's standard-bearers. A key factor in this success was the leadership provided by its longtime medical director, Dr. Sumantra Mitra.

General surgery grew steadily during these years. In 1983 the board learned of a new record: there had been 1,157 operations in one month. Fifty years earlier the hospital had boasted about 171 operations in an entire year, indicating an *eighty-fold* increase since 1935. Crowding and an inconvenient location convinced the board to approve relocating and enlarging the surgery suite as part of the hospital's building program early in the 1990s.

Already one of Memorial's major assets, the pathology department continued to excel and expand under Dr. Grant Johnson's aggressive leadership. He was determined that its equipment and services be "at the top" in laboratory medicine. Automated fluid analysis technology improved the department's efficiency, productivity and accuracy. The addition of electron microscopy was another milestone. Dr. John O. Dietrich, Johnson's senior colleague, oversaw the selection and operation of advanced computer equipment in the 1980s, making it possible to prepare cumulative lab reports on individual patients.

The department's continuing growth promoted a nearly insatiable appetite for space. One solution was dispersal of laboratory units to better serve their various medical clients. In 1991, for example, the entire surgical pathology unit moved to space adjoining the new surgical suite in E building, thereby ensuring faster and more reliable service. Similarly, an outpatient laboratory unit received space in the new Baylis Building west of Rutledge Street.

Pathology's payroll also grew, rising above 200 by 1994, and including ten physicians. Among the outstanding specialists were Drs. Barry W. Dick, Travis L. Hindman and Natwar J. Mody. One notable addition was in the field of neuropathology, and that in turn stimulated an increase in the hospital's neurology and neurosurgery services. One simple measure of staff depth was the presence, by 1990, of four photographers and a medical illustrator.

Johnson reluctantly retired in 1992, ending a career of remarkable achievement. In a fitting gesture, Memorial's board acted to name the department in his honor. Succeeding him as director was Dr. Dietrich, who oversaw a department that was much more integral to successful hospital medicine than its 1950s precursor. In earlier days physicians necessarily relied principally on direct patient examination for their diagnoses.

Subspecialization and advanced technology now made the pathologist a full partner in medical diagnosis and treatment.

Psychiatry had been a problem in earlier years, but now Memorial captured more than 50 per cent of the community's hospital inpatients. To expand that edge Clarke recommended several projects. One, at a cost of several million dollars, was to renovate the Psychiatric unit on the fourth and fifth levels of A building. Another was the 1984 decision to establish an adolescent psychiatric service, which at that time did not exist between Chicago and St. Louis. National data and findings identified this as a rapidly growing field. Memorial administrators and doctors surveyed the regional demand and prepared the necessary Certificate of Need. Regulatory approval led to construction of a 23-bed space on the third floor of A building. Upon opening late in 1985 it was filled to capacity.

Inpatient psychological care was only part of the story. New behavioral therapies were available in addition to (or in place of) the traditional medical approach. Tracking the professional literature, Clarke saw outpatient and community based counseling programs as a ripe opportunity for Memorial. Accordingly, in 1996 he successfully negotiated the hospital's affiliation with Mental Health Centers of Central Illinois (MHCCI), a system that provided residential, outpatient and crisis care in four sites serving residents of Logan, Mason, Menard and Sangamon counties.

Radiology had long been an institutional strength, with excellent staff and modern equipment. In 1991 the department performed 145,000 examinations and generated $19 million in revenue. Its equipment was worth $9 million, excluding leased items. Dr. David Porter headed a team of 13 radiologists and 60 technicians and clerical staff. Their work was streamlined by new technology, and the groundwork was laid to transmit diagnostic images from outlying facilities to Memorial, and even the homes of radiologists.

The contagions and pandemics of earlier decades no longer haunted hospitals, with one alarming exception, AIDS. Directors received the first official report of this modern plague in 1986, when the board discussed current procedures for AIDS screening, consent issues and liability questions. A special hospital committee monitored legal and regulatory implications, in order to ensure that admittance and other policies were current. With nationwide reports of a contaminated blood pool, board members in 1988 sought legal advice on Memorial's liability as a partner in the Community Blood Bank. Meanwhile, the hospital began admitting its first

AIDS patients. Several years later these worries proved prophetic, when hospital officials learned that a patient who received a blood transfusion back in 1985 had contracted AIDS and died. The procedure had occurred before laboratory tests were available to detect HIV in blood supplies. Nevertheless, Memorial shared in the liability, and had to pay a portion of the lawsuit award. AIDS remained a relatively manageable challenge in central Illinois, but hospital officials observed rigorous rules and procedures to protect patients as well as nurses and other staff.

Underlying all the glamour and technology of modern medicine and surgery was the tedious and mundane work of patient recordkeeping. Maintaining current medical records at Memorial was an administrative headache as old as the hospital. It was a chronic topic of discussion among doctors, nursing directors, administrators and board members. Periodically there would be a concerted effort to reduce the number of delinquent files, then gradually the list would begin expanding again. Almost invariably hospital accreditation teams issued stern warnings, and sometimes even threats.

Officers of the medical staff and others regularly debated how to enforce deadlines and how to discipline the worst offenders. In a city like Springfield with two or three competing hospitals, the ultimate sanction of denying admitting privileges was a double-edged sword. A physician barred from one hospital could take his business to another, hurting the former without personally suffering any loss. Levying fines proved no more effective.

Frustrated by a seemingly uncontrollable problem, Memorial's board worried about the monthly delinquency figures: 1,274 incomplete records in January of 1974, 1,682 in November of 1976, a record-breaking 2,060 in December of 1978, and so forth. Such numbers did not go unnoticed by JCAH inspectors. In 1982 Memorial's accreditation was limited to one year due to excessive delinquencies.

One possible solution was a coordinated approach with St. John's Hospital. Accordingly, the SAM committee explored developing a uniform policy in 1982. A sliding scale of suspended privileges was another policy proposal. Characteristically, Jack Cook preferred the carrot approach to the stick. He instructed medical staff officers to award free golf balls to those saintly physicians who completed their records on time. Still, the problem persisted, and it became a financial issue because Memorial needed complete records before it could apply for Medicare reimbursement.

Nursing in the Nineties

During the late 1980s, a serious nursing shortage developed nationally and at Memorial. Local efforts to improve recruitment and retention included higher pay, flexible scheduling and the services of a staff child care center. These steps succeeded in reducing the RN turnover rate below the national average and improving the quality of nursing care, as measured by patient and physician surveys. A new Nursing Strategic Plan included professional advancement and shared governance structures. In 1992, Vice President of Patient Care Services Marsha Prater led the implementation of the Clinical Practice Model (CPM) as the framework for professional nursing practice at Memorial.

Rapid change in the health care environment has continued to affect staffing needs, notably the dramatic shift from inpatient to outpatient and community based service. As the need for acute care nursing positions has declined, nurses both locally and nationally have been restive about the future. Memorial has responded with a tuition reimbursement program and on-site conferences and workshops aimed at helping nurses gain new skills and professional opportunities. However, if past history is any guide, the ebb and flow in nursing demand will continue to challenge hospital administrators and nursing personnel.

One breakthrough occurred when CEO Clarke reassigned veteran nurse Ed Quarry to tackle the immense backlog. His personal acquaintance with staff physicians and his knowledge of DRG reporting requirements enabled him to tutor physicians on using the proper form and terminology. He went to extraordinary lengths to facilitate the process, visiting doctors in their offices, faxing data to them, working with their nurses, and poring over records in advance to spot gaps. This special effort steadily shrank the backlog, and was a fitting capstone to Quarry's long career, which ended in 1993.

To institutionalize this one-time gain required development of a truly streamlined medical records program. In mid-decade Memorial officials invested in a state-of-the-art electronic system that included remote data-entry sites in doctors' offices. Acquisition and installation costs were high, but the system's comprehensive data base and user convenience showed promise—once and for all—of solving the medical record-keeping challenge.

Wellness, Inc.

Like the petroleum, automobile and other growth industries in earlier times, American health care institutions developed to a point late in the 20th century that organizational expansion became not just desirable but essential for survival. Whether by horizontal integration (hospital mergers) or vertical integration (comprehensive services), medical institutions rapidly transformed from traditional acute care facilities into complex and far-flung health emporiums. A simple measure of the scope of this change was the speed with which hospital letterheads, logos and organization charts substituted nouns like "center," "system," "alliance," "network" and "affiliate" for the once-standard "hospital." The rise of medical conglomerates was a centerpiece of health care's quiet revolution.

There were compelling reasons for this profound change. Declining bed occupancy was a major factor, forcing hospital officials to search for alternative patient and revenue sources. Tightening DRG and third-party reimbursement formulas intensified the quest for new income streams. Tax laws, liability concerns and regulatory constraints made it necessary to compartmentalize an institution's various endeavors into separate legal and financial entities, all within a holding company structure. Mergers and networks could yield easier capital formation, more efficient management and lower purchasing costs.

Americans were spending an enormous amount (over ten per cent of the Gross National Product) on health care, but the allocation of those funds was changing radically: less on inpatient hospital care, more on everything else. The challenge for governing boards and officials was to nimbly follow the money with what amounted to "health care service malls."

Outreach and diversification had their modest origins at Memorial before the revolution took hold in the 1980s. Through the "Shared Services Program" it had offered management contracts to small hospitals in neighboring towns. In return for fees that included some overhead profit, Memorial agreed to hire managers and help them with purchasing and other responsibilities. A central purpose was to develop a regional referral system to bring seriously ill patients to Springfield.

The program worked well for a while, and when Clarke arrived in 1983 there were arrangements with hospitals in Beardstown, Pittsfield, Carlinville and Hillsboro. But problems developed as the DRG system strained rural hospitals with an excess of costly convalescing patients. These struggling institutions lagged in paying their management fees and resisted the difficult choices facing them. The Carlinville arrangement ended in 1985, presaging an end to the Shared Services Program.

Another, more successful early initiative was the establishment of satellite dialysis units in area communities. Bringing the convenience as well as the blessings of dialysis to thousands of central Illinois kidney patients was an inspired move. By 1996 there were seven such Memorial outposts within a 100-mile radius: Decatur, Effingham, Jacksonville, Lincoln, Litchfield, Mattoon, Taylorville and Springfield itself.

This success led to similar installations for other medical services. In 1984 Memorial opened a mammography center on the city's west side, and 12 years later announced plans for an outpatient clinic with various convenient services still further west. Recognizing the larger logic of this approach, administrators in 1995 announced a new Community Health Advisory Group to assess and meet the needs of citizens on such disparate concerns as lead poisoning, teen pregnancy, infant mortality and cultural sensitivity.

Eager to join the national trend toward revenue-producing diversification, Memorial's board in 1984 approved Clarke's proposal to add the

Visiting Nurse Association of Central Illinois (VNA) as a controlled subsidiary. VNA officials welcomed this opportunity to gain greater stability
and visibility. The newly organized entity had its own board, named and
directly represented by Memorial directors. From the outset this arrangement served all parties. In its first year under hospital auspices, VNA
enjoyed a 52 per cent surge in home visitation. Described as "a wonderful
relationship," Memorial's VNA soon became the region's dominant provider of home care services, with over 100,000 visits a year.

Vertical rather than horizontal integration now became a Clarke byword
at board meetings. What had begun incrementally as a series of unre-
lated initiatives now took the form of a systematic and strategic search
for outpatient and wellness services to counterbalance declining acute
care revenues. Clarke was careful, however, to limit Memorial's appetite
to those opportunities serving the basic mission of health care, education
and research. Elsewhere expansion-minded hospitals made unwise investments in shopping malls and cattle ranches, but prudence dictated keeping
to what one best understood.

Thus was born "a whole new era" in the scope and structure of Memorial
Medical Center. With several auxiliary activities in place and others on
the horizon, it was time to redesign the corporate structure like a holding
company, to safely accommodate distinct enterprises, both for-profit and
not-for-profit. In his preparations for board consideration, Clarke relied on
models from the literature in hospital administration plus consulting advice
from a Chicago law firm. During a series of meetings in 1986, directors
agreed to create Memorial Medical Center System (MMCS), a parent corporation for the hospital, the foundation, the Friends organization, and its
other entities. New bylaws provided for the composition, authority and
election of corporation members, its board, and subsidiary boards.

The newly constituted MMCS board met monthly, just before hospital
board meetings. Its standard agenda differed sharply from its forerunner, with foundation and joint venture reports plus analyses of state and
national developments replacing hospital operational matters. CFO Paul
Smith developed separate financial systems for the proliferating corpora-
tions, and served as treasurer of nearly all of them.

What began as a fairly simple structure of four boxed entities on the system organization chart quickly sprouted new rectangles and other shapes,
as Clarke and his team conjured new acquisitions and joint ventures. Two
notable initiatives occurred in radiology and plastic surgery. Anxious

A New Front Door

Rapid growth of outpatient services and an expanding regional market for Memorial's "centers of excellence" produced another building boom during the late 1980s and 1990s. Hospital officials also were anxious to relocate the entrance and lobby, which were obscured on Rutledge Street behind a parking deck.

What began 40 years earlier as a single hospital building had evolved into a sprawling medical complex or "campus" filling ten blocks. Once a quiet and stable residential neighborhood, the near northwest side area had profoundly changed. Hospital officials were sensitive to the concerns of area residents, striving to offer fair market land prices, construct landscaped parking areas as a perimeter buffer, and generally be a responsible neighbor.

The principal construction projects were the Baylis Building, a unique cooperative venture, and Building E, a large structure whose diagonal placement (facing the intersection of Miller and First Streets) echoed the original 1943 facility. E was a costly and complex construction effort that took three years to complete. Functionally it created expansive new space for the Regional Cancer Center, lobby, offices, patient rooms, conference facilities and a state-of-the-art surgical area. This last unit reflected changing hospital design concepts through its location below ground level, to provide a hermetically sealed environment for surgery. Fifty years earlier the preference had been for a top floor location, to maximize access to natural light and fresh air.

Symbolically, E Building gave Memorial an impressive new "front door" facing downtown Springfield, and readily visible to arriving patients and visitors. It thus underscored fulfillment of the decades-old quest for hospital parity and Memorial Health System's regional stature.

to bring Magnetic Resonance Imaging (MRI) to Springfield, local radiologists knew that an investment of this magnitude ($3 million for the equipment and installation) would require cooperation between Memorial and St. John's. Accordingly, they prodded both hospitals to break their competitive tradition by signing a contract for joint usage of a new MRI facility located nearby. The tripartite arrangement with area radiologists was spearheaded by Drs. Charles Williams and William Sherrick.

Partly to retain Springfield's outstanding group of plastic surgeons, led by Dr. Elvin Zook, Memorial's administration joined forces to construct the Baylis Medical Building, housing the Institute of Plastic and Reconstructive Surgery. This complex arrangement enabled physicians to build on the hospital's land and lease a portion of the building's space back, for Memorial's expanded outpatient services.

A novel initiative that tested the outer limits of Clarke's health-only rule was the decision to jointly develop a "Best Inns of America" motel a few blocks away. At first glance an odd choice, in fact this development was vital to Memorial's marketing goals. Twenty per cent of the hospital's patients lived beyond the nine-county region around Springfield. Families who could not commute needed a convenient temporary residence, as did recovering patients who required close monitoring by doctors and visiting nurses. The novel agreement specified that Memorial would guarantee a minimum of 16 health-related guests a night, seven days a week. Occupancy over 65 per cent would entitle MMCS to rebates. The venture was a success both in attracting area patients and generating a small profit.

To both serve doctors and reap their loyalties, a new management consulting service was established. Designed to relieve physicians of their office management burden, this company offered a full menu, from billing to space acquisition and staffing. By 1996 it boasted over 90 clients in Springfield and other locations. Linking central Illinois primary care physicians was Health Care Network Associates (HCNA), with primary sites in Jacksonville, Lincoln, Springfield, Chatham and Petersburg.

There were other projects and partnerships as well: a child care center for families of Memorial employees, pharmacies, a medical supplies and equipment company, the previously mentioned mental health network, joint ownership or leasing of equipment for doctors and a skilled nursing care facility. A major expansion occured in the mid 1990s, when Abraham Lincoln Memorial Hospital (Lincoln) and St. Vincent Memorial Hospital (Taylorville) decided to affiliate within Memorial Health System.

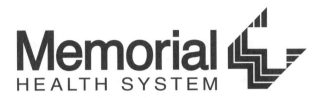

2007

Havana ■
Lincoln ★●■♦
Petersburg ●■
Jacksonville ♦●■
Springfield ★●■♦▲
Chatham ●
Taylorville ★♦

★ **MHS Hospitals**

● **HealthCare
Network Associates**

■ **Mental Health Centers
of Central Illinois**

♦ **Memorial Home Services**

▲ **Heritage Manor**

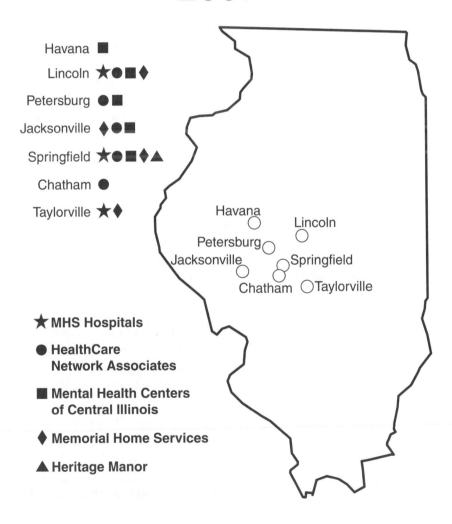

Memorial's Lutheran forebears would have been incredulous over the affiliation with Taylorville's Catholic institution. By 1996 the system's table of organization resembled a "Rube Goldberg" device, with 16 boxes or ovals and a maze of connecting lines.

By 1993 MMCS already was a misnomer, because the word "medical" was too narrow a description. The industry's emerging capitation payment system meant that hospitals received a flat pre-paid fee for each covered patient's total care. This not only intensified cost-containment steps at hospitals, but also suggested that preventive and other forms of non-acute care would be vital sources of future revenue. "Health" and "wellness" were more inclusive and accurate descriptors of the system's scope.

Accordingly, the board agreed to rename the parent company "Memorial Health System" (MHS), another sign of the rapidly changing times. Under this ever-widening umbrella, hospital care was steadily losing its historic primacy and other services were flourishing. The growth segments in America's massive health industry were sub-acute care, skilled care, home care, and so forth.

While Memorial created its own ventures and networks, it also followed a national trend toward multi-hospital cooperative alliances. At his inaugural board meeting in 1983 Clarke signaled his interest in joining one of the emerging national health systems. The next month he revealed his top choice, Voluntary Hospitals of America (VHA), which then represented 400 hospitals (110,000 beds) in 41 states. Clarke's prior job had been with a VHA institution, and he liked their decentralized structure.

Recognizing the high startup and continuing costs, Memorial's board reacted cautiously but positively. A VHA representative answered questions later that fall, and Clarke monitored VHA's progress in developing a central Illinois group. The immediate benefits would be substantial savings from the consolidated purchase of medical supplies, and easier access to capital for construction. Staff analysts conducted impact studies, and a special board committee explored the idea in depth.

Late in 1984 directors voted to join the ten-member "VHA Illinois" with a $200,000 purchase of VHA stock. Annual assessments were projected at $50,000. Ronald Krause began a lengthy term as its president in 1985, and he regularly met with Memorial officials and directors to explore promising ventures. The alliance shifted westward to add hospitals in eastern Iowa and Missouri, resulting in a name change to VHA Great Rivers in

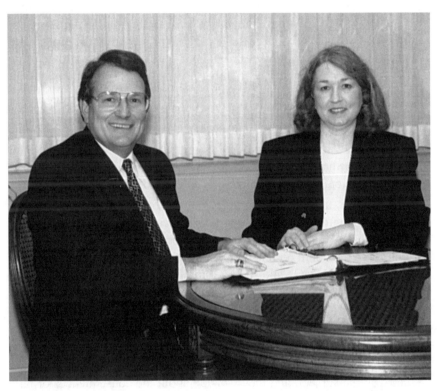

Robert Clarke (left) with Linda Culver (right), who served as Chair of Memorial's Board of Directors from 1993 to 1995. She was the first woman to serve in that role since Mildred Bunn's tenure in the 1940s.

1989. Bob Clarke served as its first board chairman. By 1996 it had grown to 16 owner members and a total of 65 hospitals, ranging in size from the sprawling Barnes-Jewish Hospital in St. Louis to small rural facilities.

The annual assessment rose somewhat, but to Clarke and others it was "a great financial investment." One study indicated that it saved or yielded $4 to Memorial for every $1 invested, counting intangible as well as tangible benefits. Moreover, it gave the institution a strategic edge in packaging health care contracts with large-scale area employers. For example, state workers or a utility's employees throughout central Illinois could be more readily served by an alliance of member hospitals that served Springfield, Quincy, Macomb, Normal, Jacksonville, Decatur and Belleville.

There seemed to be no limit to the cooperative possibilities. Among those implemented were regional purchasing agreements, joint marketing analyses, a community oncology program, and mobile lithotripter and MRI services. Short of a problematic merger of 65 disparate hospitals, VHA Great Rivers was an effective way to pool ideas and resources.

HMOs were another dynamic force on the health care horizon. Nationally, the number of such programs increased ten-fold from 1970 to 1984, reaching 250, and the tempo accelerated thereafter. Bob Clarke regularly briefed the board on this high-stakes phenomenon, as it debated the relative merits of HMOs and the less comprehensive Preferred Provider Organizations (PPOs). Central Illinois hospitals and physicians lagged behind the vanguard of programs on the east and west coasts, making any local trial ventures risky. Various initiatives surfaced and died during this exploratory period.

Board chairman Robert Lanphier and Clarke were the best-informed directors on the subject, and they worried about the consequences of failing to take the initiative. Doctor resistance persuaded them to wait, but then St. John's Hospital announced its plan for a new HMO in 1986. At stake was Memorial's share of state employee business, which then comprised a full ten per cent of its billings. It was time, all agreed, to act, if only as a tactic to protect existing market share.

There followed a bidding war between St. John's and Memorial that became a painful lesson in HMO dynamics and economics. The crosstown rival submitted a bid that Memorial analysts predicted would lose money. Clarke and his board faced a Hobson's choice: either compete at bargain-basement rates or lose ten per cent of their patients. Either option, according to projections, could cost Memorial as much as $3 million in revenues.

With misgivings but his characteristically aggressive manner, and with the board's full consent, Clarke opted to gamble with a matching bid. It was, he later recalled, "my biggest mistake." Memorial launched "Pro Health Illinois" in mid-1987, and soon was losing $100,000 a month. As predicted, premiums were too low. Worse, area doctors were not yet sufficiently pressured by competitive forces to control costs by limiting hospital usage and seeking patients from their colleagues. Struggling to motivate physicians was "an administrative disaster." In one year the projected $3 million loss ballooned to $5 million, compelling Memorial to terminate its HMO in 1987. Expecting sharp board criticism or worse, Clarke was heartened by its support and acceptance of mutual responsibility.

So burdensome was this lesson that Clarke despaired whether Springfield ever would accept HMOs, with their restrictions as well as their virtues. Consequently several years later he decided against extending Memorial's state license to offer HMOs. The combination of 1987's "sour pill" and the costly licensing paperwork convinced him. Hindsight proved this to be a second if less traumatic error, because preparing a new license application required even more time and "horrendous effort."

Within a few years area doctors and patients were ready to make HMOs work. Once again Memorial entered the sweepstakes, this time under more favorable conditions. Springfield Clinic, a large organization with considerable leverage in the local medical community, signed an agreement with the hospital for "Health Alliance Illinois." Heralded as "a milestone" in Springfield health care, the HMO enlisted state workers and other groups, and proved to be a financial success. The road had been bumpy, but central Illinoisans now joined 58 million Americans, and three out of four doctors, who have "seen the future, and it works." While President William Clinton's national health insurance, or "managed competition," failed in 1994, "unmanaged competition" thrived in the vacuum.

As traditional hospital revenue sources diminished, the Memorial Medical Center Foundation correspondingly rose in importance. Income from its steadily growing assets supported discretionary but valuable hospital activities. In its second decade the foundation accelerated development efforts on various fronts. Its holiday Festival of Trees proved to be popular and fruitful; the 1996 event drew over 24,000 visitors and raised $95 thousand. The annual giving campaign showed healthy growth, and in 1995 yielded one-half million dollars.

Planned giving is a slow and uncertain development source, but once undertaken it has great potential. One notable example occurred in 1989, when Memorial received title to land worth $1.2 million, from the estate of Opal Wedeberg. Directors decided to apply the proceeds to construction of a much needed but costly education center in the new E building. This modern complex of auditorium and meeting rooms became an immediate success, drawing over 5,000 participants in 1992. In 1995, for another example, the foundation received five bequests totaling $1.3 million.

Foundation directors and officials decided to mark the hospital's centennial with a special endowment effort, "The 1997 Society." Seeking gifts of $1,997 or more, and a grand total of $4 million, this campaign boasted nearly 300 members by 1995, with two years to go.

In 1992 the foundation recruited a new executive director, David Jahn. He, his staff and board were responsible for allocating as well as soliciting foundation funds. Its sponsored programs included free colon cancer screening, scholarships for nursing students, cardiology research, new cancer diagnostic equipment, support for in-home and hospice care, and various educational activities. In 1995, for example, the foundation awarded 23 separate grants.

In one decade Bob Clarke, his colleagues and governing board fundamentally changed the name, shape, purpose and appearance of Memorial Medical Center. Now a highly diversified health system with a dizzying list of affiliations and enterprises, it had managed to ride the successive waves of change in health care's quiet revolution. Comprehensive in its scope and fully integrated in its corporate structure, Memorial Health System was a major player in downstate medical care.

A Century's Legacy

If anything, the fast pace of change even quickened further throughout the nation's health care industry during the final years of the century. As Memorial Health System's 1995 annual report put it, "tumultuous and uncertain" conditions had reached the point that "change is constant in today's environment." Americans long ago had become accustomed to the almost daily announcements of medical and pharmaceutical break-throughs, but now even the most stable and familiar health care habits and institutions were under assault. The revolution in "managed care" pro-duced radical alterations in the traditional doctor-patient relationship, in the roles, respectively, of primary care providers and specialists, and in deeply ingrained public assumptions about the hospital as an acute care facility. A continuing national debate over the services and funding of Medicare and Medicaid left tens of millions of Americans uncertain about their own circumstances.

At Memorial the signs of change were unmistakable. One retired phy-sician observed, "It's a health care plant. It's not a community hospital anymore." The sprawling MHS campus consumed ten square blocks, within which the familiar acute care facility was but one large component. For another example, inpatient surgery, a traditional staple of hospital ser-vice, now lagged well behind outpatient surgery in volume. During 1996, 62 per cent of all surgical procedures at Memorial were performed on an outpatient basis. At the medical center alone there were more than 300,000 outpatient visits yearly. For the entire system the volume rose well above 500,000, due principally to outpatient care provided by the Visiting Nurse Association and Healthcare Network Associates.

To Bob Clarke and his administrative staff these rapid changes and uncertainties were an exciting but uncomfortable fact of daily life, as they struggled to stay abreast if not ahead in their field. Each week brought new perils and new opportunities, and therefore fateful new decisions. Clarke put it succinctly and dramatically: "Everyone's nervous, including me." Sometimes the news was good, as with the figures accompanying a 20th anniversary observance for the Regional Cancer Center. During 1995 Memorial was the hospital of choice for over 1,100 cancer patients, and the survival rate continued to improve. Sometimes it was bad, as when the city of Springfield negotiated an exclusive agreement with St. John's in 1996 to provide all elective hospital services for city employees, thereby reducing Memorial's share of the local market.

The institution that they directed had grown into a medical behemoth. There were more then 3,100 employees at Memorial Medical Center, and many of them were anxious about job security. Total system revenue in 1997 was budgeted at nearly $500 million, making Memorial a dominant area employer and spender.

To survive and even prosper in such conditions called for administrative skills that Clarke's predecessors had not been required to possess. The successful hospital administrator now needed political skills to negotiate and mediate, a bent for strategic planning, the ability to educate lay board members on complex issues, the courage to take risks in order to protect or augment market share, access to and mastery of timely and accurate data, nimble responsiveness to changing circumstances, and habits of proactive leadership.

In this maelstrom of rapid change, a "brave new world" for Memorial Health System, it would seem dangerously anachronistic to pause for a look backward. Nevertheless, Clarke and his board deliberately kept an eye on the past even as they peered into an unclear but rapidly arriving future. Their 1995 annual report to the public, after noting all the changes underway, assured citizens that "our basic values and commitment to high quality patient care remain unchanged." The most conspicuous evidence of this historical consciousness lay in Memorial's careful and ambitious plans for recognizing the hospital's centennial anniversary.

Never before in its 100 years had Memorial paused to celebrate its past. There was no fanfare accompanying its establishment in 1897, nor on its 25th, 50th and 75th anniversaries. In several instances, as previously noted, there had been little, if anything, to celebrate. The centennial was another matter, because Memorial now was a robust institution with annual surpluses in the millions of dollars and regional prestige for the quality and variety of its services. That alone was cause for self-congratulation with a series of centennial festivities. Clarke had even more in mind, however. He viewed the milestone as an occasion not only for ceremonies, but for serious reflection as well.

With characteristic foresight and focus, he initiated systematic planning for Memorial's centennial observance six years in advance. What most interested him were activities that would underscore, in an enduring fashion, the hospital's existence as a living, changing institution. That meant commissioning a comprehensive and serious centennial history, one intended to educate rather than simply celebrate. In turn, this required collecting and organizing the institution's voluminous and widely scattered records. Accordingly, Memorial established and staffed its own archives in 1996. By this simple but fateful act, officials were declaring that ongoing institutional history is important even if (or especially because) their organization is changing rapidly.

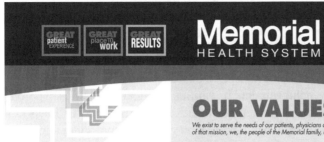

GREAT patient EXPERIENCE · GREAT placeTO work · GREAT RESULTS

Memorial
HEALTH SYSTEM

OUR VALUES:

We exist to serve the needs of our patients, physicians and the community at large. In pursuit of that mission, we, the people of the Memorial family, commit to the following values:

Service to Humanity

To care for life's precious gift of health is a calling of the highest order. We recognize the vulnerability that accompanies fear and hope. We accept the responsibility, entrusted to us every day, to serve humanity.

Excellence in Performance

By bringing together talented, dedicated people and advanced technology, we strive to provide quality healthcare. We take pride in ourselves, our colleagues and our workplace. We demonstrate that pride in the quality of service we deliver each day.

Respect for the Individual

We treat all people with dignity, respect and compassion. We believe that every person is unique and has the right to participate in decisions that affect them.

Value of Employees

More than buildings and equipment, people are Memorial Health System. Our success depends on an atmosphere of fairness and mutual respect. We are committed to provide equal opportunity for employment, growth and advancement. Furthermore, all employees are provided the opportunity to make a meaningful contribution to the fulfillment of our mission and are recognized for their accomplishments.

Integrity in Relationships

We are committed to fairness and honesty in all of our relationships. We recognize that our ability to sustain relationships, based on mutual trust, is the foundation of our success.

Community Responsibility

We hold our assets in public trust and recognize that continued financial viability is essential to fulfill our mission within the context of this statement of values. We believe that our community service obligation can best be met as a not-for-profit organization. Furthermore, we accept the responsibility to support research, education and public service programs that enrich the quality of life in our community.

Equal Access

We believe all people deserve equal access to care and services. In our pursuit of this belief we are constrained by our financial resources. We must balance our commitment to provide equal access to care and services with our obligation to ensure the continuing availability of quality healthcare for the future.

OUR MISSION:

To help maintain, restore and improve the health of the people and communities we serve.

OUR VISION:

To be the leading healthcare system that people choose over all others.

In addition to the history book, a series of special events in June marked Memorial's 100th year. First was a day-long reception honoring all employees, then a party for members of the medical staff, followed by a public open house. The hospital's conference area was decorated with artifacts and panels of text and photographs that depicted milestones in Memorial's history and notable achievements in various medical specialties. The climactic event was a formal dinner dance with hundreds of guests. Press kits and feature stories ensured that the occasion would receive wider attention. With the end of these celebrations, Memorial began its second century.

Memorial Milestones

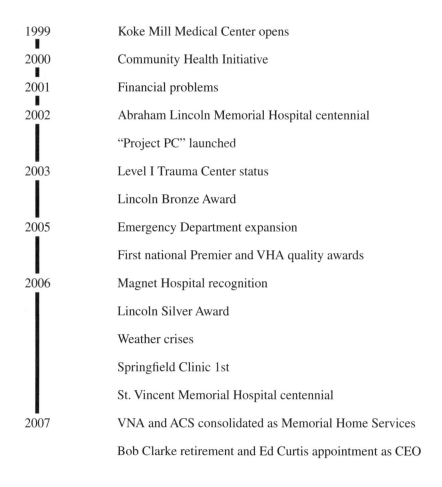

1999	Koke Mill Medical Center opens
2000	Community Health Initiative
2001	Financial problems
2002	Abraham Lincoln Memorial Hospital centennial
	"Project PC" launched
2003	Level I Trauma Center status
	Lincoln Bronze Award
2005	Emergency Department expansion
	First national Premier and VHA quality awards
2006	Magnet Hospital recognition
	Lincoln Silver Award
	Weather crises
	Springfield Clinic 1st
	St. Vincent Memorial Hospital centennial
2007	VNA and ACS consolidated as Memorial Home Services
	Bob Clarke retirement and Ed Curtis appointment as CEO

Chapter Nine

21st Century Health Care

The celebration of Memorial's centennial in 1997 was a proud but brief moment in the institution's history. Nationally and locally the health care environment was changing too rapidly for hospital administrators, physicians, and medical personnel to pause long for reflection or self-satisfaction. MHS had expanded and diversified into a network of thirteen affiliated entities and 5,400 employees. It was among the 100 largest regional health care systems in the United States, and its 1997 gross revenue was $500 million. Although some elements of this growing network have already been noted briefly, its magnitude and complexity, as well as the resulting benefits and challenges, warrant a more detailed review.

Partnerships and Ventures

"Partnerships" was the theme of MHS's 1997 annual report, and with good reason. Memorial Medical Center, a large and comprehensive hospital in Springfield, was the system's hub and headquarters. Thirty miles northeast, in historic Lincoln, was Abraham Lincoln Memorial Hospital, a financially sound and respected medical provider for residents of the community and environs. Sensing the difficult future for small rural hospitals, the ALMH board (at the urging of CEO David Sniff) cautiously entertained affiliation overtures from CEO Bob Clarke, who assured them

Paul Smith and Ed Curtis

Top officials at large hospitals typically boast the profession's standard qualification, a graduate degree in hospital administration. Two of Memorial's most accomplished executives of the modern era stand out as notable exceptions to this rule. Former CFO Paul Smith and newly named CEO Ed Curtis climbed the administrative ladder in unconventional ways. Their success stories reveal much about them individually and also about a supportive environment at Memorial for personal advancement.

Paul Smith came to Memorial in 1969 with only limited financial experience and education. Toiling quietly, he rose steadily in rank and the esteem of his peers to senior vice president. He mastered the latest and most complex issues: budgeting, cost allocation, bond financing, federal payment changes, and revenue forecasting. This "self-made star" retired in 2002.

Thirty two years ago Ed Curtis started work at Memorial on the basis of his college nursing education. Attracting favorable notice, he won several management promotions in the kidney department, and also found time to earn his MBA degree with honors from the University of Illinois. There followed three increasingly responsible vice-presidencies and his appointment as second-in-command in 1993. Both popular and highly respected among employees, physicians, board members, community leaders and his health care peers, Curtis was the natural choice in 2007 to succeed Robert Clarke. His remarkable success is the product of natural gifts of leadership and problem solving, deep loyalty to the organization, sound judgment, acute intelligence, and great people skills.

that it could survive and even thrive as a part of MHS. Lincoln banker and ALMH board member Terry Brown distinctly recalled those negotiations, which concluded successfully in September 1994. He also remembered the smooth transition, the ongoing attentiveness of Clarke and his Springfield colleagues, and the sensitive leadership of their new CEO, Forrest "Woody" Hester. To ensure dialog at the board level, Terry Brown also served for a term on the MHS board.

Whatever anxieties some Lincoln townspeople may have had about consolidation quickly dissolved, as ALMH remodeled its facilities, added new equipment and services, and celebrated its own centennial in 2002. This success story continues, as plans are well underway to replace the aging hospital structure with a new building on 57 acres that are more accessible to community residents. While the partners to this affiliation differ enormously in size, their relationship is one of mutual respect and satisfaction.

The year 1995 brought a second hospital into MHS. St. Vincent Memorial Hospital in Taylorville (30 miles southeast) was founded in 1906 by the Adorers of the Blood of Christ. Sister Meg Kopish, the order's Provincial, understood that small hospitals were in peril, so she invited Catholic health networks to explore an affiliation. When no offers came, she took a chance and spoke to Bob Clarke, who was both interested and understanding. Joining a religious institution to a secular one required great care, which both Clarke and Sister Meg exercised. MHS would provide management and financial controls, and also pay an annual stewardship fee, while SVMH would continue owning the property and preserving its religious identity.

The affiliation worked very well. Under MHS management the hospital converted most of its underutilized inpatient rooms to outpatient facilities, which by 2006 boasted 60,000 visits annually. Sister Meg served on the MHS board until her retirement and move to Rome in 1999. Her successor was Sister Barbara Jean Franklin, who also enjoyed cordial relations with Clarke and his staff. By 2006, the hospital's centennial year, she and others realized that the order's humanitarian mission needed to focus beyond hospitals. Her conversations with MHS officials resulted in an agreement to cede the hospital's property (valued at $4.9 million) to MHS, and convert it to a secular institution, Taylorville Memorial Hospital. This was a major change, but owing to the partnership's history of trust and goodwill, Sister Barbara Jean concluded, "it seemed like a natural thing." MHS paid its last annual stewardship fee and also made a contribution of $100,000 to the ongoing work of the Adorers of the Blood of Christ.

In addition to affiliating with small regional hospitals, CEO Clarke sensed an opportunity to recruit central Illinois primary care physicians to join a service network that would safeguard them in the approaching "managed care wars" of the1990's. The strategy was to launch the alliance in smaller communities where the anxiety was greatest before competing with existing group practices in Springfield. MHS officials hosted a series of informational meetings for selected primary care physicians, initially from Lincoln, then Jacksonville, and later Petersburg and Taylorville. There were follow-up discussions in each community, where Clarke and others identified the advantages of an area network: united strength in negotiating with insurers, MHS expertise and training in office and financial management, updates on the latest medical practices, and improved benefits for non-physician personnel. They also reassured doctors that Memorial would never interfere in each group's patient services.

For small town physicians this was a fateful step, and they deliberated at some length. After carefully reviewing national developments, Jacksonville's Dr. Marshall Hale concluded that the proposal made sense, and persuaded his partners to enlist. Thus was born HealthCare Network Associates (HCNA) in 1995. The alliance grew steadily until it was strong enough to enter the larger and more competitive Springfield market. Hale became leader of the Jacksonville group, and later served a productive term as an HCNA representative on the MHS board.

There were several nerve-racking experiences early in HCNA's growth, but the outcomes validated its effectiveness. One was a managed care company's effort in 1997 to drop Memorial as a provider. After some nervous deliberations, HCNA physicians decided to call the insurer's bluff with a counter threat to drop them. Their leverage worked, demonstrating the power of numbers. Several years later another provider imposed steep payment cuts, and once again HCNA and Memorial mounted enough influence to reverse the action. Just as Clarke had foreseen, MHS's alliance with area primary-care physicians—numbering 39 and growing by 2007—was mutually advantageous.

Nicely complementing this recruiting venture was Memorial's substantial investment in a large new clinical facility on Springfield's rapidly growing west side. Construction of the Koke Mill Medical Center began in 1998, and doors opened the next year. The handsome building at an accessible intersection comprises 96,000 square feet on a nine acre site, making it nearly a full service outpatient hospital. There are quarters for HCNA, Memorial ExpressCare, mammography, radiology, physical and occupational therapy, Memorial's Sportscare, the Orthopaedic Center of Illinois, and a pharmacy.

An unusual but fruitful 1996 initiative was Memorial's affiliation with Mental Health Centers of Central Illinois (MHCCI), a highly regarded six county system that offers a full range of behavioral and rehabilitation services. As with each of these new partnerships and ventures, the key to agreement and success lay in the support of MHCCI's CEO, Brian Allen, its board, and the synergy of mutual benefits. Another common ingredient was the continuing attention and commitment exhibited by Bob Clarke and his senior associates.

MHCCI retained its institutional and financial autonomy, but the relationship with MHS is close and productive. Mental health personnel enjoy access to Memorial's excellent training facilities and services. They also depend upon the system's depth of expertise in such areas as financial management, data operations, and human resources. MHS benefits from its close ties to a strong and widely respected mental health provider, increased patient referrals, and much improved screening of inpatient admissions. A comprehensive five-year review by MHCCI credited the partnership with significantly improving mental health care and dramatically enhancing the diagnosis and treatment of behaviorally complicated patients who are brought to the Emergency Department. Janet Stover, a member and former president of the MHCCI board, credits Memorial's Ed Curtis and Bob Clarke with sustained interest and support. Brian Allen also plays a vital role in his dual capacities as CEO of MHCCI and Memorial's Vice President for Behavioral Health.

For over 30 years Memorial Medical Center has been a teaching hospital and close neighbor of the Southern Illinois University School of Medicine. Their relationship cannot be described as a partnership, but for most of those years it has been friendly and mutually beneficial. Both Bob Clarke and Dr. Richard Moy, founding dean of the medical school, met often and welcomed joint ventures. As their respective physical plants expanded, so did the need and the opportunity for cooperation. For example, in the early 1990's Moy could not get capital funds for needed clinical space from the financially stretched state, so Clarke offered to have Memorial construct a new building and then lease the clinical quarters to SIU. The agreement was designed to facilitate state purchase once the fiscal picture improved. The new structure opened in 1993, the year Dean Moy retired, with Memorial's new, adjacent Baylis building housing plastic surgery and other Memorial offices. The SIU wing (aptly named in honor of Moy at Clarke's suggestion) relieved the medical school's overcrowding.

For the next nine years the bilateral cooperation weakened, as Dean Carl Getto took pains to avoid special ties with either of Springfield's two large hospitals. A detailed MHS board report and discussion early in 2000 noted traditional areas of cooperation, and encouraged better communication. Banker and civic leader A.D. Van Meter cared deeply about this, and was in a position to help by virtue of his service both on the MHS board and as president of the SIU Board of Trustees. Getto resigned the next year for a Wisconsin health care position, leading to the appointment of Dr. Kevin Dorsey as dean. Dorsey had earned his MD at SIU, had served on its faculty since 1983, and had won many friends and admirers.

Clarke and Dorsey were temperamentally suited to interact well, but in 2001 they had to overcome several issues, including those pertaining to financial support and the recruitment of SIU medicine/pediatricics practices. Once these problems ended, and with the active help of Van Meter, the interpersonal and inter-institutional relationship flourished. Dorsey agreed to join the MHS board, ensuring regular contact at the highest level. Clarke and his board found ways to allocate several million dollars annually in support of the medical school. Recognizing SIU's incalculable value as a neighbor, they regarded the transactions more as an investment than an expense. It is largely thanks to the medical school that health care is Springfield's largest economic activity, with 700 physicians (two-thirds of whom are SIU faculty or medical graduates). Dean Dorsey's presence at Memorial's board meetings has demonstrated to him the depth of their commitment.

Construction that is presently underway on SIU's $21 million SimmonsCooper Cancer Institute, adjacent to Memorial, is further evidence of cooperation. MHS helped obtain several of the small land parcels for this building, and will construct a pedestrian bridge linking it to the Baylis Building, Memorial Medical Center, and the medical school.

As noted in the previous chapter, Memorial became the sponsor of the ten-county Visiting Nurse Association of Central Illinois (VNA) in 1984, helping it expand its region and also its home services to include hospice care and other programs. Early in 2000 system officials considered constructing a residential hospice facility, but concluded that home care was the preferred option for most patients. Another useful affiliate was Alternative Care Services (ACS), which maintained facilities in Springfield, Lincoln, Jacksonville, and Taylorville to distribute medical equipment and supplies to home-based patients throughout MHS's service area. In 2006 these affiliates logged 31,000 hospice care days and 32,000 home health visits. Recognizing their close operating relationship and common regional boundaries, Memorial officials decided in 2007 to consolidate VNA and ACS into one unit, Memorial Home Services.

Memorial took the lead in 2000 to form the Community Health Initiative (CHI), a not-for-profit organization aimed at addressing serious and preventable health problems of Sangamon County residents. Helping with start-up funding were the MMC Foundation, St. John's Hospital, and private donations. This charitable venture was in response to mounting local and national evidence that unmet medical needs of adults and children caused serious and costly health problems for society. Qualifying for federal assistance, CHI was able to obtain funding for North Star Clinic (11th Street) and later the Capitol Community Health Center (Cook Street). MMC and St. John's Hospital continue to provide a growing volume of free clinical services for the Capitol Community Health Center, but the CHI program itself is less active, owing to uncertainties over proposals for a large state effort. One possible niche for the future would be to better coordinate the provision of short-term medication for needy people.

One final MHS venture took several years and protracted discussions, but eventually surpassed the expectations of each partner. As early as 1997 there were exploratory conversations between officials at Memorial and Springfield Clinic, an established medical group based on South 7th Street. At that time, the clinic already had 129 physicians on its staff, and partly due to the distance of its campus from either large hospital, it viewed them neutrally, as simply the yellow brick one (St. John's) and the red brick one (Memorial). The subject of institutional cooperation was sensitive for many reasons, including MHS's competitive ventures with HealthCare Network Associates and Koke Mill Medical Center. After several false starts, negotiations focused in 2002 on acute crowding at Springfield Clinic, which had led to spreading some of its physician offices elsewhere, including the Baylis Building. The patience and creativity of Bob Clarke and Ed Curtis paid off with an agreement in 2003 to consolidate Springfield Clinic's scattered outposts in a new four-story building on the

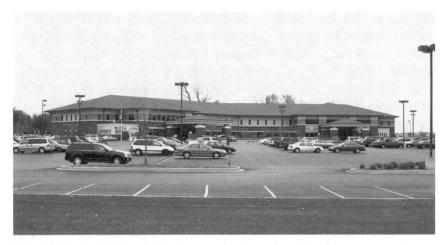

Koke Mill Medical Center.

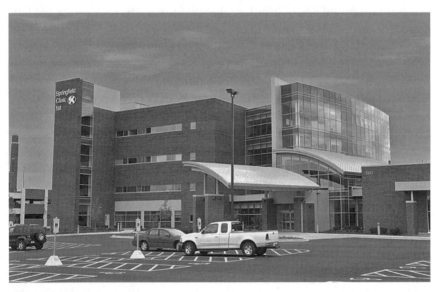

Springfield Clinic 1ˢᵗ.

east edge of Memorial's campus. The 70 Clinic surgeons and their office staffs wanted the convenience of hospital proximity, and they preferred the operating rooms, technicians, and convenient scheduling at Memorial Medical Center. Choosing "red over yellow" broke longstanding Clinic policy and represented major progress in Memorial's decades-long rivalry with St. John's Hospital.

Springfield Clinic 1st, which opened on North 1st Street in 2006, contains over 100,000 square feet of offices and examining rooms for surgeons and their staffs. Memorial Health System purchased the land and constructed the $27 million building, which it leases exclusively to Springfield Clinic. Thanks in part to this building's proximity and the confidence it reflects, MMC currently receives 67 per cent of all Clinic hospital referrals. Incidentally, Springfield Clinic continues to grow, with some 200 physicians under contract and a major construction project at its base facility.

At this writing, all of the partnerships and ventures of the past 15 years have survived and even succeeded. That alone is a notable accomplishment. Contributing to the success have been numerous MHS employees and administrators and a responsive board, but critical leadership came from Bob Clarke and his executive colleagues. They noted national trends, scouted growth opportunities, carefully developed proposals that would be mutually beneficial, and tirelessly worked to persuade potential partners of their sincerity and reliability.

Challenges and Opportunities

Acquisitions and partnerships, no matter how successful, cannot insulate a modern hospital system from difficult financial conditions, a problem that Memorial Health System faced in the early years of the millennium. Net income plummeted from $7.4 million in fiscal year 2000 (October 1, 1999 to September 30, 2000) to a loss of $25.1 million in 2001. After years of smooth financial sailing, this was a severe jolt that demanded both analysis and action. The analysis revealed two causes, one internal and the other external. Internally, there were serious delays and mistakes in the installation of new billing and collection software, which badly stretched the hospital's ordinary collection cycle, and also raised the level of bad debt write-offs. CFO Paul Smith and his financial specialists had to work overtime for months to iron out the problems and get the new system operating properly. Externally, the state of Illinois abruptly and significantly reduced its Medicaid reimbursements, greatly impacting the organization's bottom line.

Bob Clarke kept this subject at the forefront of monthly board meetings until the crisis passed. He also took all reasonable steps to mitigate the problem through a cost containment campaign. Inevitably, there were some employee layoffs, 42 in all, which were very difficult for everyone. Board members also approved Clarke's recommendation to defer or even cancel several promising initiatives that had been under active consideration. Memorial had to reduce its annual financial support of a residency clinic at SIU School of Medicine, which was unwelcome news to the new dean, Kevin Dorsey. MHS also terminated a costly and outdated mobile mammography unit that served Sangamon and surrounding counties. Reacting to the state's sudden and drastic cuts, Clarke reported to the press, "I'm enraged." He and several associates joined many members of the Illinois Hospital Association in denouncing Governor George Ryan's arbitrary and costly behavior. COO Ed Curtis testified before a state senate committee about the burden to Memorial, and Senior Vice President for Marketing and Planning Mitch Johnson offered similar remarks to a house committee. Eventually the state relented, but the damage was substantial for fiscal year 2001 and much of 2002. At a time when so many good things were happening for MHS, this setback was a sobering reminder of fortune's fickle ways.

Governance of both Memorial Medical Center and the entire Memorial Health System rests in two separate boards of directors that meet seriatim every other month. There is some overlap of participation and agenda in the two meetings, but their respective areas of authority naturally differ. Bob Clarke envisioned governing boards that would be diverse in composition, representative of as many Memorial constituencies as possible, focused on large planning and policy issues, well-informed in advance on agenda items, orderly in their deliberations yet open to full discussion on every issue, and comfortable with consensus decision making. By all accounts and measures these are, in fact, the characteristics of both boards, which draw praise from those who serve or have served. The MHS board of directors numbers 17, and is diverse by gender, race and age. There are two active physicians to represent their profession's concerns, plus (on a rotating basis) representatives of the numerous affiliates and partners described in detail earlier in this chapter. Current policy permits members to serve up to nine one-year terms, but it was not imposed retroactively on incumbents. There also is an age limit of 72.

Several former board members (Terry Brown, Marshall Hale, A.D. Van Meter) and two incumbents (chairman Dwight O'Keefe and Kevin Dorsey) agree that the MHS board is a model of productivity and collegiality. Its meetings rarely last longer than 90 minutes, but manage to address all agenda issues fully. To begin the meetings Clarke typically has a Memorial official or an outside expert report on some timely and important subject. A standard monthly focus in the past several years has been monitoring progress on MHS's strategic plan. Successful governance structures and behavior are one measure of a healthy organization, and they are a conspicuous plus at Memorial.

A perennial issue in Memorial's 100-plus year history has been its relationship with the older and for many years larger and better respected St. John's Hospital. In modern times that story has comfortably settled into a mixture of cooperation and competition, and these practices continue today. While carefully avoiding any actions that might draw antitrust litigation, MMC and St. John's have found many areas of mutual interest. For example, they coordinated planning and implementation of the partial and then total ban on smoking, developed joint efforts to battle hospital infection, and cooperated to launch the previously mentioned Community Health Initiative (CHI). In addition they conferred on the daunting task of automating their respective medical records systems, knowing that area physicians would be more compliant when faced with a united approach.

A novel initiative was the decision to jointly apply to state authorities for Level 1 Trauma Center status. Neither hospital acting alone could cite sufficient volume to qualify, or afford the added staffing expenses, but by combining forces and agreeing to rotate the designation annually, Memorial and St. John's won this important recognition on July 1, 1999. The center receives state financial support, and accepts approximately 1,000 critical care cases annually, from 15 hospitals in central and southern Illinois. Typically these trauma patients are transported by helicopter to approved landing areas at either hospital. The annual transfer of center status needs refinement, but overall this has been a model of inter-institutional cooperation. Finally, Memorial and St. John's each agreed in 2004 to be a 25 per cent partner in Prairie Cardiovascular's venture for a separate Prairie Diagnostic Center, which opened in 2006 on Carpenter Street, roughly midway between the two hospitals.

The other side of this relationship, competition, has remained strong and in some cases intense. Memorial's Mitch Johnson observes that their

From Smoke-Filled to Smoke-Free

One measure of society's changing health habits has been Memorial's policy on smoking. Lutheran strictures against tobacco on moral grounds somewhat deterred smoking during the hospital's first forty years. For the next half century Memorial officials, staff patients and visitors were free to smoke as much as they wished, and virtually anywhere on the premises. Ashtrays were available in waiting rooms, patient rooms, all staff lounges, the cafeteria, corridors, and even the surgical area. The only restricted locations were where oxygen usage created a serious fire risk. Cigarette vending machines were available as a convenience.

One lonely but determined voice against smoking was that of Dr. Stuart Yaffe. Beginning as early as World War II, when GIs were receiving free cigarettes from a patriotic tobacco industry, Yaffe campaigned to place signs on the vending machines, disavowing hospital endorsement of an unhealthy practice. His annual appeals to fellow physicians and directors fell on deaf ears, even after the Surgeon General's critical report on smoking, issued in. By then he was pressing to remove vending machines and limit smoking to designated areas.

Yaffe's persistence, plus gradually changing public opinion finally persuaded hospital officials in the 1970s to begin imposing restrictions. Sparse and ill-enforced at first, and yet still intensely unpopular with smokers, the "No Smoking" zones steadily expanded until May 7, 1990, when Memorial and St. John's jointly proclaimed their facilities as "SmokeFree" environments.

competitive focus is not so much on St. John's, but rather a variety of national quality benchmarks, but in a city with two good hospitals, people inevitably will compare experiences and reputations. Each institution has longstanding strong suits (e.g., pediatrics and cardiac care at St. John's; plastic surgery, the renal unit, and rehabilitation services at Memorial), but no specialty is sacrosanct in their rivalry or the marketing they employ. Such competition is healthy for both hospitals, and it increases the options available to patients.

There is widespread acknowledgement in the medical community and elsewhere that, over the past fifteen years or so, Memorial generally has outperformed its "yellow brick" rival. In its programs, relationships, and initiatives MHS has been more energetic, entrepreneurial, and progressive than St. John's. While such opinions are necessarily subjective, they also are well-informed and supported by market share changes. Memorial's share of hospital admissions has risen from 42 per cent in the late 1980's to 55 per cent in recent years. Among the reported factors are governance and administrative differences, plus a rising preference among area surgeons for the efficiency, timely scheduling, and staff responsiveness in Memorial's surgery department.

St. John's continues to be an excellent hospital, but it has often lagged because it lacks a local governing board with the authority to respond quickly to issues and opportunities. The same applies to its on-site executives and administrators, who have been able people but lacked the power to act without time-consuming clearance from above. The leadership circumstances also have differed. Robert Clarke spent 24 years as Memorial's CEO; at St. John's there were four different executive vice presidents over that period. Clarke had both administrative latitude and board backing to explore and negotiate new ventures. His counterparts, highly capable and respected as they were, lacked such authority. People at Memorial who have met Stephanie McCutcheon, the new CEO of the Hospital Sisters Health System (which governs St. John's) are impressed by her ability and goals, so this existing disadvantage may change in coming years. Furthermore, St. John's is now recovering from a serious income shortfall in 2006 (similar to Memorial's problems in 2001), and likely will be in a position to sharpen its competitive efforts.

For some years another local competitor was the much smaller Doctors' Hospital, but it closed in 2003. Interestingly, plans are well underway to open two small and specialized proprietary institutions. "Kindred Healthcare" will serve long-term acute care patients, and "Psychiatric Solutions, Inc." will convert the Doctors' Hospital building into a children's psychiatric facility. Far from objecting on competitive grounds to these niche hospitals, both Memorial and St. John's have registered their approval. Kindred Healthcare will relieve the pressure on MMC's intensive care beds, and Psychiatric Solutions will be a welcome partner in concert with Memorial and Mental Health Centers of Central Illinois (MHCCI).

Disaster readiness is a perennial concern for hospitals as well as public safety and public health organizations. But in the modern era the variety of real and potential disasters has significantly increased, from seismic and weather crises to pandemics and now terrorism. The events of September 11, 2001 and the Katrina hurricane flooding are but the most dramatic examples of this challenge. It is a truism that hospitals can never be fully prepared for mass emergencies, but Memorial has worked hard to be ready for anything. In 2004 it and St. John's received state funds to assist terrorism response planning in an 18 county area of central and southern Illinois. From those meetings there are advisory checklists and advance arrangements to streamline response time. That same year the MHS board received a special presentation on a threatened influenza pandemic.

To date, the actual emergencies have not been global, but local. A tornado carved a destructive path through Springfield in the early spring of 2006, leaving many people homeless and many streets impassable. Later that year an early winter ice storm left much of the area without electricity or easy transportation. Just two months later a heavy blizzard had similar consequences. In all three of these natural disasters many Memorial employees either could not return home from work or get to work, so providing space for the stranded workers and substitutes for the others was a major challenge. Moreover, both MMC and Koke Mill Medical Center handled a large volume of emergency and Express Care patients. Thanks to advance planning and much personal effort, Memorial handled these three emergencies effectively. The hospital's large conference center became a temporary shelter for stranded employees, and the cafeteria produced meals at a volume well above normal. Disaster planning is an imperfect science, but MHS has learned from each past crisis, and expects to be better prepared for the next one.

Recruiting and retaining a capable work force is a challenge to any organization, and especially in the modern health care industry, which continues to experience growing pains. With over 5,400 workers, Memorial

Health System is a leading area employer, and like its peers faces some temporary labor shortages and others like nursing that are almost constant. Good personnel management includes in-service educational programs, avenues for advancement, periodic and constructive evaluation, regular communication through publications and/or meetings, two-way dialogue with supervisors, recognition of lengthy service, and reasonable levels of salary and benefits. All of these requisites (and more) at Memorial are the responsibility of Senior Vice President and Chief Human Resources Officer Forrest "Woody" Hester. A 30 year employee himself, Hester previously served eleven very successful years as CEO of the MHS affiliate, Abraham Lincoln Memorial Hospital. A senior associate calls him "one of our strongest leaders."

Memorial Memo is a four-page weekly employee newsletter, with program announcements, construction updates, benefits news, United Way appeals, recognition of honored employees, and often a message of congratulations or thanks from CEO Clarke. In recent years it has included a monthly insert, **Stars of Memorial,** to identify newcomers, salute special achievements, and quote patient testimonials. There also is an annual recognition dinner to honor employees who have served for five years or multiples of five. In 1997, for example, there were 426 honorees, including one 40-year veteran, two at 35 years, and seven at 30 years. These and other programs make Memorial an attractive workplace, as measured by various surveys. One, a study of 500 American hospitals, placed MHS in the 87th percentile of employee "satisfaction and engagement." The high morale reflected in this measure comes from the many programs and benefits administered under the direction of Woody Hester and the system's entire human resources team, plus the example set by administrators up to the executive level. Bob Clarke keeps his door open as much as possible, welcoming employees who want to visit. His successor, Ed Curtis, makes daily trips around MMC and greets most employees by name. Such personal attention makes Curtis a highly respected and popular figure.

The above-noted survey mentioned "engagement" as well as satisfaction. The word was well-chosen, because there is persistent effort to communicate Memorial goals and values to all employees, through meetings, posters, newsletter reminders, wallet cards, and other means. It is very unusual for a large and diverse labor force to absorb institutional values to the point that they actually apply those values in their daily work practices. Skeptics might question whether Memorial really could accomplish this,

Leonia Cole's Record of Service

Early in 2007 surgical technologist Leonia Cole observed the **53rd** anniversary of her employment at Memorial Medical Center. As the 54th anniversary approaches, she has no desire to slow down or retire.

Leonia was born in Mississippi and grew up in Tennessee. Soon after moving to Springfield with her young family, she was hired by Memorial Hospital, which had begun employing African-Americans only a few years earlier. She lacked professional training, so the best job available was as a nurse's aide. In those baby boom years Memorial Hospital's one building (constructed in 1943) was overcrowded much of the time, which kept Leonia busy with the many housekeeping tasks assigned to her. She also took every opportunity to learn the demanding work of operating room nurses, and after fifteen years of experience was promoted to surgical technologist.

Leonia rises daily at 5:00 a.m., and is at work by 6:30. A woman of great loyalty and many accomplishments (but few words), she calls Memorial, simply, "a nice place to work."

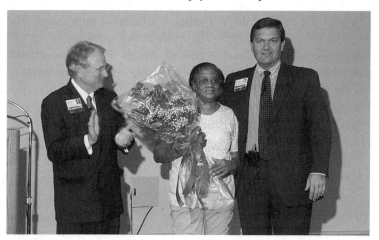

President and CEO Robert Clarke, left, and executive vice president and COO Ed Curtis congratulate Leonia Cole for her 50 years of service in 2004.

but surveys and numerous interviews validate the claim. Reinforcing staff dedication is monetary recognition; MHS awards success sharing bonuses to all employees (full and part time) following any year in which it has met or exceeded certain financial goals.

Like all hospitals, Memorial faces a chronic shortage of nurses, in the range of fourteen per cent. It uses the familiar recruiting methods: close contact with nursing schools, targeted advertising, job fairs, and also works hard to retain those already on staff. One unusual advantage in these efforts is its designation in 2006 as a "Magnet" hospital by the American Nurses Credentialing Center. This prestigious award for "Excellence in Nursing Services" is based on rigorous criteria, voluminous data, and an intensive site inspection. Through 2006, only four per cent of American hospitals had earned Magnet status, which places MHS in an elite category and gives it an edge in recruitment.

Great Expectations

Expansion and diversification were two overriding objectives in Memorial's centennial years; a third was to develop and achieve the highest possible standards of performance throughout the system. To focus on this effort, Bob Clarke created two new ranking positions: Medical Director and Vice President of Quality and Organizational Development. The latter job title might seem amorphous to the layman, but it had great impact throughout MHS. Jim Bente, who was appointed to the post in May 2000, had the responsibility to generate broad performance goals and measurements that could be employed by every department and unit within the system. In concert with other administrators, he produced the MHS Performance Excellence Model, which identified three vital objectives for patients: Safety (freedom from risk or harm), Clinical Effectiveness (evidence-based care), and Quality (process consistency). Explaining and promoting this model through meetings, posters, annual reports, and issues of **Memorial Memo** and other employee newsletters took both effort and time, but within a few years it was familiar as a blueprint for improved performance.

In 2004 CEO Bob Clarke spearheaded a second, complementary approach to making quality a Memorial byword. By evaluating the best strategic planning practices of other high-performing organizations, he concluded that a successful plan must be simple and concise, focused on

front line employees, and reinforced constantly. After extensive staff deliberations, it was agreed that excellent performance should (1) create a **great**
patient experience, (2) make MHS a **great** place to work, and (3) get **great**
results. Pruning many ideas and words into this simple mantra was difficult
but effective, and permeating the message with a familiar and feel-good
word, "great," made it easier to promulgate among 5,000 employees. With
a performance model emphasizing excellence and strategic goals stressing
great, Memorial's leaders could proclaim a succinct but vital message to
every employee. Organization-wide employee meetings, plus newsletter
features and even a handy wallet "Great" card combined to strengthen a
sense of common purpose. Valuable in its own right, this effort also led to
a series of national awards that are covered later in this chapter.

Striving for excellence and greatness applies to every facet and function
of an organization. For example, MHS embarked in 2002 on "Project PC,"
a multi-year plan to convert all medical records to an electronic format
in a fully integrated system. If implemented successfully, it will improve
the quality of patient care, enable qualified users to access data easily and
anywhere, further safeguard the privacy of patient records, provide off-site
redundancy in the event of a disaster, streamline the work of physicians
and nurses, and help control hospital costs. An effort of this magnitude
and complexity required expert consultants, a careful plan and timetable,
new equipment and space, extensive staff training, and a large ($20 mil-
lion) budget. Within one year the Emergency Department conversion was
completed, and progress continued on other units. Various other comprehensive electronic medical records programs have been successfully
launched. In 2006 Memorial acquired large office quarters several miles
west of the system campus, and moved its entire data center there. Project
PC is scheduled to complete its work by 2010.

In modern America there are two familiar public institutions, hospitals
and airports, that always seem to be under construction. Consequently they
grow into oddly shaped and expansive structures that easily become bewildering mazes to visitors. Signage tends to become ad hoc and inconsistent.
Recognizing that MMC was close to becoming such a labyrinth, officials
decided in 2001 to entirely rethink and revamp the designation of various
hospital wings, and the directions to visitors. They engaged "wayfinding"
experts at Aesthetics, Inc., a consulting firm that employs a multi-sensory
approach and artistic values in its work. Their first recommendation was
to identify three zones of the sprawling complex, give each zone a familiar but distinctive name, and use colors, photographs, artwork and icons

as well as text to guide visitors. Memorial Medical Center now has three zones, Lincoln, Capitol, and Garden, each with its own bank of elevators, maps, directories and identifying images in signs, at hallway intersections, and on the tile floors. Distinctive colors and artwork at regular intervals easily guide people to their destinations. The overall effect is informative and aesthetically pleasing, demonstrating that the quest for quality can take many forms.

Early in his years as CEO, Bob Clarke identified six centers of excellence, which were medical specialties of notably high quality and reputation at Memorial. They were cancer care, plastic surgery (including the burn unit), the kidney program, women's health, cardiopulmonary medicine, and physical rehabilitation services. More than 20 years later the list is largely unchanged, except for several additional areas. The following pages briefly recount developments during the past fifteen years in the original six specialties, then turn to the later ones.

Cancer research is vital to improved care, and in 2002 Memorial Medical Center shared a National Cancer Institute research grant with two other Illinois hospitals. That same year MMC became the first Illinois hospital to introduce a fully integrated approach to detecting lesions that are precursors to cervical cancer. It also was a leader in combining PET (positron emission tomography) and CT (computed tomography) for superior cancer diagnosis. Thanks to these initiatives and others, Memorial is a leading provider of breast biopsy procedures in central Illinois and Missouri.

The Institute of Plastic Surgery remains highly valued as a department at SIU School of Medicine and a program at MMC. It was chaired for over 30 years by Dr. Elvin Zook, who enjoyed a close social and working relationship with Bob Clarke. Their mutual respect was central to the unique partnership that constructed and leased the Baylis Building. Institute offices and examining rooms occupy the entire first floor, with surgery facilities one level below, which is a great convenience for patients and doctors alike. Memorial officials responded quickly and consistently to requests for research support, new operating room instruments, and new procedures such as liposuction and gene therapy. Appreciating these improvements, plastic surgeons have directed 80-90 per cent of their elective surgeries to MMC. In accordance with their original agreement, Institute surgeons sold their majority interest in Baylis to Memorial Health System in 2004, making it sole owner and landlord. Two years later Zook retired as chair, and was succeeded by Dr. Michael Neumeister, a specialist in hand and microsurgery. The Institute and its physicians hold a highly respected national reputation.

The highly regarded kidney department marked a milestone in 2001, its 500th transplant. This came 28 years after founding director Dr. Alan Birtch performed the first procedure. Upon retirement Birtch received a Lifetime Achievement Award for his efforts to promote organ donor awareness. His successor was Dr. Timothy O'Connor. Another Memorial leader is Rehabilitation Services, which has grown in volume and personnel to the point that its existing quarters are crowded. In 2007 it was awarded a rare, fivefold accreditation for its rehabilitation services from the Commission on the Accreditation of Rehabilitation Facilities (CARF). Memorial is one of only four health care organizations in the world, and the only one in Illinois, to receive full three-year accreditation for five program areas of rehabilitation services. These program areas are (1) inpatient rehabilitation—adults and children; (2) brain injury inpatient rehabilitation—adults and children; (3) spinal cord system of care—adults and children; (4) multiple service outpatient medical rehabilitation—adults and children; and (5) stroke inpatient specialty.

Cardiac surgery is among the most profitable specialties available to hospitals, so naturally there is sharp competition among those large enough to have their own heart programs. In Springfield, St. John's Hospital has Prairie Heart Institute on its campus, making it the largest program in the state. Memorial Medical Center follows right behind, a respectable position but one that hospital officials have worked for years to reverse. One method is to concentrate on certain distinctive specialties: women's health and vascular medicine. Women's cardiac health is more important than most people appreciate, because heart disease is the leading cause of death in females. Memorial targets women with some of its cardiac advertising, and occasionally sponsors women's heart fairs and publications. It also made sense in 2006 to rename its cardiac program the Heart and Vascular Institute. One problem in the last several years has been turnover in the position of executive director, held on an interim basis in 2007 by Doug Rahn. Looking ahead, there are tentative long range plans to reinforce the MHS commitment to cardiac care with a major construction project.

The Emergency Department joined the existing centers of excellence by virtue of its shared Level 1 Trauma Center status, plus Memorial's investment in expanded facilities and streamlined attention to patients. The year 2002 was MMC's turn as Trauma Center, and its record was impressive.

There were over 47,000 emergency visits, including 764 trauma cases. A $1 million expansion and remodeling occurred late in 2005, doubling the department's space, creating fourteen more beds for a total of 44, and increasing staff support by ten. The purpose was twofold: to respond to growing volume (60,000 cases in 2007), and to improve both patient care and response time. Triage procedures and patient intake steps were streamlined, and these combined improvements reduced by one-third the average duration of an emergency patient's stay.

One reason these commitments and investments have been possible year-in and year-out is the formula MHS employs to budget capital improvements (construction, remodeling, equipment). It allocates 90 per cent of operating income every year for capital purposes, ensuring steady and significant expansion and improvement. The remaining ten per cent, plus all non-operating income, are treated as surplus, which grew by a generous $120 million between 2001 and 2007.

When any public organization is both expanding and improving, it wants to broadcast the good news, so that its consumers (patients), employees, benefactors, peers and community leaders will appreciate and support the asset they have. Memorial officials believed that its performance excellence and great results warranted wider notice, which it has sought through candidacy for a variety of state and national awards, plus a generous budget for advertising.

In the keen competition among hospitals for recognition, MHS has enjoyed a string of gratifying announcements. Earlier in this chapter there was mention of the prestigious "Magnet Hospital" recognition in 2006 by the American Nurses Credentialing Center. In 2003 the Joint Commission on Accreditation of Healthcare Organizations (JCAHO) awarded Memorial a preliminary score of 97 (out of 100), and then ranked it in the top 20 per cent of 16,000 American hospitals. There was special commendation of an increased emphasis on patient safety and care. That same year the Lincoln Foundation for Performance Excellence honored MHS with its Bronze Award, then in 2005 its Silver Award, one of only nine in Illinois. In addition, MMC and its partner to the north, Abraham Lincoln Memorial Hospital, earned a Premier Award for Quality in joint replacement and open heart surgery.

Memorial's membership in the cooperative association, Voluntary Hospitals of America, led to a series of awards. For three years in a row it received the VHA Leadership Award for Supply Chain Management, in

Who Owns Memorial?

Originally, and for its first third of a century, Springfield Hospital and Training School was the property of stockholders who met annually to elect a board of directors responsible for governing the institution. Ownership shares were closely held by Lutheran leaders and later the Evangelical Lutheran Hospital Association of Central Illinois.

This arrangement changed abruptly and permanently with the new charter and bylaws adopted in 1931. Since then, ownership has diffused so broadly as to be practically amorphous; today Memorial Health System (MHS) and the original hospital, Memorial Medical Center (MMC), are the property of the communities they serve. These communities are not the familiar incorporated cities like Springfield, but the people and human institutions that inhabit them. Representing hundreds of thousands of "owners" is a body (the "corporation") of citizen volunteers ("members") who elect the MHS board of directors, and also separate boards for many of its organizational subsidiaries like MMC. The boards have fiduciary responsibility and thus serve as stewards of these valuable community assets.

Because MHS and MMC are not-for-profit charitable institutions, they pay no dividends to stockholders. Instead, any excess revenue over expenses is reinvested in facilities, equipment and jobs, all intended to serve the health and medical needs in their communities. Moreover, as a community-owned system, MHS provides many necessary but not self-supporting services, helping ensure that quality care is available to everyone, regardless of ability to pay.

Who owns Memorial? You and your neighbors do.

recognition of streamlined purchasing procedures. The year 2007 brought VHA's top honor, the President's Award, and MHS was the only hospital in the country to receive such recognition. Also that year it submitted an application and documentation for the coveted Malcolm Baldrige National Quality Award, a goal that was targeted for 2010.

Among senior vice president Mitch Johnson's various oversight responsibilities is advertising, and working closely with him is vice president of communications and marketing Ed McDowall. Over the past 20 years, Memorial has had three primary audiences or markets: patients, doctors, and insurers. The relative importance of them has changed with time, and in recent years the focus has sharpened on reaching patients, whose hospital choices directly affect operating income. The total marketing budget (under $1 million) has not changed greatly, but a sharply increased portion has addressed patients, the consumers of health care. Vying with other health care organizations for patients, Memorial has shifted from institutional or goodwill advertising to bolder and more direct appeals, all produced by a medical marketing firm in Champaign. The highest potential specialties get the most advertising attention: cardiovascular care, emergency services, pain management, stroke treatment, and joint replacement surgery.

Ads for "JointWorks" touted Memorial Medical Center's hip and knee replacement program as "No. 1 in Illinois" in 2006 and 2007, according to HealthGrades, a national health care quality measurement company. Consumers were urged to choose MMC's Emergency Department because it was "FastER, StrongER, and SmartER." Paralleling this marketing has been an intensified public relations effort, with frequent press releases and encouragement of print and electronic media coverage.

Overall, Memorial Health System entered its 110th year with a clear vision for the future, great energy, excellent employee morale, the good will of area physicians, a modern and attractive physical plant, high quality medical and surgical departments, a wall or two of award citations, and an aggressive marketing strategy.

Leadership Transition

By 2007 Robert Clarke had been at the helm of a large and complex regional health care system for 24 years, an unprecedented duration for Memorial and an unusually long stint for any public or private institution.

He was in his early 60's and enjoyed good health. But privately he had mused for several years about retiring. The work was still rewarding, but it was tiring and deprived him of adequate attention to his elderly mother, wife, children, and young grandchildren. The top administrators he had recruited and groomed were capable of performing without his oversight. Accordingly, he quietly notified board chairman Dwight O'Keefe and then the full MHS board in January, promising an orderly transition before his retirement December 31. The public announcement came in mid-March.

Inevitably people will speak of the "Clarke era" at Memorial, because of its long duration, its many successes, and his strong imprint. The CEO recognizes this reality, but is uncomfortable about it, insisting that all of the accomplishments on his watch were "a team effort." When pressed about his record, he takes particular satisfaction in building an excellent management team, pursuing a clear strategic vision, envisioning the need to expand the system's borders and services, and concentrating employee attention on quality and performance excellence. Indeed, these are the hallmarks of the Clarke legacy, but they do not fully describe the mental and temperamental gifts that made him a superb executive. The tributes have flowed from staff colleagues, board members and community leaders. A.D. Van Meter called him "an outstanding chief executive in a time of great challenge and opportunity," and O'Keefe noted his remarkable self-discipline in always focusing on the big picture in medical care.

COO Ed Curtis, who worked closely with Clarke for nearly fifteen years, reported that his mentor had all four requisites of "an extraordinary leader": a strong and cohesive executive team, a clear and steady vision, the habit of repeatedly communicating that vision, and a genuine commitment to personnel welfare. Others commented in greater detail on his vision, which seemingly empowered Clarke "to anticipate the future around corners." Several people described his administrative style, which was always impatient for results, intellectually honest, as comfortable receiving as offering criticism, and patient in seeking consensus but willing to act in its absence. He freely delegated authority to subordinates, but held them to high performance standards.

Several current and former MHS board members agreed that it was Clarke who gently shaped its focus on large policy and planning issues, its reliance on consensus decision making, its orderly yet comfortable conduct of business, its diversity and representativeness, its courage to embrace change, its collegiality, and its productivity. Van Meter also admired his aptitude for effective communication with elected officials at the local, state, and national levels.

In response, Bob Clarke was quick to remind listeners of some setbacks among the successes: a failed HMO initiative and the fiscal crisis of 2001. In retrospect, what is interesting about both events is the personal responsibility he accepted for them. It will be many years before the appraisal of Clarke's leadership can be gauged in perspective, but there will never be doubt about its success by every appropriate measure. The 2007 fiscal year will be Memorial's most profitable ever and more than seven times greater than 1983, the year Clarke arrived. Total assets have multiplied seven-fold and cash and investments ten-fold. All of the many entities under the MHS brand, from affiliates to partnerships to physician networks to home care and mental health services, are healthy and productive. Employee morale is high, and the health care campus is bustling. Some admiring colleagues, with nervous humor, note that Bob Clarke's greatest talent may be his sense of timing: all trends are favorable, and they are converging at this transition point.

For the MHS board, identifying the best successor to Bob Clarke was both simple and swift, though propriety dictated that the announcement be deferred for a month. Clarke had recommended his COO, Ed Curtis, who was well known and highly respected in the boardroom. For fourteen years he had been managing Memorial on a daily basis, and had demonstrated all of the necessary executive skills. He and Clarke had formed a close working partnership, and had never disagreed on an important issue.

As noted earlier, Curtis was a very popular figure at Memorial, where he knew most employees and physicians by name. At meetings and on his regular walks around the hospital, he displayed an affable temperament that inspired respect as well as good will. At the same time, in the difficult job he held, Curtis could be "hard as nails" when the circumstances warranted it. He demonstrated both the velvet and the steel qualities in daily interaction with physicians, peers, employees, vendors, and others. He never shrank from the messy problems that inevitably surface in any large organization, and he handled them promptly and wisely. Along with his mentor, Curtis had maintained good communications with officials of the many affiliates and partnerships of Memorial Health System. Directors and the entire Memorial working community knew that no elaborate national search could do better than promoting the Chief Operating Officer.

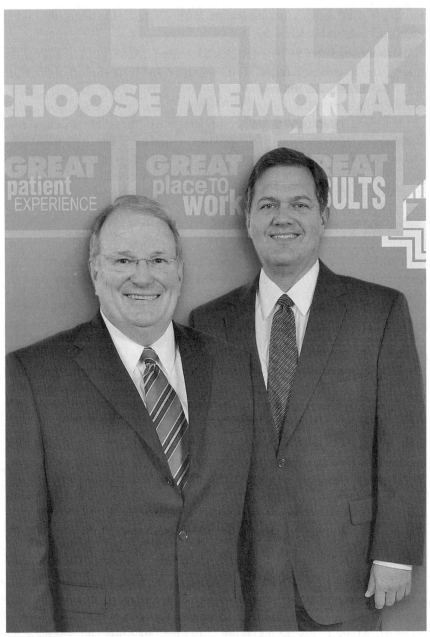

Bob Clarke , left, and Ed Curtis.

Happily, Ed Curtis was pleased to accept this opportunity, which was announced in mid-April. His entire career had been with Memorial, which he considered "a very special institution." Chief among his professional aspirations was always to provide the best patient care possible. True, for many years his nominal job was as "Mr. Inside" to Bob Clarke's "Mr. Outside," but that delineation was inaccurate in practice. Active in the civic community as well as the wider health care field, he was on good terms with individuals in the private and public organizations that are important to MHS. His volunteer services have included leadership positions with the Springfield Urban League, the Central Illinois Food Bank, and United Way of Central Illinois. He is chairman of the Mid-America section of Voluntary Hospitals of America.

Executive transitions can be awkward, but this one has been practically seamless. Most of the senior management positions are held by people with years of experience at Memorial and with Curtis. By late August there were efforts underway to fill a few vacancies, including his successor as COO. He and Bob Clarke, whose offices are perhaps 20 feet apart, confer frequently on all matters. One continuing subject is the evolving terminology and definition of MMC's centers of excellence. New to the list is Peri-operative Services, a category that covers the full surgical continuum from preparation and anesthesia to recovery. Neuro Sciences embrace both rehabilitation and orthopedics, and cancer care has become Oncology and Research. Cardiovascular Medicine is unchanged, and Behavioral Health has joined the list. The separate specialties may be very different, but Curtis is determined to keep performance excellence and great quality their common hallmarks.

At the end of 2007, Ed Curtis will succeed Bob Clarke as President and CEO of Memorial Health System. One chapter ends and a new one begins, but the story continues.

The 1997 centennial marked Memorial's humble beginnings, years of struggle, and dramatic postwar growth into a modern, comprehensive hospital system. The passage of only ten years ordinarily would seem insufficient for an updated history. However, many important challenges and accomplishments occurred in that decade, and with the leadership succession from Bob Clarke to Ed Curtis, a new edition was in order. It still remains to be seen, as it did in 1997, what practical and enduring value can be served by Memorial's published history. Skeptics might argue that the dead hand of history is at best a distraction and at worst a dangerous habit for hospital leaders who must look ahead, not backward. To them the 110th anniversary might be more a millstone than a milestone. For this view they could invoke the words of Springfield's most famous citizen, Abraham Lincoln, who had warned Congress in 1862, "as our case is new, so we must think anew, and act anew." But in that same message Lincoln added, "Fellow citizens, we cannot escape history. We ... will be remembered in spite of ourselves."

With publication of this book, the efforts, accomplishments and failures of Memorial's leaders, employees and friends have indeed been remembered in spite of themselves. The institution that they struggled to create and sustain has grown beyond anyone's prophetic imagination. It has evolved from a jerrybuilt religious infirmary into a sophisticated tertiary care health system that covers the spectrum of health services, and extends throughout central Illinois and beyond. Its pious founders could not have envisioned even the faintest outline of their hospital at age 110, nor can today's directors fully appreciate the challenges their forebears confronted. What lies between Memorial's perilous founding and its current stature is revolutionary medical change, and the daily acts of countless personnel. Those efforts are a legacy, the institutional foundation for Memorial's future. It can inform what lies ahead not in the narrow sense that "those who cannot remember the past are condemned to repeat it," but as a set of ingrained values and notions of behavior. Whatever changes may lie ahead, officials of Memorial Health System can beneficially draw upon an institutional history that reminds them to adhere to an ethic of dedication and service, aspire to excellence in all things, forge community and regional partnerships, display courage and resilience in the face of adversity, and always respect the individual patient and physician.

Sources and Notes

Two preliminary archival steps preceded and significantly served the preparation of this written history. The first was a survey of extant Memorial Health System records, scattered in many locations among 25 hospital departments, a warehouse and a bank vault. Kathryn Wrigley conducted the audit in 1992, describing a variety of records that included more than 1,000 volumes and filled over 2,000 linear feet of space. Her detailed report provided the authors with a vital guide to their research. It also laid the groundwork for a subsequent decision by Memorial officials to consolidate all records into an institutional archive, headed by a professional archivist.

The second step was to enrich the documentary holdings with a series of oral histories by selected present and former Memorial officials, directors, physicians, employees and nursing school alumnae. Cullom Davis and Kathryn Wrigley conducted the interviews, producing nearly 3,000 pages of transcript from 36 individuals. These oral histories proved especially valuable for the post-1943 period of Memorial's history.

As these two activities suggest, documentary evidence was generally plentiful for a careful and comprehensive assessment of the institution's history. In fact, the authors often felt immersed in a sea of data and details. There are only a few record gaps, and even then there were alternative sources that told the story. What follows is a classified description of the principal research sources, followed by detailed notes for each chapter.

The primary archival material consists of a nearly complete set of hospital and system governing board minutes. Except for some missing records covering 1907-13, one can trace the policy and decision-making acts of successive boards, executive committees, and other governance groups for the entire century of Memorial's existence. For the hospital's first 25 years, most of the minutes are in German, so hospital officials arranged to have Gerlinde Coates and Christine Purtell translate them. In the chapter notes, *Minutes* refers to meetings of the board of directors, *Exec Minutes* to the board's executive committee, *MHS Minutes* to the Memorial Health System board, *Nurs Minutes* to the Nursing School Alumni Association, and *Med Minutes* to the medical staff executive committee. Minutes, memoranda and proceedings of other hospital groups, such as special committees, are specified in their respective citations.

Accumulated hospital records also contain occasional letters, programs, reports and plans. Most notable are the *Minutes of the District Medical Society of Central Illinois,* 2 vols, 1875-1940 *(Dist Med Minutes);* William H. Walsh, *Report of a Study of the Hospital Situation in Springfield with Special Reference to the Future Development of the Springfield Hospital and Training School,* April 30, 1932 *(Walsh Report);* Walsh, *Memorandum of a Conference with the Building Committee of the Springfield Hospital and Training School,* April 20, 1937 *(Walsh Memo);* A.T. Kearney & Company, *Memorial Hospital of Springfield: Cost Reduction and Improvement Study,* 1957 *(Kearney Study);* Herman Smith, *Memorial Hospital of Springfield,* 1963 *(Smith Study); Medical School Location Capital City Springfield, Illinois,* May 1967 *(Med Sch Location);* James A. Campbell and W. Randolph Tucker, *Education in the Health Fields for the State of Illinois,* Board of Higher Education, 1968, vol 1 *(Campbell Report);* E. D. Rosenfeld Associates, *Memorial Hospital of Springfield, Illinois: Long-Range Master Plan,* 1973, 3 vols *(Rosenfeld Plan);* and Nursing School Alumnae, *Scrapbook (NSA Scrapbook).*

Springfield and then Memorial Hospital issued various newsletters and other publications under various titles. The most frequently cited publication is Memorial's *NewsCenter (NewsCenter).* Others are fully indicated in the chapter notes.

Other Springfield area libraries contain valuable documentary material. At Lincoln (public) Library's Sangamon Valley Collection, the vertical and obituary files are useful. It also houses the only known copy (a fragment) of Rev. Louis Hinnsen, "Selfdefense vs. The Springfield Hospital" [1900?] *(Selfdefense).* More generally accessible is its copy of Shelby M. Harrison (ed.), *The Springfield Survey: A Study of Social Conditions in an American City,* 3 vols (New York: Russell Sage Foundation, 1914-20), cited as *Springfield Survey.* Other institutional collections are at the Sangamon County Medical Society and the Southern Illinois University School of Medicine archives. Springfield city directories provide limited but often vital biographical information about hospital directors and personnel.

Public knowledge about notable hospital events is available in the files of the city's two venerable daily newspapers, The *Illinois State Journal (ISJ)* and the *Illinois State Register (ISR),* later merged as the *State Journal-Register (SJR).* Another useful periodical is the *Bulletin of the Sangamon County Medical Society (BSCMC).*

During 1992-96 the authors conducted oral history interviews with a representative group of 36 current and former employees, directors and physicians. There are memoirs by the following individuals: Russell Beckwith, Kathy Bird, William Boyd, Robert Clarke, Jack Cook, Dr. John Denby, Jessie Finley, Dr. Humphrey Fluckiger, Wilma Fricke, Dr. G. K. Greening, Dr. Grant Johnson, Norman Jones, Helen Justison, Geraldine Lee, Dr. Arthur Lindsay, Walter Lohman, Dr. Chauncey Maher, Dr. Richard Moy, Rev. Lewis Niemoeller, Mary Noseck, Robert Oxtoby, Dr. Robert Patton, Dr. Ann Pearson, George Phillips, Dr. Robert Prentice, Ed Quarry, James Rigby, Dr. Donald Ross, Margaret Schirding, William Schnirring, Eunice Scott, Helen Shull, Paul Smith, Betty Snedigar, Harvey Stephens and Dr. Glen Wichterman. In addition, the University of Illinois at Springfield has memoirs of Hallie Kinter (1977), Dr. Robert Patton (1993) and Anna Tittman (1980) in its large collection. Citations to these oral histories will be by surname (e.g., *Scott Memoir,* 16).

The field of American medical, nursing and hospital history is blessed with a variety of monographs and several excellent syntheses. Among the latter are Charles E. Rosenberg, *The Care of Strangers: The Rise of America's Hospital System* (New York: Basic Books, 1987), Rosemary Stevens, *In Sickness and in Wealth: American Hospitals in the Twentieth Century* (New York: Basic Books, 1989), Philip A. and Beatrice J. Kalisch, *The Advance of American Nursing*, 3rd ed (Philadelphia: Lippincott, 1995), and Paul Starr, *The Social Transformation of American Medicine* (New York: Basic Books, 1982). Chapter notes will refer to them, respectively, as Rosenberg, *Care of Strangers*, Stevens, *Sickness and Wealth*, Kalisch, *American Nursing*, and Starr, *Social Transformation*.

Specialized studies include Daniel Callahan, *The Troubled Dream of Life: Living with Mortality* (New York: Simon & Schuster, 1993), Sr. Mary Francis Cooke, *Doors that Never Close: A Centennial History of St. John's Hospital* (Springfield: Sangamon County Historical Society, 1975), Cooke, His *Love Heals: A History of the Hospital Sisters of the Third Order of St Francis, Springfield, Illinois 1875-1975* (Chicago: Franciscan Herald Press, 1977), Alfred W. Crosby, *America's Forgotten Pandemic: The Influenza of 1918* (New York: Cambridge University Press, 1989), Phillip V. Davis, *Practice and Progress: Medical Care in Central Illinois at the Turn of the Century* (Springfield: The Pearson Museum, 1994), Tony Gould, *A Summer Plague: Polio and its Survivors* (New Haven: Yale University Press, 1995), Everett A. and Richard L. Johnson, *Hospitals Under Fire: Strategies for Survival* (Rockville, MD: Aspen Publishers, 1986), Sr. Agnes McDougall, *Duty: The History of St. John's Hospital School of Nursing, Springfield, Illinois* (Springfield: School of Nursing, 1986), James T. Patterson, *The Dread Disease: Cancer and Modern American Culture* (Cambridge: Harvard University Press, 1987), Isaac D. Rawlings, *The Rise and Fall of Disease in Illinois,* 2 vols (Springfield: Illinois Department of Public Health, 1927), Baxter K. Richardson, *History of the Illinois Tuberculosis Association* (Springfield: Illinois Tuberculosis Association, 1967), Frank Ryan, *The Forgotten Plague: How the Battle Against Tuberculosis Was Won-and Lost* (Boston: Little, Brown & Company, 1992), and Michael E. Teller, *The Tuberculosis Movement: A Public Health Campaign in the Progressive Era* (Westport, CT: Greenwood Press, 1988).

Local and other general histories supply a valuable context for Memorial's evolution. Notable among them are Bruce A. Campbell, *The Sangamon Saga* (Springfield: Phillips Brothers, 1976), Stuart Fliege, "Springfield Hospital and Training School" and "The Use and Demise of the German Language at Trinity" (Springfield: Trinity Lutheran Church, 1991), Erich H. Heintzen, *Prairie School of the Prophets: The Anatomy of a Seminary 1846-1976* (St. Louis: Concordia Publishing House, 1989), John Higham, *Strangers in the Land: Patterns of American Nativism 1860-1925* (New York: Atheneum, 1963), Thomas S. Hines, *Burnham of Chicago: Architect and Planner* (New York: Oxford University Press, 1974), Stanley and Eleanor Hochman, *A Dictionary of Contemporary American History: 1945 to the Present* (New York: Penguin, 1993), Robert P. Howard, *Illinois: A History of the Prairie State* (Grand Rapids, MI: William B. Eerdmans Publishing Company, 1972), George A. Larson and Jay Pridmore, *Chicago Architecture and Design* (New York: Harry N. Abrams, Inc., 1993), David McCullough, *The Path Between the Seas: The Creation of the Panama Canal 1870-1914* (New York: Simon & Schuster, 1977), Hugh T. Morrison, *Logan Place* (Springfield: privately printed, 1938), and Edward J. Russo, *Prairie of Promise: Springfield and Sangamon County* (Woodland Hills, CA: Windsor Publications, 1983).

Source citations that follow are grouped by paragraph, with each such paragraph identified by its concluding phrase (in italics). Sources for each chapter's vignettes appear at the end of that chapter's citations. The following abbreviations apply: SH for Springfield Hospital and Training School; MH for Memorial Hospital; MMC for Memorial Medical Center; MMCS for Memorial Medical Center System; MHS for Memorial Health System.

Chapter One: An Act Of Faith And Courage

The title comes from SH *Bulletin,* 2:4 (June 1926); *a shooting victim: ISJ* 4/20/1897; *fortune of the founders: Walsh Report,* 1.

as among physicians: Stevens, *Sickness and Wealth,* 14; *efforts could contain disease:* McCullough, *Panama Canal,* 410-13; Patterson, *Dread Disease,* 19-20, 33, 36-37, 64; *than the bonafide* drugs: see *ISR,* 1/10/1897 for typical patent medicine advertisements of the age; *training and development:* Patterson, 29.

interaction with peers: Starr, *Social Transformation,* 30-31, 47, 65; *American medical profession: Dist Med Minutes; rigorous accreditations standards:* Starr, 90, 102-09, 118; *status and income:* Starr, 117, 124.

heading the list: Starr, 145, 169; Patterson, 48; *hygiene and patient care:* Rosenberg, *Care of Strangers,* 97-98; *job-related injuries:* Rosenberg, 104-05, 113-15, 148, 157, 178; Starr, 145; *in the 19th century:* Starr, 173-75; *most commonly, physicians:* Stevens, 20-25, 33; Starr, 164; *other therapeutic baths:* Russo, *Prairie of Promise,* 39-40; *Patton Memoir,* 41; *a time of rapid change:* Rosenberg, 290-93; Starr, 145-46.

many deaths every year: Russo, 40; James Krohe, *Midnight at Noon: A History of Coal Mining in Sangamon County* (Springfield: Sangamon County Historical Society, 1975), 6, 8; *during the crisis: ISJ,* 1/29/1897; *Wheeler as mayor: ISR,* 4/20/1897; *Mason and Eighth: Cooke, Doors Never Close,* 1-2, 6, 10-11; *Oak Ridge Cemetery:* Campbell, *Sangamon Saga,* 230-31; *throughout the Middle West:* Heintzen, *Prairie School,* 78-79, 85, Fliege, "German Language;" *alternative for hospital care:* Heintzen, 91, 95-97, 100-01; Fliege, "Springfield Hospital;" *Fifth and North Grand streets:* Henrietta Herndon, *My Grandpa* (Springfield: privately printed, 1971), 2:26-27, 34-36.

in bitter invective: ISJ, 1/20/97; *due for payment in June: Minutes,* 2/8/97; *ISJ,* 2/9/97; *Zapf as treasurer: Minutes,* 2/15, 17, 24, 3/1/97; *ISJ,* 2/18/97; *Ralph C. Matheny: Minutes,* 3/19/97; *ISJ,* 3/3, 9/97; *are against her: ISJ,* 4/20/97; Helena Hanser to Rowena Kirkwood, 6/20/47 (in Memorial Archives); *legislature was in session: Tittman Memoir,* 21; *Minutes,* 5/13/98; Rosenberg, 262-63; *payable in advance: Minutes,* 3/26, 5/14, 28, 6/18/97, 2/10, 5/13, 6/17/98; Stevens, 4: *space and equipment: Minutes,* 5/28/97; *fragile hospital's future: Minutes,* 4/29, 10/29/97, 1/13/98.

1,129 in 1910: Rosenberg, 213, 220, 225; Starr, 156; *what students learned: Minutes,* 9/17/97, 10/2/99; *alumna of the training school: NewsCenter* (Fall 1978), 27-28; Helena Hanser to Rowena Kirkwood, 6/20/47; *Tittman Memoir,* 77; *split equally with the nurse:* "School of Nursing, (unpublished manuscript, Memorial Archives), 2; *Minutes,* 2/10/98; *for the operating rooms:* Starr, 146-47, 161.

with its Protestant rival: Campbell, 132, 169; *Polk's Springfield City Directory 1898* (Springfield: R. L. Polk & Co., 1898), 1:642-43; *grown slightly, to 15: Med Minutes,* 1/22/99, 1/16/00; *Minutes,* 3/8/97, 11/6/99; *ended with a prayer: NSA Scrapbook,* 5; *board at Concordia Seminary:* Fliege, "Springfield Hospital;" *destroyed the embryonic institution: Minutes,* 2/8, 3/26/97, 2/97-2/98; *ISJ,* 2/9/97; *financial reports in English: Minutes,* 1/18/99; *hostility that had developed: Selfdefense,* 1-7.

District Medical Society of Central Illinois: Dist Med Minutes.

Martin Luecke, Founding Father: SH Bulletin, 2:4 (June 1926); Fliege, "Springfield Hospital."

Elizabeth Matthews, M.D.: Susan Harmon, "Dr. Elizabeth Matthews: An Illustrative Career," 3-18 in Davis, *Practice and Progress.*

Anna Tittman, Notable Nurse: Tittman Memoir, 16-17, 27, 52; *ISJ,* 12/5/37; *SJR,* 5/11/75, 9/11/77.

Chapter Two: Innocuous Desuetude

"innocuous desuetude": Walsh Report, 2; *College in Fort Wayne: Minutes,* 7/8/00, 8/5/01; *an appeal for gifts: Minutes,* 4/19/00, 5/6, 7/16/01; *voted to dismiss her: Minutes,* 1/7, 7/16/01, 1/6/02; *loans to cover costs: Minutes,* 11/15, 26/98, 1/18/99, 4/20, 8/31/03; *of these overtures: Minutes,* 4/19/00, 9/3, 11/3, 12/1/02, 3/2/02, 3/7/04, 9/4, 10/2, 11/6/05, 1/8/06, 5/6, 6/3/07; *totaled ten: Minutes,* 1/9, 8/1/99, "School of Nursing" (unpublished manuscript, Memorial Archives), 2-4, *Minutes,* 3/2/02, 1/5/03.

beginning in 1909: Minutes, 2/5/00, 11/7/04, *Med Minutes,* 1/21/07; *medical services: Patton Memoir,* 4; *management of hospitals:* Patterson, *Dread Disease,* 52-53; Stevens, *Sickness and Health,* 19, 57-64; Rosenberg, *Care of Strangers,* 209, 325; *were more successful: Minutes,* 2/4/07; *Med Minutes,* 8/17, 9/27, 10/2, 11/4/12; *the new century: Med Minutes,* 1/8/13, 12/7/14, 1/19, 5/31/16.

and fee collection: Starr, *Social Transformation,* 177-78; *in the records: Minutes,* 2/6/99, 7/16/01, 9/4, 11/6/05; *City Directory 1900,* 244; *next several years: Minutes,* 1/4/04, 6/5, 7/17/05; Hanser to Kirkwood, 6/20/47; *nearly seven years: Minutes,* 11/6/05, 1/8, 9/10, 10/8/06, 1/7, 7/8, 8/5, 9/9/07.

over eighty years): Rosenberg, 264, 276; *Minutes,* 1/13/98; *to succeed her: Minutes,* 1/7, 7/16/01, 1/4/04; *ISJ,* 1/1/04; *less than 27: Minutes,* 1/6, 2/3/02, 9/9/07; *end of that debt": Minutes,* 4/15, 7/7/14; *a tiny darkroom: Patton Memoir,* 2; *its empty beds:* Stevens, 25-26; *Minutes,* 3/5/06; *in the 1970s: Minutes,* 10/6/14, 7/14/15; Fliege, "Springfield Hospital;" *Tittman Memoir,* 18; Campbell, *Sangamon Saga,* 217.

the State Armory: Springfield Survey, I:5-7, III:353-56; *of such conditions: Springfield Survey:* "Public Schools," 104-05; "Mental Defectives." 30, 33-34; "Housing," 6-8; "Public Health," 82, 129; *one third were preventable:* "Public Health," 3, 11, 128; *indigent patients:* "Charities," 41, 43, 47.

full-time medical doctor: "Public Health," 58; Rawlings, *Disease,* 315-17; *"pest house:"* Rawlings, 322-23; *NewsCenter* (Fall 1978), 32; *funds were solicited:* Rawlings, 323-24; *Tittman Memoir,* 32; *Springfield Survey:* "Public Health," 45-46; *The Palm Leaf* (June 1938), 1-4; *ISJ,* 12/11/56; *Cooke, Doors Never Close,* 16.

to 40 million: Crosby, *Forgotten Pandemic,* 205, 207, 216; *hundreds of deaths:* Crosby, 5, 21, 57, 60-61; Thomas D. Masters, "Springfield Newspapers Report the Influenza Epidemic of 1918," 57-63 in Davis, *Practice and Progress; ISJ,* 10/16-17/18; *from related tuberculosis:* Masters, 64-66; *Kinter Memoir,* 43-44; Campbell, 223; *NewsCenter* (Fall 1978), 32.

including violence: Higham, *Strangers,* 175-80, 195, 204; *newsletter in English:* Fliege, "German Language;" *Minutes,* 7/10/18, 5/9, 7/13/21, 1922-23 generally.

the hospital's storeroom: Minutes, 5/9/21; *and research institutions:* Rosenberg, 10, 341; Stevens, 13; *new decade began:* Stevens, 57, 114; *Minutes,* 8/9/20; *non-sectarian entity: Minutes,* 7/9/19; *these difficult years: Minutes,* 7/21/20, 9/21/22; Fliege, "Springfield Hospital;"

hospital's Lutheran identity: Minutes, 7/21/20, 2/14, 4/11, 6/14/21, 9/11/22, 9/30/24; *seemed intractable: Minutes,* 7/21/20, 7/20/21.

demanded payment: Minutes, 1/19, 3/8/20; *raise was denied: Minutes,* 8/9, 9/13/20, 10/8, 12/11/22, 8/4, 9/13/24; *local volunteers: Minutes* 9/13/20, 3/12, 4/9/23; *financial deterioration:* flyer in *NSA Scrapbook; Minutes,* 9/13/24; *could save charity: Minutes,* 7/18/23, 7/16/24; *suffering as a result: Minutes,* 4/10/16, 5/15, 22/16, 3/11/18; *much in evidence": Minutes,* 11/9, 12/11/22; *at the hospital: Minutes,* 11/5/13, 4/12/15, 5/15, 22/16, 3/11/18.

Hospital Hyperbole: State Topics: Springfield in the Twentieth Century (Springfield, IL: 1903), 41.

Reporting the News: Hospital News Sheet (November 1900); *Minutes,* 9/2/01, var/02, 2/13/20.

Hospital Discipline: Minutes, 9/13/15.

Nursing School: Minutes, 3/8, 4/12, 5/10/20, 7/20, 9/14, 10/19/21.

Medical Staff, 1923: Minutes, 8/13/23.

Chapter Three: An End And A Beginning

several thousand dollars: Minutes, 4/6, 5/11, 6/8, 8/22/25, 7/21/26; *the next year: Minutes,* 9/21/27; *mid 1930s: Minutes,* 6/11/23, 5/10, 5/21, 10/11/26, 1/10, 3/14, 8/15/27, 4/16, 5/21, 6/18, 8/21/28; *kitchen, and anesthesiology: Minutes,* 4/11/27, 5/21, 6/4, 6/18, 8/21/28; *place of home care: Minutes,* 11/9/25, 1/10, 2/14, 5/17, 6/13, 5/28, 7/11, 8/15, 9/12/27, 11/29/29, 1/27, 2/17/30; *plan was deferred: Minutes,* 1/21, 7/11, 10/24, 12/21/27; *Exec Minutes,* 4/4/38; Stevens, *Sickness and Health,* 176; *Patton Memoir,* 34-35; *ISJ,* 10/6/35.

hospital as needed: Shull Memoir, 10-12, 17; *area coal mines: Minutes,* 11/21/27, 2/13/28; *Shull Memoir,* 40; *Springfield Hospital Bulletin* 2:4 (June 1926); *hospital board: Ibid., Med Minutes,* 1920-26, 10/25/27; *Minutes,* 3/8/26, 3/14/27; *transformation of 1931: Minutes,* 4/11, 9/12, 12/12/27, 1/16, 2/13/28; *decision was irreversible: Minutes,* 4/25, 5/9, 6/26, 7/20/27; *the emergency room: Minutes,* 10/24, 12/12/27, 3/12, 6/30/28; *Shull Memoir,* 45-46; *new, larger building: Minutes,* 3/18, 4/22, 5/22, 8/19/29; *ISJ,* 5/6/29; *perilous condition: Minutes,* 8/19, 11/18, 12/2/29.

or county governments: Minutes, 4/26, 5/11, 8/18, 8/21, 9/15/30; *nearly ten years: Minutes,* 10/29, 11/24, 12/15/30; *hospital's existing debt: Minutes,* 1/19/31; *ISR,* 2/8, 15/31; *institution non-sectarian: ISR,* 4/21, 5/15/31; *Minutes,* 4/21, 5/15, 18/31; *Memorandum of Meeting,* 5/1, 15/31; *the troubled institution: Minutes,* 5/18, 6/5, 10/27/31; *ISR,* 6/6/31; *for personal reasons: Minutes,* 11/16/31, 6/20, 7/12/33.

Social Security coverage: Starr, 295, 312; Stevens, 142-47, 150, 164-72; *conclude the meeting: Minutes,* 1/12, 2/23/32, 2/19/34; *Patton Memoir,* 12; *Springfield Hospital's future: Minutes,* 12/15/31; *meeting in May: Minutes,* 1/12, 2/15, 3/25/32; *in the hospital: Minutes,* 2/16, 3/23, 4/21/31, 4/5/32; *Exec Minutes,* 4/5, 11, 18, 25/33; 4/2, 5/23/34; *trend was favorable: Exec Minutes,* 5/31, 11/21/33; *Where it Counts": Exec Minutes,* 11/1, 28/32; *down to $23,500: Exec Minutes,* 6/27/33, 2/28, 10/3/34, 10/21/35; *health care institutions:* Starr, 269-70, 298; *a diathermy machine: Exec Minutes,* 4/18, 11/21/33, 7/10, 17, 31/34, 11/11/35; *171 clean operations: Exec Minutes,* 2/21/35, 3/11/36.

staff dining area: Walsh Report, 23-24, 36; *Shull Memoir,* 19, 21, 80-81; *Patton Memoir,* 15-16; *Scott Memoir,* 6; *adequate financial cushion: Walsh Report,* 2, 4-8, 10-14, 19-20, 22, 29-30, 37-42, 47, 50-52; *new Memorial Hospital: ISJ,* 5/29/32; *the new hospital: Exec Minutes,* 3/25/32, 7/22/36; *Walsh Memo,* 2-5; *x-ray facility:* Starr, 167, 177; ACS, *Manual of Hospital Standardization,* 5-7; *incompetent staff members: Exec Minutes,* 7/26, 11/21, 12/13/32; *Patton Memoir,* 7, 42-43; *ACS standardization: Exec Minutes,* 12/5/33, 2/13, 6/5, 7/3/34; *job in New Jersey: Exec Minutes,* 10/29, 12/3, 12/10/34, 1/28, 7/8/35, 6/1, 7/20/36; *monitor staff performance: Exec Minutes,* 7/28, 10/15, 11/19/36; *Shull Memoir,* 42.

of inestimable value: Exec Minutes, 12/16/35, 3/2, 10/4/37; *and cigarette breaks:* Stevens, 172-73, 175, 196; *ISJ,* 3/26/38; *Shull Memoir,* 64; *Snedigar Memoir,* 4-6; *kitchen and laundry:* "Emergency Room Routine Procedure" (MMC Archives); *NSA Scrapbook* (1939-42); *bequest the next year: Exec Minutes,* 3/15/37, 12/5/38, 2/6, 9/25/39; *for surgical privileges:* Starr, 229-31; *Exec Minutes,* 3/4/35; *with his peers: Patton Memoir,* 44-45; *Shull Memoir,* 38.

as much as $250: Starr, 204, 210, 212; Russo, *Prairie of Promise,* 98; *Patton Memoir,* 26, 28-29; *undertake clinical research:* Starr, 340-42, 346-47; *attracted much interest: Exec Minutes,* 7/19/32; Stevens, 177; *Patton Memoir,* 16-18; Patterson, *Dread Disease,* 71-76, 94, 112, 114-15; *head of the laboratory: Patton Memoir,* 21-23; Campbell, *Sangamon Saga,* 262; *Exec Minutes,* 10/21/35; *over 300 graduates:* Kalisch, *American Nursing,* 293; *NSA Scrapbook* (1939-42); *ISJ,* 10/24/37; *Shull Memoir,* 3-9, 13-19, 25-26, 75; *Minutes,* 5/19, 7/28/30, 2/16/31.

lucrative fund-raising event: Minutes, 12/15/31, 2/21/33; *NSA Scrapbook* (1939-42); *Shull Memoir,* 51-52; *Exec Minutes,* 7/5/32, 2/19/34; *on family health: Bulletin* 4:3 (April 1928); *literature on infant care: Exec Minutes,* 7/10, 7/17/34, 10/28/35; *NSA Scrapbook* (1939-42).

Two Generations in Medicine: Denby Memoir, 27-28; *Minutes,* 1/14/81; *ISR,* 9/14/35; *SJR,* 7/18/76; *Patton Memoir.*

The Palmer Legacy: Minutes, 10/26/67; George T. Palmer, *A Conscientious Turncoat: The Story of John M. Palmer 1817-1900* (New Haven: Yale University Press, 1941); "Jessie Palmer Weber File," Illinois State Historical Library.

Fred W. Wanless: Jones Memoir, 42-43; *SJR,* 9/5/49.

Mildred Bunn: Minutes, 2/27, 10/27, 12/29/47; *NewsCenter* (Nov 1974); *ISJ,* 8/5/58; *Jones Memoir,* 41-42.

Mitzvah at Memorial: Polk's City Directory 1937; ISJ, 12/8/60; *SJR,* 1/9/85.

Chapter Four: Building A Future

decade of general development: ISR, 5/12, 10/17/38; *Walsh Report,* 30; *SJR,* 9/26/43; *the pre-war years: Walsh Report,* 22; *of those funds:* Russo, *Prairie of Promise,* 62-63; Stevens, *Sickness and Wealth,* 210; *Americans by 1940:* Stevens, 7, 159-160, 170, 182; *from 1940 to 1946:* Kalisch, *American Nursing,* 413; Stevens, 204; *modern hospital building:* Stevens, 172-73; *Snedigar Memoir,* 45-46.

The subheading comes from Hines, *Burnham,* 401; *leader in modern architecture:* Stevens 161-62; *the hospital directors: ISR,* 10/37/38; *Minutes,* 12/10/38; Hines, 158; Stevens, 162; *vegetables on the lot: Walsh Memo,* 6; Morrison, *Logan Place,* 74; *North Grand Avenue: Exec Minutes,* 5/12/38; *ISR,* 10/27/38; *a striking exception: Exec Minutes,* 6/12/39; Stevens, 209; *hospital's distinguishing moniker: Sarah Nelson Scrapbook; matched that level: BSCMS* 6 (June 1941): 39; *ISR,* 11/23/41; *ISJ,* 7/27/41, 11/23/43, *Oxtoby Memoir,* 9; *SJR,* 7/18/76.

to $1.25 million: ISJ, 11/23/41; *ISR,* 9/21, 11/23/41; *floor for $9,000: Shull Scrapbook; ISR,* 7/27/41; *ISJ,* 9/21/41; *rely upon donations: Sarah Nelson Scrapbook; ISJ,* 1/29/42; program, *The Women's Auxiliary of Springfield Memorial Hospital and the Illinois State Journal-Register Present Lily Pons in Recital,* April 1, 1943; *operated in the black: Exec Minutes,* 3/4/47.

The subheading *Shining Citadel* comes from Stevens, 162; *the construction contract: Exec Minutes,* 10/6/41, 1/19/42; *BSCMS* 8 (November 1943): 167; *the hospital entrance: BSCMC* 8 (November 1943): 167-68; *Exec Minutes,* 3/9/43; *ISJ,* 11/14/43; *of private rooms: Maher Memoir,* 18; *BSCMC* 8 (November 1943): 167-8; *Exec Minutes,* 5/11/43.

the surrounding communities: SJR, 9/27/43; *ISJ,* 9/26/43; *Shull Scrapbook; bag of cornstarch: Shull Memoir,* 59; *Shull Scrapbook; Scott Memoir,* 19; *St. Louis and Ohio: Scott Memoir,* 19; *McKelvey resume, filed with 1940-1942 Board Minutes; resignation with regret: Exec Minutes,* 2/9, 5/11/43; *and the elevators: Exec Minutes,* 5/18, 6/21/44; *the dietary department: Exec Minutes,* 9/11/42, 1/12/43; *and managerial personnel: Exec Minutes,* 11/26, 12/14/43; *teapots had arrived: Exec Minutes,* 5/18, 6/8, 8/10/42; *Scott Memoir,* 19-21.

the Women's Auxiliary: Scott Memoir, 13; *Exec Minutes,* 6/21/44, 11/29/48; *ISJ,* 4/8/51; *Patton Memoir,* 40; *within its walls: Wichterman Memoir,* 13; *Exec Minutes,* 5/7/51; *for her effort: Med Minutes,* 4/24/51, 5/28/53; *Exec Minutes,* 4/26/51, 12/15/53; *Boyd Memoir,* 17; *Patton Memoir,* 40; *Shull Memoir,* 60; *Fricke Memoir,* 14; *Scott Memoir,* 32; *Exec Minutes,* 6/26, 12/15/53.

the hospital hallways: Exec Minutes, 12/8/41; *a $5,200 expense: Exec Minutes,* 1/28/48; *radiologist's pay increase: Exec Minutes,* 5/11, 6/8/43, 10/26/44; *instead of two: Exec Minutes,* 3/9/42, 1/12/43; *NewsCenter* (February 1978): 33; *dietary sugar rations: Exec Minutes,* 4/13, 11/9/43; *Scott Memoir,* 23-4; *from the army:* Russo, 64; *Exec Minutes,* 3/12/43, 6/21, 9/27/44, 3/29/45; *SJR,* 9/26/43; *your noble endeavors: Exec Minutes,* 1/18/45; *Kalisch,* 344-45; *Nursing School Alumni Association Papers.*

there were 145: Kalisch, 344, 349; *Exec Minutes,* 8/9/43, 9/24/45; *with red epaulets: Exec Minutes,* 11/26/43, 8/31/44; *Nursing School Alumni Association Papers; Sangamon County salute you: BSCMC* 9 (1944): 4; *contribution to peace: Exec Minutes,* 2/9, 3/9/43; *SJR,* 9/26/43; *sharply declined:* Russo, 65, 67-68; *ISJ,* 8/15/45.

during visiting hours: Exec Minutes, 3/24/47, 2/27, 12/2/52, 3/25/53; *for patient use: Exec Minutes,* 3/29/45, 3/24, 8/7/47, 2/27, 3/25/53; *under no indebtedness: Exec Minutes,* 3/24/47, 3/20/50, 8/21/52; *medical laboratory technicians:* Stevens, 220; *Kalisch,* 378; *Exec Minutes,* 3/24/47, *supply never materialized: Exec Minutes,* 7/26/45; *take blood pressures:* Kalisch, 372; *Shull Memoir,* 65-66.

296 by 1954: Kalisch, 135, 407; *Exec Minutes,* 3/24, 9/30/47, 1/28/48, 1/28/52; Kalisch, 407; *1946 and 1952:* Kalisch, 359, 408-09; *was not intense: Snedigar Memoir,* 23-26; *later that year: Exec Minutes,* 4/13/43, 5/18/44, 11/28/47, 1/28, 9/27/48, 1/31, 7/27/49; *Med Minutes,* 5/1/51; *fit for nursing: Shull Memoir,* 53; *Exec Minutes,* 2/4, 6/8/43; *much they owed: Exec Minutes,* 8/9/43, 9/27, 10/26/44, 5/8/46, 5/26/52, 11/26/54.

early religious affiliation: Exec Minutes, 11/28/50, 5/25/52; *Justison Memoir,* 29-30; *Snedigar Memoir,* 21; *Shull Memoir,* 60-61; *at subsequent meetings: Exec Minutes,* 2/27, 3/18/48; *for gradual implementation: Exec Minutes,* 9/29/50, 3/28/52, 8/28/53; *benefits in 1951: Fricke Memoir,* 29-30; Stevens, 237; *this teaching type:* Stevens, 65-67; 238; *competition too keen: Exec Minutes,* 2/9, 4/24/45, 12/17/46, 12/27/51, 12/13/55, 9/6/57, *Patton Memoir,* 33; *Fluckiger Memoir,* 3; *Med Minutes,* 4/25/50, 3/27/52, 1/3/56; *Minutes of the Intern Committee of the Medical Staff:* 4/20/51; *at St. John's: Exec Minutes:* 5/20, 8/15/48; *Wichterman Memoir,* 6, 7, 11.

58 Springfield victims: ISJ, n.d, 8/10, 12/29/49, 2/13/50; *ISR,* 8/10, 8/13/49; *isolate infectious diseases: Med Minutes,* 8/1/50; Cooke, *Love Heals,* 47; *Exec Minutes,* 7/27/50; *Fricke,* 34; *ISJ,* 8/14/48; *Pearson Memoir,* 8-9; *Fluckiger,* 24-25; *of individual muscles: ISJ,* 8/4/49; Stevens, 233; *Exec Minutes,* 7/17/46; Gould, *Summer Plague,* 97; *for stand-by service: Med Minutes,* 3/6/51; *Exec Minutes,* 1/22/51; *an extreme disaster: BSCMS* 20 (February 1955): 39; *Exec Minutes,* 1/25, 11/1/62; *million by 1960:* Starr, 341, 343, 347.

Link to a Legend: Hines, *Burnham,* xviii, xix, 156, 247, 257-258, 268, 352, 401; Albert N. Marquis, ed., *Who's Who in America: a Biographical Dictionary of Notable Living Men and Women of the United States 1940-41* (Chicago, Marquis, 1940) 21:475; *Guide to*

Illinois State Buildings, 22-23; *ISR,* 12/11/38; *newspaper clipping,* 5/11/48; John Bartlett, *Familiar Quotations: a Collection of Passages, Phrases, and Proverbs Traced to their Source in Ancient and Modern Literature,* 15th ed. (Boston: Little, Brown, 1980), 661.

Masonic Support: Alfred F. Becker, *Description of masons' roles in laying Memorial Hospital cornerstone and accounting monitory contributions,* June 1, 1942; *Exec Minutes,* 6/5, 7/1/69.

Dedicated to Service: ISJ, 3/29/41; *Exec Minutes,* 9/16/43; *Memorial Hospital of Springfield Dedication Program,* September 26, 1943; *ISR,* 3/26/43.

Littler Legacy: ISJ, 10/?/38, 9/21/41; *NewsCenter* (July 1974): 5-7; reported by Paul Smith as $8,807,799 on 9/30/96; Morrison, *Logan Place.*

Summer Plague: Gould, xi-xii, xiv, 135; Starr, 86-87, 346-347; *ISJ,* 3/27/53.

Chapter Five: Expansionary Drift

nation's largest industries: Starr, *Social Transformation,* 335-36; Stevens, *Sickness and Wealth,* 227; *an expansionary spiral:* Starr, 311, 313, 329, 334-35; Russo, *Prairie of Promise,* 70; Stevens, 229, 257; *changing technologic industry:* Stevens, 296; Kalisch, *American Nursing,* 425; *their hometown hospitals:* Stevens, 239; *lose their jobs:* Kalisch, 416; Starr, 146; *Exec Minutes,* 5/8/46, 12/27/56, 1/20/58, 9/30/65; Stevens, 238; *Snedigar Memoir,* 51.

a pension plan: Exec Minutes, 2/3/56, 5/23/57, 3/6/58, 4/1/60, 3/30/61, 1/17, 10/26/67; *times were changing: Exec Minutes,* 5/28/59, 4/27/61; *Boyd Memoir,* 23; *Smith Study,* II-18; *in August 1952: Exec Minutes,* 8/21/52, 10/25/54; *Johnson Memoir,* 15; *Boyd Memoir,* 8; *led the expansion:* Stevens, 237-38, 240, 248, 249; *Snedigar Memoir,* 43.

projects were completed: Russo, 70; *Oxtoby Memoir,* 5; *associated with Shank: Scott Memoir,* 61; *Boyd Memoir,* 17; *them by name: Boyd Memoir,* 16; *Scott Memoir,* 61; *Snedigar Memoir,* 48-49; *under Lanphier's leadership: Exec Minutes,* 7/30/53; *rates 50 cents: Oxtoby Memoir,* 15; *Lanphier visited theirs: Med Minutes,* 10/29/53.

the nursing school: Johnson Memoir, 55-6, 58-62; *a nurses' home: Boyd Memoir,* 23-24, 91; *cost of $11,140: ISR,* 11/29/53; *Evans Construction Company: Exec Minutes,* 5/4/72, 3/30/67; *victims and paralytics: ISR,* 7/10/58; *an electroencephalography technician: Exec Minutes,* 4/3/58; *180 patients daily: Johnson Memoir,* 10; *Exec Minutes,* 3/9, 3/12/43, 5/7/70; *ahead of his time: Exec Minutes,* 4/13/46, 5/19/52; Stevens, 231; *Johnson Memoir,* 10; *Land Community College: Exec Minutes,* 1/10, 9/26/46, 11/28/47, 1/30/58, 2/29/68, 2/6/69, 5/7, 6/4/70; *Maher Memoir,* 142; *Wichterman Memoir,* 8.

were African Americans: Kalisch, 380; Stevens, 254; *their favorite hangout:* McDougall, Duty, 141-42; *Shull Memoir,* 54; *surgery at Memorial: Exec Minutes,* 3/28/58; *Finley Memoir,* 4, 7, 13-14, 19; *without any fanfare: Fricke Memoir,* 45; *Lee Memoir,* 12, 17; *admitted in 1963: Quarry Memoir,* 1-2, 12-13; *Shull Memoir,* 71; *in automatic dismissal: Justison Memoir,* 61; McDougall, 145, 152; *Justison Memoir,* 16-17.

pool had disappeared: Kalisch, 362-63, 417; *Justison Memoir,* 4; *baccalaureate nurse training:* Kalisch, 410; *Memorial's Lutheran founders:* Kalisch, 417, 419; *SJR,* 2/9/64; *shortage of patient rooms:* Kalisch 433; *Exec Minutes,* 1/11/55, 3/29/62; *Smith Study,* II-26; *Exec Minutes,* 2/27/64; *Boyd Memoir,* 87-89; *to be admitted:* Stevens, 229; *Fluckiger Memoir,* 25-26; *Exec Minutes,* 1/27/66; *Smith Study,* I-21; *advice in planning:* Oxtoby *Memoir,* 24-25; *Smith Study,* I-4; *Exec Minutes:* 9/27, 11/1/62, 1/19/65; *Justison Memoir,* 14; *Exec Minutes,* 3/28/63.

into bunk beds: Smith Study, I-3; *Exec Minutes,* 6/27/63, 1/19/65; *razed in February 1967: ISJ,* 10/1/64; *ISR,* 2/10, 2/13/67; *Exec Minutes,* 10/29/59, 1/17/67; *SJR,* 9/19/66; *the B building: Exec Minutes,* 2/27/63; *Boyd Memoir,* 92-93; *professional kitchen planner: ISJ,* 1/20/66; *Exec Minutes,* 1/18/66, 1/21/69; *Scott Memoir,* 17, 40; *pay its radiologist: Exec Minutes,* 3/5/58, 1/20/59, 8/26/65; *few of the recommendations: Kearney Study,* VIII-2-4, VIII-12; *Intensive Care Unit: Minutes,* 1/16/62, 6/4/63, 10/26/67; *NewsCenter* (July 1974): 6; *Exec Minutes,* 1/22/63, 8/9, 9/28/67; *Smith Study,* II-6; *Smith Study,* Appendix B, 4.

on coronary care: Stevens, 231, 251-52; *such a facility:* Patterson, *Dread Disease,* 171; Starr, 355; Stevens, 228, 231, 252; Russo, 69; *Denby Memoir,* 15-16; *Exec Minutes,* 11/10/55; *repair than cancer:* Patterson, 216, 221; Stevens, 230-31, 277; *patient in surgery:* Stevens, 231; *Denby Memoir,* 5-6; *Fluckiger Memoir,* 54; *Exec Minutes,* 3/28, 5/23/57; 5/1/58; *performed at Memorial: Denby Memoir,* 3; *Exec Minutes,* 3/25/53, 2/23/61; 1/16/62; *Fluckiger Memoir,* 52-54; *Denby Memoir,* 7; *Smith Study,* I-4; *jurisdiction and fees: Exec Minutes,* 10/31/57; 3/26/59; *services and equipment: Denby Memoir,* 4.

to outright hostility: Stevens, 234-35; *the board agreed:* Oxtoby *Memoir,* 27; *Boyd Memoir,* 28, 33; *Exec Minutes,* 3/28/57; *on unpaid bills:* Fricke *Memoir,* 21; *Shull Memoir,* 78-79; *Snedigar Memoir,* 41; *Scott Memoir,* 46; *Exec Minutes,* 5/26/60; *ensured escalating costs:* Stevens, 228, 232; *of raising these:* Kalisch, 417; *Exec Minutes,* 3/24/47, 12/29/54, 4/3/58; 10/26/67; *Justison Memoir,* 52-53; *Exec Minutes,* 12/27/56; 11/7/78.

cost of medical care: Stevens, 228, 255; *hire at will:* Starr, 337-338; *Exec Minutes,* 1/18, 12/1/66, 1/17/67; *Fluckiger Memoir,* 26; *Smith Memoir,* 15; *begun to erode: Exec Minutes,* 1/27/66; *succeeded at Memorial:* Starr, 177; *Exec Minutes,* 1/11/55; Stevens, 247; *board as members: Exec Minutes,* 5/23/57, 1/28/68; *Med Minutes,* 4/25/57; *of community dedication:* Stevens, 249; *somewhat rambunctious institution: SIU School of Medicine: a Chronology,* June 1976 (in SIU School of Medicine Archives); Richard H. Moy, *The Origins and Conceptual Development of the Southern Illinois University School of Medicine,* May 1972, 1, 3 (in SIU School of Medicine Archives).

Charles H. Lanphier; III: vertical files (Sangamo Electric) in Sangamon Valley Collection, Lincoln (Public) Library, Springfield, Illinois; Robert Carr Lanphier, *Forty Years of Sangamo, 1896-1936* (Chicago: privately printed, 1949), v.; John H. Schact, *Sangamo, 1949-1959,* part three (Springfield: Sangamo Electric Company, 1960), 2, 7; *Denby Memoir,* 21, 27; *Moy Memoir,* 6; *Lohman Memoir,* 10; *Phillips Memoir,* 19-20; *Exec Minutes,* 4/12, 11/8/78.

Grant Johnson, M.D.: Johnson Memoir, 1-6, 38, 51, 79, 81, 84; *Rigby Memoir,* 90; *Moy Memoir,* 82, 86; *Cook Memoir,* 88; *Maher Memoir,* 32; *SJR,* 2/18/97.

Mid-Century Nursing School: Exec Minutes, 9/15/49, 7/27/50, 4/29, 5/27, 7/30/54, 9/13/55; *Justison Memoir,* 38-39; *NSA Scrapbook; Snedigar Memoir,* 3, 11-13, 21.

The Great Whale Hunt: Johnson Memoir, 35-36, 40-42.

William Boyd: Exec Minutes, 3/6/58, 9/10/70; *Boyd Memoir,* 1-3, 5, 56, 152; Eunice Scott correspondence following interview, 9/1/93; *Quarry Memoir,* 51.

Chapter Six: Turmoil And Transformation

housing and education: Kalisch, *American Nursing,* 444; *and Menard counties:* Howard, *Illinois,* 570; Russo, *Prairie of Promise,* 51-52, 70-72; Hochman, *American History,* 272; Campbell, *Sangamon Saga,* 333; *as technological brinkmanship:* Starr, *Social Transformation,* 379, 382, 389-90; Callahan, *Troubled Dream:* 40-41; *and Responsibilities policy:* Kalisch, 445; Starr, 390-91; *Exec Minutes,* 4/13/77; *large progressive hospitals:* Stevens, *Sickness and Wealth,* 279; Starr, 360-61; *turmoil and transformation:* Starr, 379; 403; Stevens, 279, 380.

more than doubled: Starr, 360, 421; *by February 1968:* Campbell Report, 1: iii; *the missed hearing:* Moy, Richard H., *The Origins and Conceptual Development of the Southern Illinois University School of Medicine,* May 1972, 2; *Exec Minutes,* 1/26, 2/23/67; *Oxtoby Memoir,* 34; *Campbell Report,* 1: vii; *city council members: Exec Minutes,* 4/27/67; *excellence in Springfield: Exec Minutes,* 2/23, 4/27, 9/28/67, 6/6/68; *facilities in Springfield: Patton Memoir,* 60; *Maher Memoir,* 26-28; *Exec Minutes,* 10/26/67; *Campbell Report,* 1: 314; *Medical School Location Capital City,* Springfield, May 1967; *Denby Memoir,* 32; Moy, *Origins,* 72.

quality and success: Patton Memoir, 60; Starr, 389; *quality of care: Rosenfeld Plan,* 2:8-8; *Johnson Memoir,* 32; Dr. William Sherrick, et al., "Organizing a Community Department for Academic Radiology," *American Journal of Roentgenology,* 126:4 (April 1976): 761-64; *Pearson Memoir,* 25-26; *Lanphier represented Memorial: Maher Memoir,* 28; *Exec Minutes,* 9/26/68, 8/14, 9/4/69; *Moy Memoir,* 2; *the board agreed: Exec Minutes,* 9/26/68, 10/14/69.

that were suggested: Exec Minutes, 10/2/69, 4/2/70, 3/2/72; *BSCMS* 34 (November 1969): 303; *Med Minutes,* 11/6/70; *the teaching hospital: Moy Memoir,* 2-3, 6; *continued for years: Smith Memoir,* 37; *Rosenfeld Plan,* 1: viii, 2: iii; *Lohman Memoir,* 27; *Steering Minutes,* 6/8/71, 9/25/73; *Exec Minutes,* 1/8/74; *in siting SIU: Oxtoby Memoir,* 49-52; *Exec Minutes,* 7/7/66, 2/23/67; *Boyd Memoir,* 39; *and razing costs: Moy Memoir,* 8; *Exec Minutes,* 10/22/70, 4/1/71.

next 15 years: Maher Memoir, 24-26; *Exec Minutes,* 5/5, 25, 7/7/66, 8/9/67, 6/27, 9/26/68; *costly window dressing: Exec Minutes,* 5/6/71; *Moy Memoir,* 17; *highway direction signs: Moy Memoir,* 17; *Rigby Memoir,* 42; *and its services: Phillips Memoir,* 14; *Exec Minutes,* 7/12/72; *Steering Minutes,* 9/18/72; *and 20 nurses: Exec Minutes,* 3/21/74; *SJR,* 5/14/79; *the two hospitals: Lindsey Memoir,* 24; *Rigby Memoir,* 44; *share all calls: Exec Minutes,* 7/12, 10/5/72, 5/10/89; *Rigby Memoir,* 44; *the AMA in 1966: Exec Minutes,* 3/31/66, 9/28/67; *cardiac volume increased: Exec Minutes,* 7/7/66, 5/1/69, 2/5/70, 5/7, 10/1/70, 5/6, 7/8/71, 11/2/72; *BSCMS* 31 (September 1966): 241; Conversation with Dr. William Sherrick, 2/8/97.

and Alton Morris: Exec Minutes: 1/31/63, 10/26/67, 1/25, 11/7, 11/21/68; *Fricke Memoir,* 26-27; *ISJ,* 7/24/68; *Maher Memoir,* 24; *hospital's service region: NewsCenter;* Fall, 1978; *Maher Memoir,* 93; *Exec Minutes,* 2/1/73; *occurred at Memorial: Maher Memoir,* 90; *Exec Minutes,* 11/5/70, 1/19/71; *Fricke Memoir,* 23; *Denby Memoir,* 34-35.

under age 65: Exec Minutes, 11/5/70, 1/6/72, 12/6/73; *Maher Memoir,* 36-37, 40-42; *Denby Memoir,* 34-35; Starr, 442; *the trial period: Exec Minutes,* 1/25/68, 6/5/69, 1/8/70, 2/4/71; *Schnirring Memoir,* 39; *Rosenfeld Plan,* 2: 9-33; *still lost money: Exec minutes,* 2/4, 11/4/71; *Denby Memoir,* 37; *Rosenfeld Plan,* 2:9-36; *support to the unit: Quarry Memoir,* 11, 97; *SJR,* 7/24/77.

for the program: Exec Minutes, 7/12/76; *SJR,* 7/24/77; *Denby Memoir,* 38; *the center's director: NewsCenter;* Report to the Community, Spring 1978; *SJR,* 7/24/77, 9/24/78; *Exec Minutes,* 6/30/79, 3/10/82; *an audiology program: Exec Minutes,* 7/1/69, 11/15/73.

as Mr Inside: Exec Minutes, 4/16/70; *Maher Memoir,* 25, 49-50; *Moy Memoir,* 50; *Boyd Memoir,* 49; *Phillips Memoir,* 4-6; *was a disaster: Phillips Memoir,* 1, 4-5; *Boyd Memoir,* 49; *Moy Memoir,* 51; *the tacit criticism: Phillips Memoir,* 14, 16, 20, 47; *Boyd Memoir,* 75-76; *Oxtoby Memoir,* 74; *Maher Memoir,* 51.

of Hendrix's making: Phillips Memoir, 21, 23; *Smith Memoir,* 24; *Oxtoby Memoir,* 94-98; *resignation with regret: Phillips Memoir,* 21-22; *Oxtoby Memoir,* 77, 79, 80-81, 100-102; *Boyd Memoir,* 52-53; *Exec Minutes,* 4/5, 6/14/73; *as they arose:* Stevens, 306; *Rosenfeld Plan,* 1:4-2; *Exec Minutes,* 11/5/64; *School of Medicine: Phillips Memoir,* 9-10, 12, 28; *Steering Minutes,* 5/3/72; *Exec Minutes,* 5/3, 6/15/72; *Rosenfeld Plan,* 1:viii; 3: front matter, 10-11.

planning with Memorial: Phillips Memoir, 30, 49; *Exec Minutes,* 3/1/71, 8/16, 9/20, 29/73; *built its future: Phillips Memoir,* 32; *Rosenfeld Plan,* 2:i-ii; *raised medical standards: Rosenfeld Plan,* 1:i-ii; *Steering Minutes,* 2/15/73; *Moy Memoir,* 10, 14; *a major reorganization: Rosenfeld Plan,* 1:i, 2:9-25, 9-26; *Exec Minutes,* 5/1, 3, 9/73, 11/15/73; *Steering Minutes,* 5/9/73.

into stellar services: Exec Minutes, 3/7, 9/5/74, 2/20/75; *Moy Memoir,* 14; *Rosenfeld Plan,* 1:7-30; *Rigby Memoir,* 46-47; *face of challenge: Rosenfeld Plan,* 2:i; *this was illegal: Phillips Memoir,* 31; *Rosenfeld Plan,* 1:ii, 3:10-27; *Steering Minutes,* 2/15/73; *Exec Minutes,* 10/2/69.

need for change: Phillips Memoir, 32; Stevens, 241; *Exec Minutes,* 2/5/70; *named to the board: Exec Minutes,* 11/15/73; *Phillips Memoir,* 46-47; *Lohman Memoir,* 4-6; *or in the lobby: Phillips Memoir,* 18-19; *president was eliminated: Exec Minutes,* 4/6/72, 5/3, 12/6/73; Stevens, 304; *Phillips Memoir,* 16; *Rosenfeld Plan,* 3:10-44, 10-51.

ties to Memorial: Exec Minutes, 5/4/72, 7/5, 9/6/73, 1/14, 15/74, 11/20/75; *Smith Memoir,* 31-34, 46; *Phillips Memoir,* 33, 40; *Maher Memoir,* 24, 29; *employee Betty Carder: Phillips Memoir,* 40; *Smith Memoir,* 4-7; *the trust $888,388: Exec Minutes,* 11/7/68, 3/6/69, 1/8, 20, 4/2, 9/10, 10/1, 12/3/70, 1/19, 9/23/71, 2/3/72; *NewsCenter* (October 1974): 7; *SJR,* 1/26/74.

and expert staff: Exec Minutes, 3/6/69, 3/5/70; *Smith Memoir,* 4, 9-10; *report in 1974: Smith Memoir,* 9-10, 14; *Exec Minutes,* 11/21, 12/7/72, 5/16/74; *Phillips Memoir,* 40, 42; *costs in the 1970s: Exec Minutes,* 2/24, 7/7/66, 1/17, 26/67, 9/4/69, 1/19, 10/7/71; *Smith*

Memoir, 16-17; *nearly $500,000 annually:* Beckwith *Memoir,* 1-2, 7-8, 12, 50, 54; *than a hospital now:* Boyd *Memoir,* 4; *ideas and change:* Jones *Memoir,* 27-29; *Exec Minutes,* 1/15/74; *SJR,* 1/16/74.

on this recommendation: *Rosenfeld Plan,* 1:3-6; *Exec Minutes,* 5/10/73; *than enough nurses: Exec Minutes,* 6/6/68, 1/18/73; *Rosenfeld Plan,* 1:5-6, 5-7, 2:ii, *Campbell Report,* 1:41; *twice as many:* Kalisch, 446-448, 450; *Rosenfeld Plan,* 1:9-13; *Maher Memoir,* 132-33.

the medical school: *Rosenfeld Plan,* 2:ii; *Oxtoby Memoir,* 106-07; *Exec Minutes,* 1/18/73; *only 24 freshman: NewsCenter;* Fall, 1978; *Exec Minutes,* 3/6, 4/3, 6/5, 8/14, 9/4/69; *matter of timing: Exec Minutes,* 9/10/70, 5/6/71; *ties to SIU: Exec Minutes,* 1/12, 9/10, 10/1/70; *Steering Minutes,* 10/13/70; *Maher Memoir,* 134-35.

to the school: *Exec Minutes,* 5/3/75; *Steering Minutes,* 5/1/73; *had ever seen: Nurs Minutes,* 3/27/73; *Phillips Memoir,* 53-54; *graduated 1,551 nurses: SJR,* 10/19/75; *Exec Minutes,* 10/16/75; *and southern Illinois: Phillips Memoir,* 37; *Rosenfeld Plan,* 3:10-12; *was a tragedy: Quarry Memoir,* 43; *Fluckiger Memoir,* 19-20; *Shull Memoir,* 67.

A Difficult Decision: The vignette title comes from Joy Gardner, *A Difficult Decision: A Compassionate Book about Abortion* (Freedom, California: Crossing Press, 1986); *Exec Minutes,* 3/8, 3/22/73; *Illinois Times,* 9/30/93; *Maher Memoir,* 106-07; *Moy Memoir,* 102; *Cook Memoir,* 66-69.

A Standard of Excellence: SJR, 5/10/86, Conversation with Dr. James Singleton, 2/22/97; *Exec Minutes,* 1/2/69, 2/4/71, 1/6, 12/2/72, 2/7, 3/21, 9/5/74, 2/20, 12/4/75.

Practice on a Pig: Maher Memoir, 22; *Exec Minutes,* 6/4/63.

Chauncey Maher; M.D.: Maher Memoir, 8-9; 14-16, 113, 126; *Exec Minutes,* 5/4/72.

George Hendrix: Lohman Memoir, 20; *Fricke Memoir,* 15; *Exec Minutes,* 10/4/73; *Cook-Memoir,* 39; *SJR,* 11/15/81.

Chapter Seven: Seeking Parity

obstetrics and gynecology: *Exec Minutes,* 1/4/74; *university teaching hospitals: Exec Minutes,* 1/4, 6/6/74; *Rosenfeld Plan,* l:v; *million fundraising campaign: Denby Memoir,* 16-17; *Exec Minutes,* 5/6/71; *Cook Memoir,* 17; *Extendicare Corporation's construction:* Stevens, *Sickness and Wealth,* 297; Starr, *Social Transformation,* 430; *SJR,* 4/3/74; *Rosenfeld Plan,* 3:10-12; *Exec Minutes,* 9/20/73; *Springfield Community Hospital:* Stevens, 319; *ISJ,* 4/3/74; *intensified their rivalry: Rosenfeld Letter;* 5/28/74; *Exec Minutes,* 2/7/74; *than the capitol: Exec Minutes,* 4/4/74; *imminent regulatory legislation: Exec Minutes,* 3/21, 7/25/74; *the planned groudbreaking:* Stevens, 301, 304, 307; Starr, 399; *Exec Minutes,* 11/21/74.

than two weeks: *Exec Minutes,* 1/28, 9/18, 24, 10/31, 12/4/75; *SJR,* 1/29/75; *Phillips Memoir,* 44-45; *Jones Memoir,* 16-17; *in the minutes: NewsCenter* (March 1975): 10, (Fall 1978): 7; Stevens, 299; *Exec Minutes,* 4/4, 5/14, 8/1/74; *the Dairy Rose: Exec Minutes,* 6/5/75, 10/19, 12/14/77, 3/8, 8/9/78; *Boyd Memoir,* 104-05; *SJR,* 10/10/78; *Maher Memoir,* 33; *1943 G building: SJR,* 10/10/78; *Exec Minutes,* 7/17/75; *NewsCenter* (March 1975):

10, (Fall 1978): 8; *September 24 open house: Exec Minutes,* 9/10/70, 4/18/78; *Steering Minutes,* 7/27/77; *SJR,* 7/24, 11/19/77, 9/24/78.

around the block: Boyd Memoir, 78-79; *Ross Memoir,* 3; *timing was perfect: Exec Minutes,* 9/4/75; *filled the news: SJR,* 9/24/78; Patterson, *Dread Disease,* 247-51, 259, 274-81; *did not participate: Exec Minutes,* 9/1, 12/4/69, 1/6/72, 12/4/75, 2/26, 11/3/76, 1/18/77, 7/25/79; *Schnirring Memoir,* 44; *SJR,* 9/24/78; *NewsCenter;* Report to the Community, April 18, 1978; *gifts exceeded $1,977,000: Exec Minutes,* 11/18/75, 7/12/76; *SJR,* 7/18/76, 9/24/78; *Schnirring Memoir,* 2.

by 102 votes: Kalisch, *American Nursing,* 445; Stevens, 303; *Exec Minutes,* 4/4, 5/2, 6/13, 8/28, 9/4, 19, 11/14/74, 1/31, 5/1/75; *SJR,* 2/15/75; *to reduce expenses: Exec Minutes,* 1/23, 5/1, 5/15/75; *Scott Memoir,* 51; *the engineering department: Exec Minutes,* 9/12/76, 7/13/77; *and then ignored: Med Minutes,* 8/7/71; *Exec Minutes,* 4/2/76; *advice for administrators:* Kalisch, 451-52; *Fluckiger Memoir,* 49-50; *insecurity among nurses: Steering Minutes,* 5/9/73; *the higher standards: Phillips Memoir,* 54-55; *have baccalaureate degrees: Rigby Memoir,* 18, *Denby Memoir,* 22; *Phillips Memoir,* 56; *Quarry Memoir,* 49.

out of control: Fricke Memoir, 57; *Snedigar Memoir,* 50; *requests as troublemakers: Cook Memoir,* 19; *Quarry Memoir,* 33; *Maher Memoir,* 59, 62-63; *in an uproar: Smith Memoir,* 45, *Phillips Memoir,* 59; *to organize nurses: SJR,* 6/24/76; *Quarry Memoir,* 39-40, 44; *Fricke Memoir,* 40; *Maher Memoir,* 64-65; *Exec Minutes,* 5/6/76; *assignments and shifts: Phillips Memoir,* 54, 56, 59-60; *Rigby Memoir,* 19; *SJR,* 7/2/76.

exceeded it by $100,000: Exec Minutes, 3/3, 6/23/76; *Schnirring Letter;* 5/18/76; *had to leave: Quarry Memoir,* 39, 46-47; *Steering Minutes,* 6/18/76; *Boyd Memoir,* 63; *SJR,* 6/24/76; *Schnirring Memoir,* 26; *or reassure people: Oxtoby Memoir,* 110; *SJR,* 6/24/76; *Lohman Memoir,* 34; *Denby Memoir,* 23; *Schnirring Memoir,* 24-26; *Cook Memoir,* 17; *and double shifts: Cook Memoir,* 15-16; *Phillips Memoir,* 54; *Quarry Memoir,* 40; *Fricke Memoir,* 55, 57; *was going wrong: Smith Memoir,* 44; *Schnirring Memoir,* 26.

the crisis conditions: Beckwith Memoir, 34, 36-37; *Exec Minutes,* 6/23/76; *NewsCenter* (April 1974); *from Duke University: Beckwith Memoir,* 38; *NewsCenter* (April 1974):14; *back to Springfield: Cook Memoir,* 28, 54-56; *that became necessary: Cook Memoir,* 17; 52-53; *calm and support: Rigby Memoir,* 21-22; *under Bill Boyd: Cook Memoir,* 58-59; *Rigby Memoir,* 23; *a miraculous job: Quarry Memoir,* 51-54, 56; *Schnirring Memoir,* 28.

priority in 1977: Exec Minutes, 6/26, 7/12/76; *Nurs Minutes,* 7/27/76; *salaries and benefits: Quarry Memoir,* 58-59, 61; *Exec Minutes,* 9/14/77, 4/29/80; *others in testing, etc.: Exec Minutes,* 8/5/76, 1/12/77; Polly Magargal, "Modular Nursing: Nurses Rediscover Nursing," *Nursing Management,* 18:11(1987): 98-104; *Quarry Memoir,* 76-77; *new post-Lanphier era: Scott Memoir,* 56.

on the board: Cook Memoir, 42; *Schnirring Memoir,* 1-2; *Lohman Memoir,* 23; *Oxtoby Memoir,* 104; *was in Michigan: Schnirring Memoir,* 13; *Beckwith Memoir,* 38; *Cook Memoir,* 43; *Schnirring to Lanphier;* 5/18/76; *the cocktail party: Cook Memoir,* 47-48; 90 *service agreements: NewsCenter;* Report to the Community, April, 18, 1978; *Cook Memoir,* 46; *Exec Minutes,* 12/13/78.

and John Denby: Cook *Memoir,* 43-44, 72-73, 76-77; Lohman *Memoir,* 42-45; Schnirring *Memoir,* 14-15; *Exec Minutes,* 11/3/73; *Schnirring to Lanphier,* 5/18/76; Conversation with Dr. William Sherrick, 2/18/97; Board of Directors List (in archives).

to tort liability: Stevens, 315-16; *lawyer Norman Jones:* Lohman *Memoir,* 50-51; *Exec Minutes,* 6/3/76, 3/11/81, 4/17/85; Schnirring *Memoir,* 35-36; *than $2 million:* Exec *Minutes,* 9/15/81, 9/8/82, 4/17/85; Lohman *Memoir,* 50-51; Jones *Memoir,* 43.

as health education: Schnirring *Memoir,* 34-35; *Exec Minutes,* 6/15/77; *of Memoiral ambassadors:* Exec *Minutes,* 10/11/78, 10/8/80, 6/9/82; Cook *Memoir,* 69-71; *NewsCenter,* Report to the Community, April, 18, 1978, 14; *School of Dietetics:* Schnirring *Memoir,* 30; *Exec Minutes,* 12/3/64, 2/23/65, 11/30/67, 6/14/73; Oxtoby *Memoir,* 30-33; Fricke *Memoir,* 36; Scott *Memoir,* 56; *as increased competition:* Quarry *Memoir,* 28-30, Denby *Memoir,* 16-17; Phillips *Memoir,* 48-50; *came from it:* Schnirring *Memoir,* 30-32; Cook *Memoir,* 61; *Exec Minutes,* 6/3/76; *Schnirring Letter;* 5/11/76.

changes in facilities: Exec Minutes, 10/31, 12/5/63; SJR, 8/25/96; *that hospital anyway:* Maher *Memoir,* 74-76; Boyd *Memoir,* 29; *in cardiac surgery:* Rigby *Memoir,* 39-40; Cook *Memoir,* 83-84; *as their ratchet: Rosenfeld Plan,* 3:10-18; Smith *Memoir,* 89; *Steering Minutes,* 6/27/79; *Exec Minutes,* 5/12/82; Beckwith *Memoir,* 45-46; Cook *Memoir,* 83, 85; *start a program:* Beckwith *Memoir,* 47; *Exec Minutes,* 4/9/80; Smith *Memoir,* 89.

in February 1980: Exec Minutes, 6/13, 10/10/79, 2/13/80; *reflect this intent: Exec Minutes,* 4/8, 5/14, 7/9/80; Schnirring *Memoir,* 30-31; SJR, 4/17/80; *eight-year-old equipment: Exec Minutes,* 11/11/81, 5/12, 9/8/82; Rigby *Memoir,* 34; *every board meeting: Exec Minutes,* 3/10, 4/14, 5/12/82; Boyd *Memoir,* 100-01; *certificate of need: Exec Minutes,* 11/11/81, 10/13/82; *the state HSA:*Beckwith *Memoir,* 45-46; Rigby *Memoir,* 31-33; *Quarry Memoir,* 82; *chamber in Jacksonville:* Rigby *Memoir,* 36-37, *Exec Minutes,* 1/12/83; Beckwith *Memoir,* 45-46.

stature to St. John's: Rigby *Memoir,* 38-40; *Exec Minutes,* 2/9, 4/13/83; Cook *Memoir,* 84; *a sharp observation:* Cook *Memoir,* 94; *Exec Minutes,* 10/13/82, Rigby *Memoir,* 26; Smith *Memoir,* 98; Johnson *Memoir,* 98-99; *out of court: Exec Minutes,* 10/13/82; Johnson *Memoir,* 100; Boyd *Memoir,* 164; Smith *Memoir,* 96; *and tough competitor:* Schnirring *Memoir,* 46-47.

Dr. Kenneth H. Schnepp, Librarian: NewsCenter (February 1978):33-34; *Exec Minutes:* 4/28/49, 6/28/54, 3/6/69, 5/4/72, 2/28, 3/8, 4/20/78; SJR, 4/20/78.

George Phillips: Phillips Memoir, 35, 61-63

Jack Cook: Cook *Memoir,* 17-20, 22, 33, 39, 86; Maher *Memoir,* 34-35; Rigby *Memoir,* 53; SJR, 7/2/76; Lohman *Memoir,* 36; Quarry *Memoir,* 68; Oxtoby *Memoir,* 116; Johnson *Memoir,* 108.

Memorial Meals: Eunice Scott Letter; NewsCenter (November 1975).

Friends: Steering Minutes, 2/15/77, SJR, 9/26/43, *Exec Minutes,* 9/28/61, 2/28, 6/4/63, 1/8/76.

Chapter Eight: Quiet Revolution

of the 20th century: Johnson, *Hospitals,* xiii-xv, 21-29, 331-32, 388-89, 411-12; *and the community:* Cook *Memoir,* 97; Rigby *Memoir,* 56-57; *Minutes,* 3/9, 4/13/83; *at Community Hospital:* Rigby *Memoir,* 57, 77; Clarke *Memoir,* 1-4; *evading tough decisions:* Schnirring *Memoir,* 55; Smith *Memoir,* 115-16; Rigby *Memoir,* 61-63; *style and goals:* Clarke *Memoir,* 15-17; Quarry *Memoir,* 92; *Minutes,* 7/13/83; *concerns and initiatives: Minutes,* 8/10, 9/14, 10/12/83; *and Alvin Becker:* Clarke *Memoir,* 19, 44-46, 67.

Lanphier's long tenure: Clarke *Memoir,* 34-35, 113-13; *medical service company:* Beckwith *Memoir,* 59-60; Quarry *Memoir,* 90-91; Smith *Memoir,* 60; *drop in income: Minutes,* 1/13/82, 12/14/83; *administration were over:* Johnson, 57; Clarke *Memoir,* 6-8, 12-14; Beckwith *Memoir,* 29; *Minutes,* 3/14, 11/14/84, 2/13/85, 2/10/88; Smith *Memoir,* 65-67; Rigby *Memoir,* 70-72.

continuing board priority: Minutes, 2/15/80, 1/14/81, 6/9/82; 11/9/83; Clarke *Memoir,* 8;

of regional prestige: Minutes, 10/9/85, 1/14/87; *his own people: Minutes,* 3/14, 4/11, 9/12, 10/10/84; Rigby *Memoir,* 65, 69, 70-72, 76; Smith *Memoir,* 79-80; *Johnson succeeded him:* Clarke *Memoir,* 25-31, 78-79, 93; *Minutes,* 8/8/90; *curb administrative growth: Minutes,* 4/8/92.

antitrust litigation: Moy *Memoir,* 26; *Doctors Hospital:* SJR, 9/1/84; *Minutes,* 9/12/84, 11/11/87; Schnirring *Memoir,* 33; Oxtoby *Memoir,* 132-34; *in modern times: Minutes,* 2/12, 9/10/86, 1/13/88; Clarke *Memoir,* 84-88; *justified the expense: Minutes,* 10/11/89, 1/10, 6/13/90, 4/8/92; Clarke *Memoir,* 108; *more creative response: Minutes,* 6/14/89, 4/8/92; Clarke *Memoir,* 70, 101, 104-05.

and St. John's: Kalisch, *American Nursing,* 482; *Minutes,* 9/9/81, 2/8, 6/13, 7/11/84, 2/8, 10/11/89; *with national trends: Minutes,* 9/11/85; *MHS Annual Report 1992; of Showing It": Minutes,* 4/9, 12/10/86; *pledge of superior service: Minutes,* 2/12, 10/8/86, 4/20/88; *adapt or wither: Minutes,* 8/12/87, 5/11/88, 4/11/90.

centers of excellence: Clarke *Memoir,* 39-42; *Minutes,* 4/11, 10/10/84, 3/12/86, 10/9, 11/13/91, 1/8/92; Smith *Memoir,* 89; Conversation with Mitchell Johnson, 12/5/96; *offered the cures:* Clarke *Memoir,* 147; *Minutes,* 8/14, 10/9/85, 5/14, 6/11/86; *COPE: Oncology News for Professionals* (November 1988), 10-13; *cancer center program: Minutes,* 5/13/87, 4/20/88; *"Cancer News,"* 1:1 (May 1989); *of downstate citizens: Minutes,* 11/2/72, 6/7/73, 11/14/79, 11/8/89; Rigby *Memoir,* 50-51.

other medical services: Conversation with Johnson, 12/5/96; *premier obstetrical service: Minutes,* 5/9, 11/14/90; Conversation with Johnson, 12/5/96; *Dr. Sumantra Mitra: Minutes,* 2/8, 5/9/84, 6/12/85, 9/10/86, 4/13, 6/8/88, 11/14/90, 8/24/96; Conversation with Johnson, 12/5/96; *in the 1990s: Minutes,* 4/13/83; *diagnosis and treatment:* Johnson *Memoir,* 48-49, 59-62, 69-72, 75-76, 112, 115-19, 123-24; *and Sangamon counties: Minutes,* 3/13/84, 9/11/85, 1/8/86, 3/14/90, 11/11/92; Conversation with Johnson, 12/5/96.

homes of radiologists: Minutes, 2/9, 6/8/83, 5/9/84, 8/14/91; Conversation with Dr. William Sherrick, 2/8/97; Conversation with Johnson, 12/5/96; *and other staff: Minutes,* 3/12/86, 3/9/88, 1/9/91; *due to excessive delinquencies:* Fluckiger *Memoir,* 39-40; *Minutes,*

12/2/65, 1/3, 2/7, 12/19/74, 11/3/76, 12/13/78, 4/14/82; *medical record-keeping challenge:* Cook *Memoir,* 75-76; *Quarry Memoir,* 108, 110-18, 124, 129-32; Conversation with Johnson, 12/5/96.

"health care service malls": Johnson, 23-9, 33, 331, 411; *Clarke Memoir,* 116-17; *Rigby Memoir,* 66; *Shared Services Program: Clarke Memoir,* 5; *Minutes,* 3/13/85; *Smith Memoir,* 82-83; *and cultural sensitivity: Minutes,* 4/11/84; *MHS Annual Report 1992; SJR,* 8/13/96; *MHS Q&A* (June 1995); *100,000 visits a year: Minutes,* 2/8/84, 4/17/85; *Clarke Memoir,* 129; *nearly all of them: Clarke Memoir,* 118; *Rigby Memoir,* 66; *Smith Memoir,* 111; *Minutes,* 2/12, var/86; *MMCS Minutes,* 2/10/88.

expanded outpatient services: Clarke Memoir, 106; *Rigby Memoir,* 66; *Minutes,* 4/9/86, var 86-88; Conversation with Dr. William Sherrick, 2/8/97; *a small profit: Minutes,* 1/13/88; *Clarke Memoir,* 118-19; *and so forth: MMCS Minutes,* 4/12/89; *Clarke Memoir,* 83-84, 89, 124-25, 128-29, 130, 132; *ideas and resources: Minutes,* 8/10, 9/14/83, 1/11, 4/11, 9/12/84, 11/13/85, 12/13/89, 3/4/92; *Rigby Memoir,* 59; *Clarke Memoir,* 141-43.

of mutual responsibility: Minutes, 1/11, 6/13, 7/11/84, 4/20/88; *Clarke Memoir,* 56-65; *Rigby Memoir,* 81; *thrived in the vacuum: Clarke Memoir,* 60-62, 64-65, 158-59; *New York Times,* 7/30/96; *23 separate grants: Minutes,* 11/8/89; *MHS Annual Report 1995,* 16-24.

Healthcare Network Associates: MHS Annual Report 1995, 15; *Fluckiger Memoir,* 32; *of the local market: Clarke Memoir,* 161; *SJR,* 6/12, 10/23/96; *employer and spender: MHS Annual Report 1995,* 15; *hospital's centennial anniversary: MHS Annual Report 1995,* 4-6.

The Clarke Imprint: Lohman Memoir, 36-39; *Johnson Memoir,* 109-10; *Boyd Memoir,* 71-72; *Fricke Memoir,* 50; *Moy Memoir,* 57.

VIP Patients: SJR, 2/16, 5/24/62, 8/3-4/78, 10/6-8/92, 6/18-19/93; Letter from Robert Oxtoby to Cullom Davis, 10/11/96.

The Modern Medical Staff: Minutes, 2/8, 7/11, 11/14/84, 4/10, 10/9/91; *Maher Memoir,* 48; *Rigby Memoir,* 28-29; *Clarke Memoir,* 32-36.

Nursing in the Nineties: Minutes, 6/9/82, 12/9/87, 7/13/88, 11/8/89; *Boyd Memoir,* 161; *SJR,* 2/25, 9/2, 10/24, 10/31/96; *Justison Memoir,* 41-45; Memorandum from Edgar Curtis to Cullom Davis, 1/2/97.

A New Front Door: Boyd Memoir, 95, 103, 112-16, 119, 130-34; *Wichterman Memoir,* 21.

Chapter Nine: 21st Century Health Care

respect and satisfaction: MHS Annual Report 1997; Brown Memoir; Minutes, 08/13/97; *Lincoln (IL) Courier,* 04/11/02; *SJR,* 12/15/06; *Minutes,* 05/10/06; *Clarke Memoir,* 2007.

Blood of Christ: Sr. BJ Franklin Memoir; Minutes, 07/12/06; *SJR,* 10/27/06; *Clarke Memoir,* 2007.

was mutually advantageous: Clarke Memoir, 2007; *Hale Memoir.*

for Behavioral Health: Minutes, 09/10/97; *Center Line,* October 1999; *MHS Annual Report 2004; Stover Memoir.*

the medical school: Clarke Memoir, 2007; *Minutes,* 01/12/00; *VanMeter Memoir; Dorsey Memoir; SJR,* 02/24/03, 06/15/04; *Memorial Memo,* 06/21/04.

for needy people: Minutes, 06/10/98, 09/09/98, 02/09/00, 04/12/00; *Memorial Memo,* 05/07/07; *SJR,* 06/02/07; *Mitch Johnson Memoir; Clarke Memoir,* 2007; *Minutes,* 02/09/00.

sincerity and reliability: Minutes, 08/12/98, 04/14/99, 08/09/00, 12/11/02; *Memorial Memo,* 03/29/04; *SJR,* 05/22/03; *Curtis Memoir, Clarke Memoir,* 2007.

fortune's fickle ways: Clarke Memoir, 2007; *Minutes,* 10/10/01, 01/09/02; *SJR,* 05/22/03, 11/30/01, 12/01/01, 02/08/02; *Memorial Memo,* 02/11/02.

plus at Memorial: O'Keefe Memoir; Dorsey Memoir; Hale Memoir; Brown Memoir; VanMeter Memoir.

its competitive efforts: SJR, 06/30/04; *Minutes,* 06/09/04; *Mitch Johnson Memoir; Clarke Memoir,* 2007; *Curtis Memoir; Zook Memoir; Dorsey Memoir.*

for the next one: SJR, 05/30/03, 06/09/07, 02/26/07; *Curtis Memoir; Memorial Memo,* 02/23/04, 02/16/07; *Minutes,* 01/14/04; *SJR,* 02/01/07.

edge in recruitment: Clarke Memoir, 2007; *Memorial Memo (2000-2007); Curtis Memoir, Dorsey Memoir, Shelbyville Daily Union,* 02/05/04; *Center Line,* Summer 2002; *Memorial Memo,* 11/16/06, 11/20/06; *Curtis Memoir.*

take many forms: Mitch Johnson Memoir; Memorial Memo, 06/14/04, 04/22/02; *SJR,* 09/22/03; *Minutes,* 06/12/02, 07/10/02, 04/12/06; *Memorial Memo,* 03/25/02.

major construction project: Memorial Memo, 07/22/02, 09/03/02, 05/19/03, 03/15/04; *Zook Memoir; Center Line, Fall 2001; Memorial Memo,* 04/22/02; *Mitch Johnson Memoir; Clarke Memoir,* 2007; *Memorial Memo,* 02/06/06, 02/05/07, 06/11/07; *SJR,* 05/24/06; *Minutes,* 07/12/00, 04/11/01, 12/13/06; *Curtis Memoir.*

2001 and 2007: Memorial Memo, 07/01/02, 01/02/06; *SJR,* 01/04/06, 08/22/07; *Mitch Johnson Memoir; Curtis Memoir; O'Keefe Memoir; SJR,* 05/02/04.

aggressive marketing strategy: Memorial Memo, 05/17/04; *Curtis Memoir; Memorial Memo,* 08/25/03, 09/01/03, 11/02/03, 11/21/05, 06/06/05, 04/24/06; *MHS Annual Report 2003; SJR,* 01/07/07; *Application for 2007 Malcolm Baldrige National Quality Award; Mitch Johnson Memoir; Minutes,* 11/12/03; *Memorial Memo,* 01/13/02.

this transition point: O'Keefe Memoir; Clarke Memoir, 2007; *SJR,* 03/16/07; *Memorial Memo,* 03/19/07; *VanMeter Memoir; Curtis Memoir; Mitch Johnson Memoir.*

Hospitals of America: O'Keefe Memoir; SJR, 04/13/07; *Curtis Memoir; Dorsey Memoir.*

patient and physician: Curtis Memoir; Roy P. Basler et al (eds.), *The Collected Works of Abraham Lincoln* (New Brunswick, NJ: Rutgers University Press, 1953), 5:537.

Paul Smith and Ed Curtis: Smith Memoir, 1-2, 38, 48, 113-14; *Rigby Memoir, 73; Clarke Memoir,* 74-75, 93; *Boyd Memoir,* 183.

From Smoke-Filled to Smoke-Free: Minutes, 12/05/63, 10/02/69, 07/12/72, 12/06/73, 08/01/74, 02/28/75.

Leonia Cole's Record of Service: Cole Memoir.

Who Owns Memorial?: Notes from Mitch Johnson, 12/18/96.

Index